Handbook of
Urological Diseases in Children

Handbook of Urological Diseases in Children

Editors

Ricardo González
Children's Hospital of the University of Zurich,
Switzerland & Thomas Jefferson University, USA

Barbara M. Ludwikowski
Hannoversche Kinderheilanstalt,
Kinderkrankenhaus auf der Bult, Germany

World Scientific

NEW JERSEY • LONDON • SINGAPORE • BEIJING • SHANGHAI • HONG KONG • TAIPEI • CHENNAI

Published by

World Scientific Publishing Co. Pte. Ltd.
5 Toh Tuck Link, Singapore 596224
USA office: 27 Warren Street, Suite 401-402, Hackensack, NJ 07601
UK office: 57 Shelton Street, Covent Garden, London WC2H 9HE

British Library Cataloguing-in-Publication Data
A catalogue record for this book is available from the British Library.

HANDBOOK OF UROLOGICAL DISEASES IN CHILDREN

ISBN-13 978-981-4287-40-1
ISBN-10 981-4287-40-7

Typeset by Stallion Press
Email: enquiries@stallionpress.com

Printed by FuIsland Offset Printing (S) Pte Ltd. Singapore

This book is dedicated to:

My mother, Clyde A. Prevettoni who supported my education and instilled the values I have to this day.

Dr. Jorge C. Taullard whose example inspired me to become a surgeon.

My mentors, Dr. Elwin E. Fraley, Dr. Hardy W. Hendren and Dr. Owen H. Wangensteen who inspired, encouraged and supported my academic pursuits.

My former fellows, too numerous to list, who constantly challenged my teaching abilities.

To my children Diego Andres, Carlos Ricardo and Alexander Serif for giving a different meaning to my life.

Prof. Dr. Ricardo González

My parents, who always supported my education.

My son Alexander who opened my eyes also for the little things in the world.

My teacher Dr. Irene Oesch Hayward who was always a mentor for me.

PD Dr. Barbara Ludwikowski

Contents

Contributors

EDITORS

González, Ricardo
Division of Urology
University Children's Hospital
Zurich, Switzerland

Consultant Paediatric Urologist
Italian Hospital
Buenos Aires, Argentina

Professor of Urology
Thomas Jefferson University
Philadelphia, USA

Ludwikowski, Barbara M.
Associate Professor
Chief of Paediatric Surgery and Urology
Kinderkrankenhaus auf der Bult
Hannover, Germany

ILLUSTRATOR

Staubli, Susanne
Scientific Illustrator
University Children's Hospital
Zurich, Switzerland

CONTRIBUTORS

Bani-Hani, Ahmad H. *(Haematuria)*
Alfred I. DuPont Hospital for Children
Wilmington, USA
Assistant Professor
Thomas Jefferson University
Philadelphia, USA

Castellán, Miguel A. *(Ureteral obstruction)*
Department of Urology,
University of Miami
Miami, USA

deBadiola, Francisco I. P. *(Tumours)*
Chief of Paediatric Urology
Hospital Italiano
Buenos Aires, Argentina

Franc-Guimond, Julie *(Incontinence)*
Associate Professor
Division of Pediatric Urology
Sainte Justine Hospital for Children
University of Montreal
Montreal, Canada

García Mérida, Manuel *(Undescended testes)*
Paediatric Urology
University Hospital Materno Infantil Carlos Haya
Málaga, Spain

Gobet, Rita *(Bladder exstrophy)*
Professor of Paediatric Surgery
Division of Urology
University Children's Hospital
Zurich, Switzerland

Horst, Maya *(Neuropathic bladder)*
Division of Urology
University Children's Hospital
Zurich, Switzerland

Hurwitz, Richard S. *(Ambiguous genitalia)*
The Center for Medical Education
Kaiser Permanante Medical Center
Los Angeles, California, USA

Jauregizar Monereo, Enrique *(Vesicoureteral reflux)*
Chief Paediatric Urology
La Paz Children's Hospital
Madrid, Spain

Lobos, Pablo A. *(Tumours)*
Chief of Paediatric Surgery
Hospital Italiano
Buenos Aires, Argentina

López Pereira, Pedro *(Vesicoureteral reflux)*
Staff Paediatric Urology
La Paz Children's Hospital
Madrid, Spain

Martínez Urrutia, María J. *(Vesicoureteral reflux)*
Staff Paediatric Urology
La Paz Children's Hospital
Madrid, Spain

Miguélez Lago, Carlos *(Undescended testes)*
Paediatric Urology
Clínica Santa Elena
University of Málaga
Malaga, Spain

Noh, Paul H. *(Lithiasis)*
Assistant Professor
Division of Pediatric Urology
Cincinnati Children's Hospital Medical Center
University of Cincinnati
Cincinnati, Ohio, USA

Piaggio, Lisandro A. *(Trauma)*
Assistant Professor of Surgery, Facultad de Medicina
Universidad Nacional del Sur
Attending Paediatric Surgeon, Hospital Interzonal General de Agudos
Dr. José Penna
Attending Paediatric Urologist, Department of Urology
Hospital Italiano Regional del Sur and Hospital Privado
Dr. R. Matera
Bahía Blanca, Argentina

Podesta, Miguel L. *(Urethral obstruction)*
Associate Professor of Urology, Medical School of Medicine
University of Buenos Aires
Head of the Urology Unit, Department of Surgery
Children's Hospital Ricardo Gutierrez
Clinical Investigator CONICET (National Research Council)
Buenos Aires, Argentina

Ramírez, José Alberto *(Renal insufficiency, Hypertension)*
Former Assistant Clinical Professor of Pediatric Nephrology
University of California, Los Angeles
Honorary Chief Paediatric Nephrology Service
Hospital Italiano de Buenos Aires
Assistant Professor of Paediatrics
Instituto Universitario Hospital Italiano
Buenos Aires, Argentina

Shlossman, Philip A *(Prenatal diagnosis)*
Delaware Center for Maternal & Fetal Medicine of Christiana Care
Associate Director
Division of Maternal and Fetal Medicine
Christiana Hospital
Newark, Delaware, USA

Traxel, Erica J. *(Lithiasis)*
Assistant Professor
Division of Urology
St. Louis Children's Hospital
Washington University School of Medicine
St. Louis, Missouri, USA

Weber, Daniel M. *(Hypospadias)*
Associate Professor
Division of Paediatric Urology
University Children's Hospital
Zurich, Switzerland

Prologue

This book carries the title of handbook. Unfortunately, many medical handbooks are used as cookbooks to follow "recipes" for the diagnosis and treatment of various diseases in a given specialty. Although we have attempted to be as practical as possible in selecting the information provided to the reader, we have resisted the temptation to oversimplify or to give answers where there are none. The treatment of most diseases in paediatric urology is far from evidence based. We have given the reader a concise summary of the information currently available in the literature and left it up to the readers to make up their own minds as how to act when the information available is conflicting. Although this is a handbook, it should not be taken as a "how to" manual. If this volume motivates the reader to search and critically analyse the literature and question common dicta such as: "this is how we do it here" or "this is the way we have always done it", we will consider that it has fulfilled its goal.

The book has two sections. In the first, we discussed the common forms of the presentation of various conditions in the clinic, the emergency department, or during hospital consultation. The second part discusses more in depth specific topics in paediatric urology, selected by the frequency of occurrence or by the uniqueness of their character. We include a chapter on acute and chronic renal insufficiency and renal replacement therapy since the knowledge of nephrology and the close collaboration with our colleagues in paediatric nephrology are essential for good patient care.

We are thankful to all our expert friends and colleagues who have contributed to this work. They bring to this volume their practical knowledge backed with experience and strong academic recognition. Without them, our task would have been impossible. We greatly respect their viewpoints and generally agree with all their statements but since this book is the product of our personal vision, we have taken the liberty to add a brief editorial comment at the end of each chapter, which were not written by us.

Finally, we wish all the readers much fun in reading and more enjoyment in the practice of paediatric urology, a specialty that originated from paediatric surgery and urology and which now holds a unique place among the surgical fields.

The Editors

Part One

Clinical Presentations

Chapter 1

Prenatal Diagnosis of Urinary Tract Abnormalities

Philip Shlossman

Urinary tract abnormalities are some of the most common abnormalities seen on antenatal ultrasound, with a reported incidence up to 7.7%. The majority, however, resolve and do not pose a significant risk to the fetus. It is important to be able to differentiate those of concern from those with little or no risk for an adverse outcome, to properly counsel the family, and to develop a follow-up or treatment plan. The antenatal assessment of the urinary tract is usually done through fetal ultrasound. The evaluation of the fetal urinary tract involves the assessment of amniotic fluid, kidneys, bladder, ureters, and gender.

AMNIOTIC FLUID

The amniotic fluid is initially not produced by the kidneys. The kidneys develop the ability to produce urine by about a 10-week gestation and by about a 16–18-week gestation, the fetal kidneys are the primary contributors to amniotic fluid production. Prior to 16-weeks gestation, a normal amount of amniotic fluid cannot be considered reassurance of an intact functioning urinary tract. A normal amount of amniotic fluid at 18-weeks gestation or later gives some reassurance that there is kidney function and that the urine flow is not completely obstructed. The presence of a normal amount of amniotic fluid does, however, neither eliminate the possibility of a urinary tract abnormality nor guarantee normal renal function after birth. An abnormally low amniotic fluid volume, however, may be due to a number of different etiologies besides abnormalities of the urinary tract. The main differential diagnosis includes the premature rupture of membranes and intrauterine growth restriction with placental insufficiency.

The most common methods to assess the amniotic fluid are the amniotic fluid index and single maximal vertical pocket of fluid. The fluid is measured for amniotic fluid index by measuring the maximal vertical pocket of fluid in each of four quadrants and adding them together. Significant oligohydramnios may be defined as either an amniotic fluid index of less than 5 cm or lack of a single maximal vertical pocket of 2 cm.

NORMAL URINARY TRACT

The fetal kidneys and bladder can first be seen by ultrasound at about 10–12-weeks gestation. The kidneys are noted in the late first trimester as paravertebral paired structures, slightly echogenic when compared to the surrounding organs, in the lumbar region. As the pregnancy progresses, the kidneys can be seen as slightly echolucent structures on either side of the spine, in the lumbar region. They can be seen in the transverse, sagittal, and coronal views of the region. Their location can sometimes be better defined by the location of the renal arteries coming off the aorta, noted with either color-flow mapping or power Doppler (Figure 1-1A). Over time, the kidneys become more easily visualized, as the renal capsule thickens and the perirenal fat pad develops (Figure 1-1B). By the third trimester, the pyramids can easily be seen (Figure 1-1C). The adrenal gland can be noted superior to the fetal kidneys. The presence of a small amount of fluid in the renal pelvis is considered normal and not a clinical concern.

By 10–12-week gestation, the bladder is noted as an echolucent structure in the fetal pelvis. The bladder wall is thin and there are no internal echoes normally seen. It can be visualized between the umbilical arteries, which wrap on either side of it, as they then join to leave the fetus in the umbilical cord (Figure 1-2). The bladder appearance, other than size, changes little throughout the last half of the pregnancy. It can be noted on ultrasound to fill and empty over time. The inability to

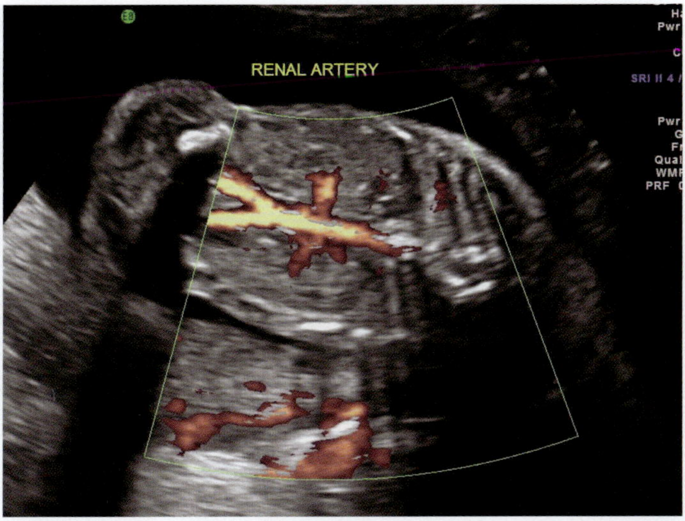

(A)

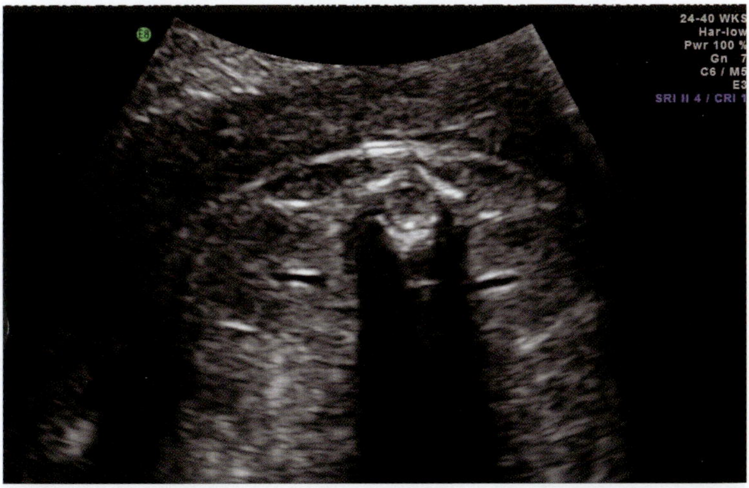

(B)

Figure 1-1. **A.** Power Doppler of normal renal arteries coming off the aorta above bifurcation into iliac arteries (thick arrows). **B.** Normal kidneys (circles surround) in 20-week fetus — transverse view, slightly hypoechoic compared to surrounding tissue. **C.** Normal kidney in 34-week fetus — sagittal view, showing echolucent renal pyramids.

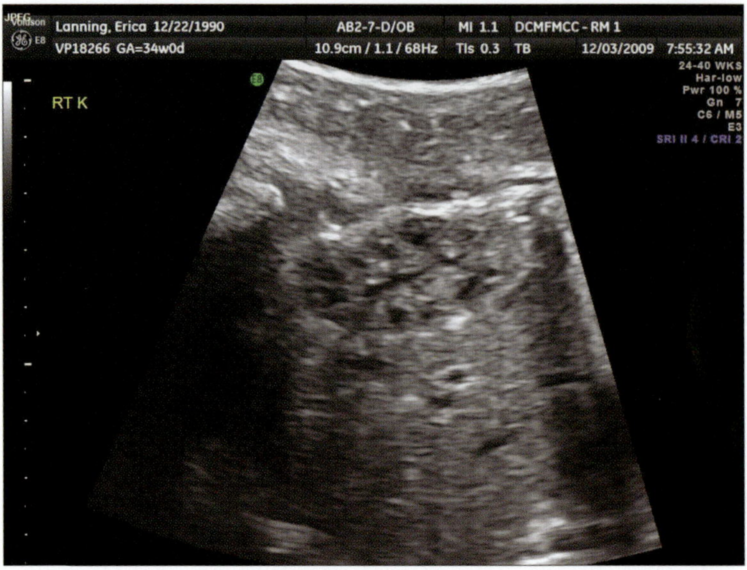

(C)

Figure 1-1. (*Continued*)

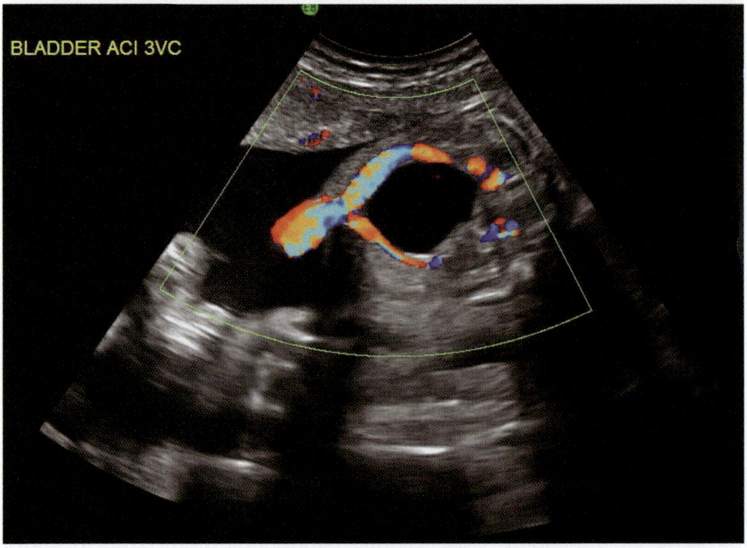

Figure 1-2. Normal bladder demonstrating umbilical arteries wrapping around bladder, then entering the umbilical cord.

visualize the fetal bladder when normal amniotic fluid is present, usually means it is empty and reevaluation at a later time will usually demonstrate its presence.

The fetal ureters are rarely seen in normal fetuses. With high-resolution ultrasound, normal ureters may be seen measuring 1–2 mm in the third trimester. Ureteral dilation of 4 mm or greater should prompt further evaluation, as it is most likely abnormal.

Normal male (Figure 1-3) and female external genital can usually be seen by the second trimester. The discussion of abnormal and ambiguous genitalia is beyond the scope of this chapter.

ABNORMAL URINARY TRACT

The antenatal evaluation of the fetus for urinary tract abnormalities includes the assessment of the presence, location, size, shape, echogenicity, and architecture; the presence or absence of dilatation of each kidney; the evaluation of the bladder for presence, location, size, wall thickness, and internal echoes; the visualization of ureters if dilated; and the assessment

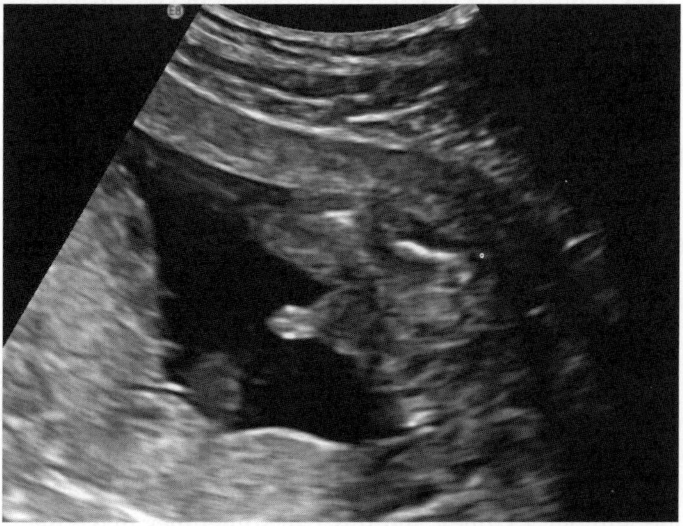

Figure 1-3. Normal 19-week male fetus, showing penis and scrotum.

of the amniotic fluid volume. The determination of fetal sex may be important, as most urinary tract abnormalities are more common in male. A careful examination for any non-renal anomalies should be performed if any urinary tract abnormality is noted.

In evaluating a fetal ultrasound for urinary tract abnormalities, they can be placed in three main groups: (1) the abnormalities of kidney number or position, (2) cystic kidney lesions, and (3) dilated urinary tract (kidneys, ureters, and/or bladder).

Abnormalities of Kidney Number or Position

The kidneys develop from the intermediate mesoderm. The pronephros and mesonephros develop and then regress. The metanephros or definitive kidney then develops from the paired ureteric buds, from the distal mesonephric duct, which grow out to the metanephric mesenchyme in the sacral region and induce kidney formation. The ureteric buds become the ureters and collecting system and the metanephric mesenchyme (blastema) becomes the nephrons. The ureteric bud reaching the metanephric blastema is necessary for the kidney formation. The kidneys then move up from the sacral region to their normal paraspinal lumbar location. The failure of the ureteric bud to reach the metanephric blastema results in renal agenesis. The failure of normal bilateral migration from the sacral region can result in ectopic kidneys.

Renal agenesis can be unilateral or bilateral. The types of renal ectopia include pelvic kidney, horseshoe kidney, and crossed renal ectopia.

Unilateral Renal Agenesis

This should be suspected when ultrasound fails to identify both kidneys in a normal location. An empty renal fossa on one side should raise the suspicion that one kidney did not develop. The use of color-flow mapping or power Doppler to assess the renal arteries will identify only one renal artery (Figure 1-4). Care should be taken to rule out an ectopic location for the suspected absent kidney. The adrenal gland can fill the renal fossae on the side without a kidney and this can sometimes make the diagnosis

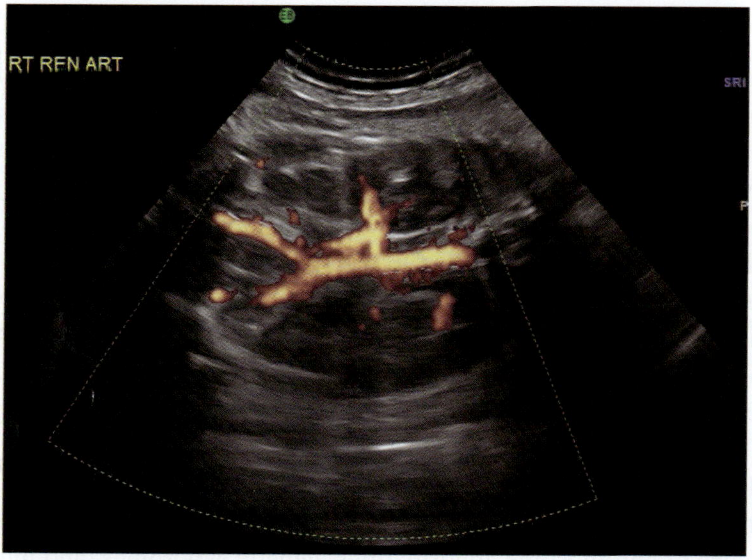

Figure 1-4. Unilateral renal agenesis — coronal view: power Doppler of arteries showing single right renal artery coming off aorta and no left renal artery.

difficult. Amniotic fluid volume is usually normal. Compensatory hypertrophy of the contralateral kidney is common.

Unilateral renal agenesis occurs in 1/500–1/1000 pregnancies. The prognosis for unilateral renal agenesis is generally good. The incidence of chromosome abnormalities does not appear to be significantly elevated, though an increased incidence of gynecologic abnormalities is reported. Fetal complications are unusual because of unilateral renal agenesis. Postnatal management should include an ultrasound evaluation to confirm the diagnosis and to assess the remaining kidney for abnormalities. An incidence of renal anomalies of up to 90% in the remaining kidney has been reported, with vesicoureteral reflux representing over half of those abnormalities. The high risk of reflux has prompted many to recommend a voiding cystourethrogram (VCUG) and prophylactic antibiotics for these fetuses. Long-term follow-up is also appropriate, as there is a reported increased incidence of hypertension, proteinuria, and renal failure in adults with unilateral renal agenesis.

Bilateral Renal Agenesis

Bilateral renal agenesis should be suspected when severe oligohydramnios is noted. Due to the severe oligohydramnios, the examination may be difficult. A careful evaluation of the renal fossae will fail to demonstrate the evidence of kidneys. The adrenal glands may be noted to fill the renal fossae and color-flow Doppler will fail to demonstrate renal arteries. The bladder will not be visualized in the fetal pelvis and this can be confirmed with color-flow mapping demonstrating no bladder between the umbilical arteries. The differential diagnosis includes the other causes of severe oligohydramnios including severe renal diseases such as polycystic kidneys, intrauterine growth restriction, and the premature rupture of membranes.

The incidence of bilateral renal agenesis is about 1/4000. Associate non-renal anomalies are common, up to 50%, and there is an increased incidence of chromosome abnormalities, genetic syndromes, and multiple malformation syndromes such as VATER association. The evaluation should, therefore, include a careful assessment for other abnormalities, which may require an amnioinfusion for better visualization. Potter's sequence is seen, with flattened facies, low set ears, beaked nose, and receding chin, with pulmonary hypoplasia and limb anomalies. The prognosis is uniformly lethal and the option of pregnancy termination should be offered. Autopsy and karyotype analysis should be considered at the time of termination or delivery.

Pelvic Kidney

A pelvic kidney should be considered anytime that one of the kidneys is not noted in its normal location. Usually, a normal contralateral kidney is seen with an empty renal fossa. Color-flow mapping will fail to demonstrate a normally located renal artery on the side with the pelvic kidney. A careful assessment of the fetal pelvis will reveal a kidney with normal renal architecture lying superior to the bladder. The differential diagnosis includes other types of ectopic kidneys and unilateral renal agenesis.

The incidence of pelvic kidneys is about 1/700–1/1000. It is the most common type of ectopic kidney. The prognosis is usually good. A careful fetal anatomic survey is appropriate as pelvic kidneys are reported to be seen with other anatomic abnormalities. Postnatal evaluation, with renal ultrasound and VCUG, for urologic abnormalities, particularly vesicoureteral reflux, is appropriate for both kidneys. There is an association with gynecologic abnormalities, which will require postnatal evaluation.

Horseshoe Kidney

A horseshoe kidney is seen when the kidneys are noted to join anteriorly in front of the spine on a transverse ultrasound of the fetus through the kidneys. The lower poles are fused. This is associated with an increased risk of both urinary tract and non-urinary tract abnormalities. It is associated with an increased risk of chromosome abnormalities particularly trisomy 18 and 45X. Evaluation should, thus, include a detailed anatomic survey and a karyotype analysis if not an isolated finding.

The incidence is 1/400–500 live births. For isolated horseshoe kidneys, prognosis is very good. In non-isolated cases, the prognosis is more reflected by the other anomalies present or by karyotype abnormality. Postnatal renal evaluation, with renal ultrasound and VCUG, is appropriate, as there is up to a 50% incidence of vesicoureteral reflux reported. Prophylactic antibiotic use should be considered.

Crossed Fused Renal Ectopia

This is a variant of ectopic kidney where the affected kidney is noted on the same side as the contralateral kidney and on the opposite side of its ureteral insertion into the bladder. Ultrasound findings include an empty renal fossa on one side and an enlarged and abnormal-shaped kidney on the other side. The kidneys are fused and the appearance is an enlarged, bilobed, and angulated or S-shaped kidney. A careful anatomic survey is appropriate as other anomalies, particularly vertebral anomalies, have been associated with this finding. The differential diagnosis includes other types of ectopic kidney, duplex kidney, and unilateral renal agenesis.

This accounts for about 27% of ectopic kidneys. The prognosis is usually very good, as long as it is an isolated finding. Postnatal renal evaluation and prophylactic antibiotics, as for a horseshoe kidney, are appropriate due to the high incidence of vesicoureteral reflux.

Cystic Kidney Disease

Cystic kidney disease in the fetus includes a varied group of disorders, from benign isolated macroscopic cysts to inherited disorders with microscopic cysts and poor prognosis. The kidneys should be assessed for the following in evaluating cystic renal disease: unilateral vs. bilateral disease; the appearance of the cysts; whether the normal renal architecture preserved to some degree; the kidney size; the echogenicity of the kidneys in relation to the surrounding organs; and amniotic fluid volume. Obtaining a family history and assessing for non-renal anomalies can also help establish the diagnosis.

Isolated Renal Cysts

Simple renal cysts are seen as solitary cysts in the fetal kidney with a well-defined border and no internal echoes. They tend to be peripherally located, but can be located anywhere in the kidney and should not connect to the renal pelvis or calyces. The prognosis is excellent. Over 90% detected in the second trimester will resolve *in utero*. It is important to differentiate this from a dilated renal pelvis or calyx. Since progression from a single cyst in the second trimester to a multicystic dysplastic kidney (MCDK) in the third trimester has been reported, follow-up in the third trimester is appropriate when the cyst is first detected in the second trimester. If *in utero* resolution is noted, no further follow-up is needed. If still present, in the third trimester, a postnatal ultrasound is appropriate. There does not appear to be a risk of contralateral renal abnormalities with isolated renal cysts.

Multicystic Dysplastic Kidney (MCDK) Disease

The most common type of fetal cystic kidney disease is MCDK (Potter type II), with an incidence of about 2.1/1000. It is easily diagnosed *in utero* with reports of up to a 100% detection rate with antenatal ultrasound. The

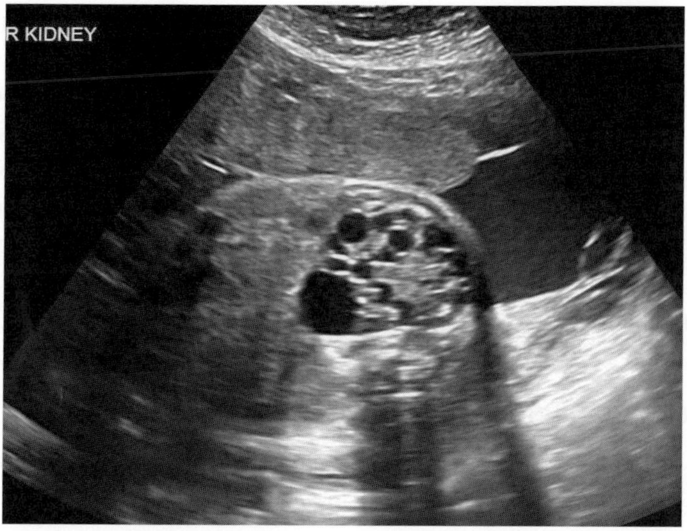

Figure 1-5. Unilateral MCDK, mostly small cysts with echodense (dysplastic) tissue between the cysts.

ultrasound appears as multiple well-defined cysts within the kidney that do not connect to each other or the renal pelvis. The cysts are variable in size (Figure 1-5). The normal renal architecture is disrupted and a normal renal parenchyma is not seen. The tissue present between the cysts is echogenic (dysplastic appearance). The kidney size can be quite large, crossing the midline and filling the abdomen. This should be differentiated from a severely hydronephrotic kidney. These kidneys are non-functioning, unless only part of the kidney is involved, for example, in a duplex system when only one pole is affected. MCDK are usually unilateral and normal amniotic fluid is noted. When bilateral, there is usually oligohydramnios. The fetal ultrasound should include an evaluation of the contralateral kidney and assessment for non-renal anomalies.

The etiology is felt to be a failed normal reaction between the development of the branching ureteric bud and the metanephros. For unilateral disease, the prognosis is good. Bilateral disease has a very poor prognosis, with no non-functioning kidneys and severe oligohydramnios; neonatal death usually occurring because of pulmonary hypoplasia. The exception would be if one side had duplex system with one pole normal. With unilateral disease, the MCDK tends to resolve either *in utero* or after birth. The rates of at least partial resolution postpartum are reported as high as 91%. The contralateral kidney should be carefully assessed after birth, as there is a 39–50% incidence of renal abnormalities reported, with vesicoureteric reflux being most common. A renal ultrasound and VCUG should be performed after birth. The use of prophylactic antibiotics is recommended by some, at least until the workup can be completed.

Obstructive Cystic Dysplasia

Obstructive cystic dysplasia (Potter type IV) presents as echogenic kidney(s) with small cortical cysts, in the presence of early severe urinary tract obstruction. It can be unilateral or bilateral and can be seen with severe urinary tract obstruction such as posterior urethral valves (PUVs) (bilateral) or ureteropelvic junction obstruction (UPJO) (unilateral). The chance for normal renal function of the affected kidney is decreased, so the overall prognosis in bilateral disease, with oligohydramnios, is poor due to the possibility of pulmonary hypoplasia. The differential diagnosis is other types of echogenic kidneys or cystic kidneys, but the presence of an obstructive lesion along with echogenic kidneys with cortical cysts is highly suggestive of this diagnosis.

Autosomal Recessive Polycystic Kidney Disease (ARPKD)

ARPKD (Potter type I) is typically characterized by the fetal ultrasound finding, in the second or third trimester of bilateral, significantly enlarged, echogenic kidneys, absent bladder, and severe oligohydramnios (Figure 1-6). It may not be detected until the third trimester; therefore, fetuses, at risk due to family history, need serial ultrasounds throughout gestation to exclude the disease. A search for non-renal anomalies should be performed, as multiple syndromes and karyotype abnormalities can be seen with enlarged echogenic kidneys. The presence

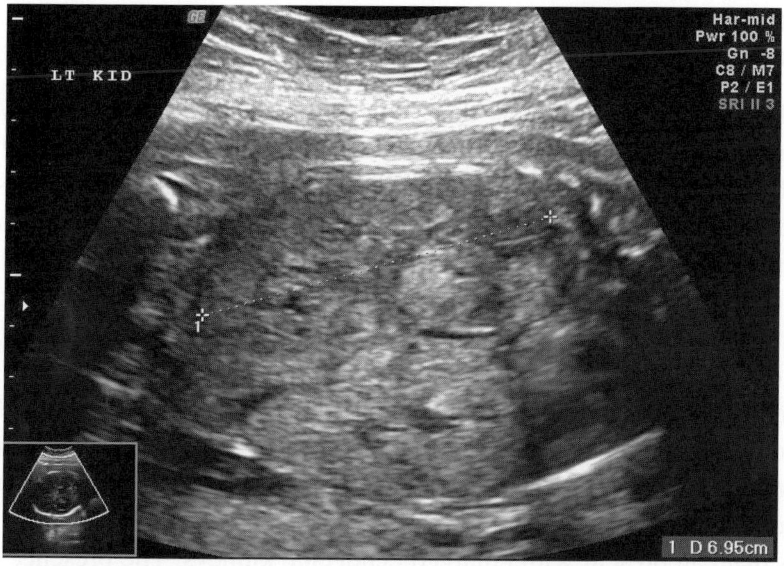

Figure 1-6. Bilateral enlarged echogenic kidneys at 26 weeks. Note the absence of large cysts and the lack of amniotic fluid. Kidney length is >6 cm both sides, which is about twice upper normal for gestational age of 26 weeks.

of a non-renal anomaly suggests a diagnosis other than ARPKD, and if present, genetic testing should be offered. The differential diagnosis includes the other causes of enlarged and echogenic kidneys (discussed under ADPKD).

The incidence is approximately 1/40,000. This is an autosomal recessive disorder usually due to a mutation in the PKHD1 gene on chromosome 6p. A family history is an important part of the evaluation. There appears to be more than one type of diseases, with the perinatal type (seen *in utero*) being the most common and the most severe. The prognosis is poor, which is usually resulting in neonatal death due to pulmonary hypoplasia (perinatal type). Hepatic fibrosis is also present, but is not seen on antenatal ultrasound. The recurrence risk is 25%. Parents should receive genetic counseling once the diagnosis is made. Due to the poor prognosis with *in utero* diagnosis, the option of pregnancy termination should be discussed.

Autosomal Dominant Polycystic Kidney Disease (ADPKD)

ADPKD (Potter type III) is the most common type of heritable cystic renal disease, with an incidence of 1/400–1/1000. It is the cause of 8–10% of the cases of end-stage renal disease in adults. The ultrasound presentation is one of bilateral enlarged echogenic kidneys with increased corticomedullary differentiation. Multiple cysts may be present and there is normal amniotic fluid. It is not uncommon for the kidneys to appear normal in the second trimester and take on an abnormal appearance later in gestation, so any fetus at risk should be followed throughout gestation. Some fetuses will have normal kidneys throughout gestation on ultrasound and not manifest changes until later in life. The kidney shape usually remains intact. A careful assessment for non-renal anomalies should be made, as there are multiple syndrome and karyotype abnormalities that can present with enlarged echogenic kidneys. The presence of a facial cleft, cardiac anomaly, and holoprosencephaly would suggest trisomy 13; an encephalocele and polydactyly would suggest Meckel–Gruber syndrome; and macrosomia and an omphalocele would suggest Beckwith–Wiedemann syndrome, as examples. If a non-renal anomaly is present fetal genetic evaluation should be offered.

ADPKD is an autosomal dominant disorder with 85% of cases localized to the PKD1 gene on the chromosome 16p and others on PKD2 gene on chromosome 4q. The neonatal prognosis is usually good. Hypertension and renal failure usually do not present until the 4–5th decade of life, but hypertension can present in childhood, in about 30% of cases. It is a disease of cyst formation in ductal organs, including the liver, pancreas, spleen, and central nervous system. These cysts are not seen prenatally. Genetic counseling should be offered to any at risk family, or if the disease is suspected by fetal ultrasound. If not already diagnosed or assessed, the parents and siblings should be evaluated, as they may have ADPKD and be asymptomatic. There is a 50% recurrence risk in children and siblings.

Dilated Urinary Tract

Dilated renal collecting systems are the most common type of renal abnormality noted on fetal ultrasound, occurring in up to 2–5% of antenatal ultrasounds. This can involve the pelvis only or extend into the calyces. Dilatation can be unilateral or bilateral. The ureters and bladder may also be dilated. In evaluating fetal hydronephrosis, the extent of dilatation as well as which structures are or are not dilated can help in making the diagnosis and assessing the general level of significance.

Some urine in the renal pelvis is normal. How much constitute abnormal changes throughout gestation and the exact cutoff values have been a subject of controversy. Prior to 32 weeks of gestation, the upper limit of normal is 4 or 5 mm. At 32 weeks of gestation or more, 7 mm should be considered abnormal. Using a cutoff of <7 mm to predict which fetuses will have no renal abnormalities, has a sensitivity, specificity, positive predictive value, and negative predictive value of 87%, 85%, 93%, and 74%, respectively. It has been demonstrated that using a higher cutoff of >10 mm to differentiate who to evaluate postnatally will miss up to 80% of the cases of vesicoureteral reflux. Thus, a renal pelvis AP diameter of ≥7 mm should be considered abnormal in the third trimester and used to identify those fetuses that warrant postnatal evaluation.

There are two different grading systems used to categorize fetal hydronephrosis to help differentiate the risk of significant abnormalities and the need for follow-up. One uses the AP diameter of the renal pelvis in the transverse view (third trimester). Most authors have used this to classify fetal hydronephrosis. Mild is an AP diameter of 7 to <10 mm; moderate 10 to <15 mm and severe ≥15 mm. The other method used is the grading system from the Fetal Urologic Society. Grade 0 is normal (Figure 1-1B). Grade 1 is mild pelvis dilatation only (Figure 1-7A). Grade 2 is moderate pelvis dilatation and some calyces (Figure 1-7B). Grade 3 is marked dilatation of the pelvis and all calyces with a normal parenchyma thickness (Figure 1-7C). Grade 4 is further pelvicalyceal dilatation and thinned parenchyma (Figure 1-7D).

Mild renal pelvis dilatation (>4 or 5 mm) in the second trimester resolves up to 80% of the time *in utero* but only up to 15% of the time if >7 mm. It is difficult to determine from a second trimester ultrasound if resolution (Figure 1-8) or worsening (Figure 1-9) will occur. Therefore, all cases of renal pelvis dilatation in the second trimester should be reevaluated in the third trimester. Dilatation of ≥10 mm or the presence of hydroureter, significant calyceal dilatation, megacystis, or oligohydramnios should be

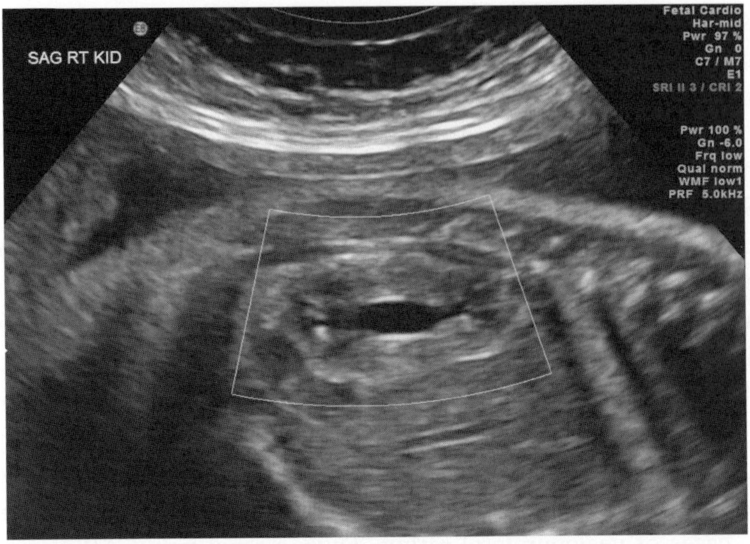

(A)

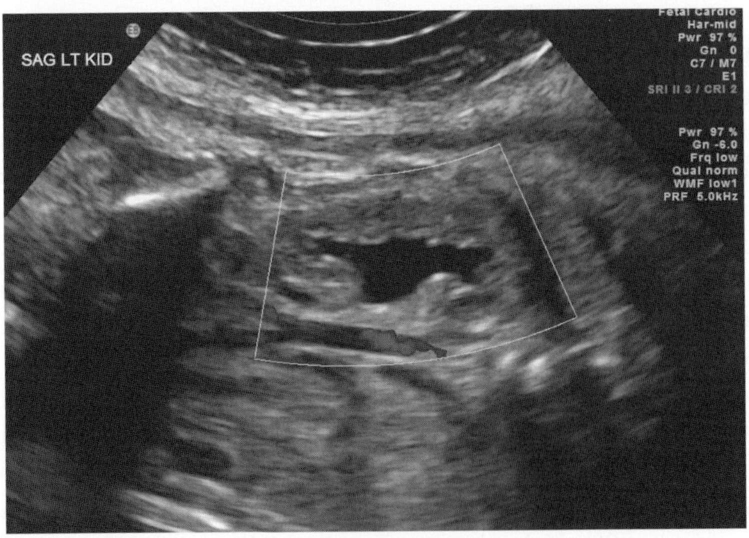

(B)

Figure 1-7. **A.** Grade 1 hydronephrosis. **B.** Grade 2 hydronephrosis. **C.** Grade 3 hydronephrosis. **D.** Grade 4 hydronephrosis.

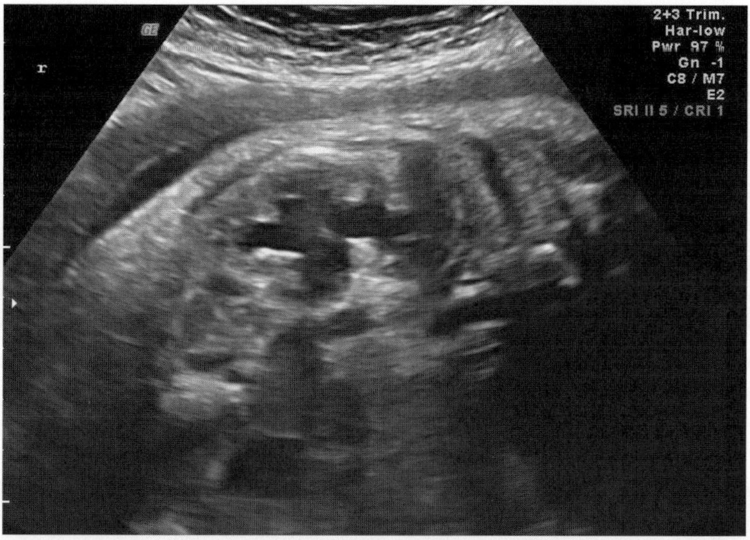

(C)

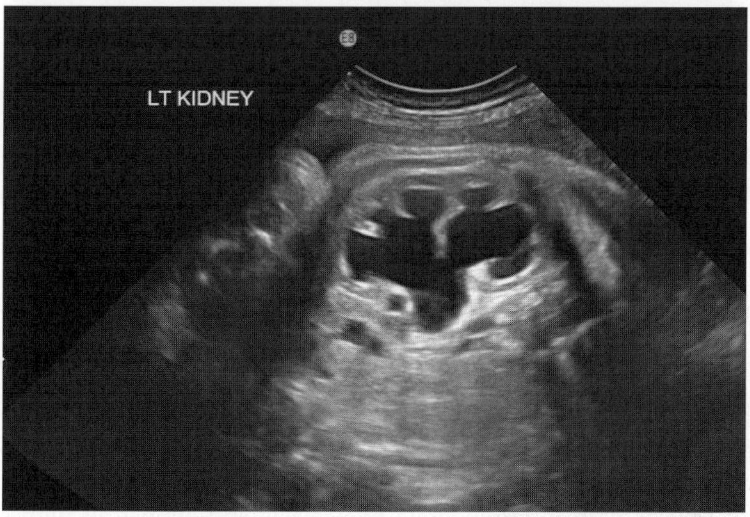

(D)

Figure 1-7. (*Continued*)

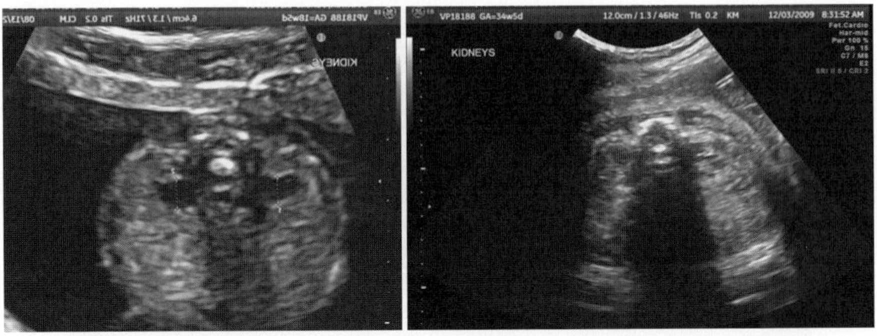

Figure 1-8. Mild bilateral renal pelvis dilatation at 18 weeks, with resolution by 34-week gestation.

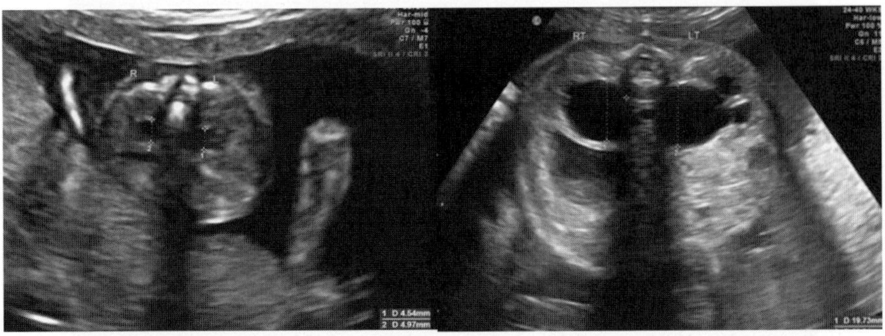

Figure 1-9. Mild bilateral renal pelvis dilatation at 18 weeks (left 4.5 mm; right 4.97 mm) that increased significantly by 30-week gestation (left 20.2 mm; right 19.7 mm) in a fetus with ureteral stenosis.

considered significantly abnormal and increased surveillance is appropriate. The greater the degree of dilatation in the third trimester, the greater the chance there will be a significant renal abnormality noted after birth. With 39% of fetuses with mild/moderate pyelectasis and almost all with severe pyelectasis having significant disease postnatally. When evaluated after birth, the most common etiologies for fetal renal pelvis dilatation/hydronephrosis are UPJO, vesicoureteric reflux, duplex system, ureterocele, ureterovesical junction obstruction (UVJO), megaureter, and PUVs.

The other area of concern in the second trimester is the risk of aneuploidy. An increased risk of aneuploidy, mostly Down syndrome, has been reported with second trimester pelviectasis. While some authors attribute an increased likelihood ratio (1.5–1.9) to this as an isolated finding, it is not universally accepted. What is agreed upon is that the presence of renal pelvis dilatation in the second trimester is a reason for a detailed anatomic survey to be performed. The presence of a non-renal anomaly in addition to the pyelectasis indicates an increased aneuploidy risk, 8% in one series, and these patients should be offered genetic counseling and testing.

Ureteropelvic Junction Obstruction (UPJO)

UPJO is the most common cause of fetal urinary tract dilatation (hydronephrosis) in most studies. The incidence is about 4.2/1000. The ultrasound appearance is a dilated renal pelvis and usually calyces, with sparing of the ureter and bladder. Classically, the pelvis is dilated more than the calyces. The dilatation ranges from mild to severe (Figure 1-10) and it is usually unilateral (61%). The amniotic fluid volume is usually normal or increased. The degree of dilatation correlates to the degree of renal impairment noted after birth, with increasing dilatation associated with decreasing renal function, in general. It does not, however, accurately predict the level of renal function. On postnatal evaluation, a physical obstruction is often not found, thus suggesting that the obstruction may be either functional or physical. The differential diagnosis includes the other causes of renal pelvis dilatation (reflux #1) and MCDK.

The prognosis is usually good, especially in unilateral disease. Neonatal evaluation should include a renal ultrasound and VCUG. It is important to evaluate the contralateral kidney for abnormalities, as their presence is reported up to 25% of the time, with vesicoureteric reflux being most common. In cases with severe dilatation or bilateral disease, a nuclear renogram may also be appropriate. Many recommend the use of prophylactic antibiotics until reflux can be excluded.

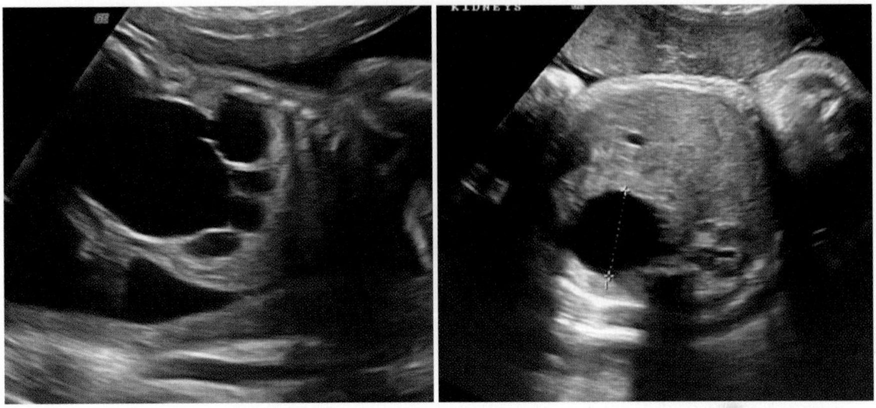

Figure 1-10. Severe unilateral UPJO — transverse and sagittal view — with classic "bear claw" appearance.

Uretrovesical Junction Obstruction (UVJO)

UVJO is a result of obstruction at the distal end of the ureter near the bladder junction. On ultrasound, a dilated kidney (pelvis and usually calyces) is seen along with a dilated ureter (Figures 1-11 and 1-12). The ureter may be dilated more than the renal pelvis. It is usually unilateral, with normal bladder and amniotic fluid volume. The differential diagnosis consists of the other causes of hydroureteronephrosis, particularly reflux.

The prognosis is usually good. If the ureter is dilated > 10 mm, there is a greater chance that surgical intervention will be required. Postnatal follow-up is warranted any time hydroureter is noted on fetal ultrasound. A renal ultrasound and VCUG should be performed. A nuclear renogram should be used if appropriate. The contralateral kidney should be evaluated due to the high incidence of anomalies reported. The use of prophylactic antibiotics until the evaluation is complete is recommended.

Vesicoureteric Reflux

Vesicoureteric reflux occurs when there is urine flow back from the bladder to the ureter and kidney. In most studies, it is one of the two most common causes of fetal hydronephrosis. The incidence is about 3.6/1000. It may be primary (discussed here) or secondary (due to another urologic

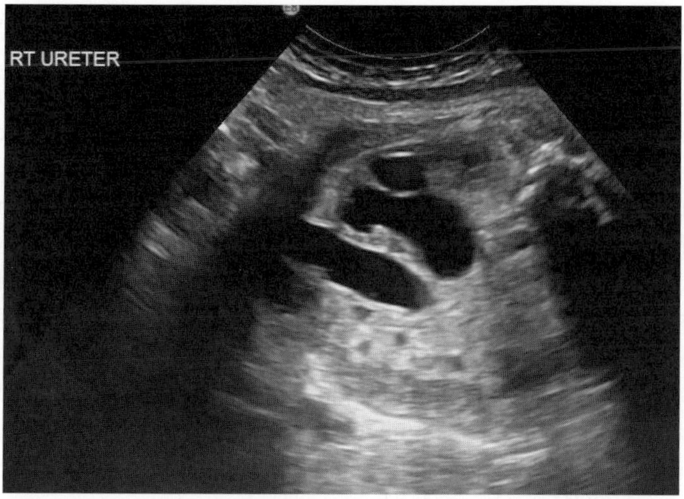

Figure 1-11. UVJO showing dilated kidney and dilated ureter.

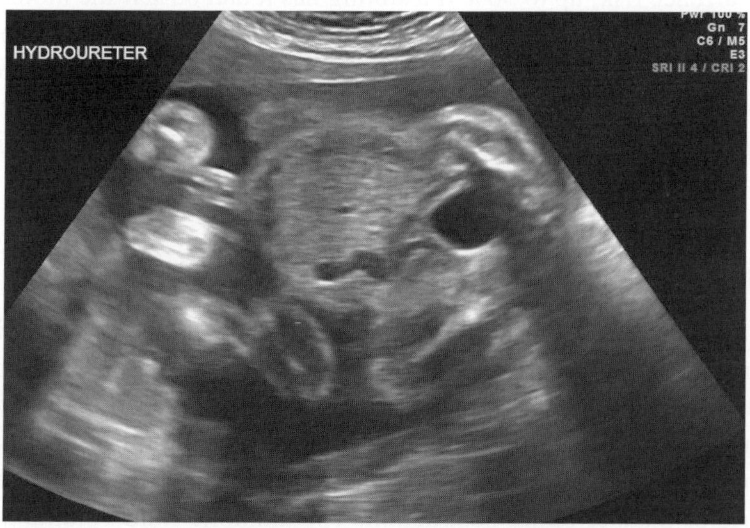

Figure 1-12. UVJO showing dilated mid and distal ureters coursing toward the bladder.

abnormality, such as PUVs). On ultrasound, it should be suspected whenever there is a dilated ureter, renal pelvis and calyces, with a normal bladder and amniotic fluid. It may be present with only kidney dilatation and normal ureters. When the renal pelvis size is noted to change during the course of an examination, it should be suspected. The degree of renal pelvis dilatation does not necessarily correlate with the degree of reflux noted after birth, so all fetuses with suspected reflux should be evaluated after birth, even if the dilatation is mild. The differential diagnosis includes the other causes of hydronephrosis.

The prognosis is usually good with postnatal resolution in 25–80% of cases, with milder cases having a better chance of resolution. Non-treated reflux can cause permanent damage and accounts for up to 25% of childhood and 15% of adult cases of end-stage renal disease. Postnatal evaluation includes a VCUG and renal ultrasound. A nuclear renogram may be appropriate, especially if severe. Prophylactic antibiotics should be used. Though no genetic markers have been identified, there is a strong familial recurrence risk, up to 30% if a sibling has it and 65% if the mother has it. In affected families, it may be appropriate to have a pediatric urologic evaluation, even if the fetal ultrasounds were normal. When a fetus/neonate is diagnosed with reflux, consideration should be given to testing siblings and parents, especially if there is a history of recurrent urinary tract infections.

Primary Non-Refluxing Non-Obstructed Megaureter

Non-refluxing non-obstructed megaureter is the presence of a dilated ureter (and kidney) with no evidence of obstruction or reflux and no evidence of bladder outlet obstruction, on postnatal examination. It is felt to be due to an abnormal ureteral innervation and function. Fetal ultrasound demonstrates dilated ureters and kidneys, but without the evidence of a ureteric or bladder outlet obstruction. The amniotic fluid volume is normal. Fetal ultrasound should look for other possible etiologies and assess the contralateral kidney. The differential diagnosis is the other causes of hydroureteronephrosis. In some studies, this may be grouped with UVJ obstruction, functional type.

The prognosis is very good. Spontaneous resolution in 72% of cases, followed conservatively, after birth, is reported. The postnatal workup is the same as for a fetus with suspected vesicoureteric reflux.

Duplex System and Ureterocele

A duplex system is present when there are two separate renal collecting systems in one kidney with separate ureters that originate from the same side. The ureters may implant into the bladder in a normal or ectopic location (trigone, bladder neck, or urethra). Duplex kidneys arise when a second ureteric bud forms and grows into the metanephric mesoderm. On ultrasound, two renal pelves are noted within one kidney. One or both poles are usually dilated; the upper one is most commonly affected, due to either an ureterocele or vesicoureteric reflux (Figure 1-13). The ureter is often dilated. If no dilatation is present, a duplex kidney will present on ultrasound as an enlarged kidney, with a contralateral normal kidney.

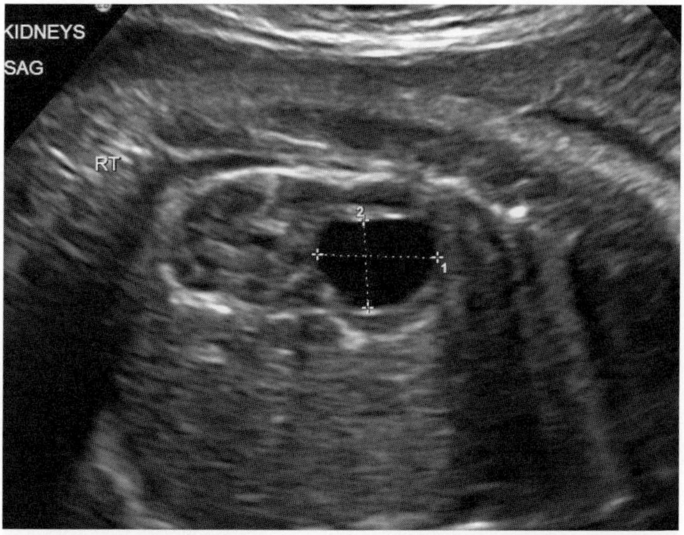

Figure 1-13. Duplex system with upper pole dilated and lower pole normal.

An ureterocele is an anomaly in which the distal intravesical portion of the ureter is dilated because of stenosis or blockage. They are usually seen in duplex systems and are more commonly associated with the upper pole. An ureterocele is seen as a dilated ureter prolapsing into the bladder. An ureterocele can easily been seen bulging into a normally filled bladder from the affected side (Figure 1-14). The amniotic fluid volume is usually normal. The differential diagnosis is the other causes of hydronephrosis, though the presence of an ureterocele bulging into the bladder is diagnostic.

When a duplex system is suspected, careful assessment for other renal abnormalities should be performed. The presence of reflux, ectopic ureter, ureterocele, or MCDK of one pole is often seen, with the upper pole most commonly affected. When the upper pole is affected with an ureterocele, the lower pole has vesicoureteric reflux in about 50% of cases. Ureteroceles and duplex systems are some of the few urinary tract abnormalities that are more common in girls. Ureteroceles without duplex systems are rarer and are more common in boys.

The prognosis is usually good. Postnatal evaluation consists of a renal ultrasound, VCUG, and nuclear renogram. The contralateral kidney

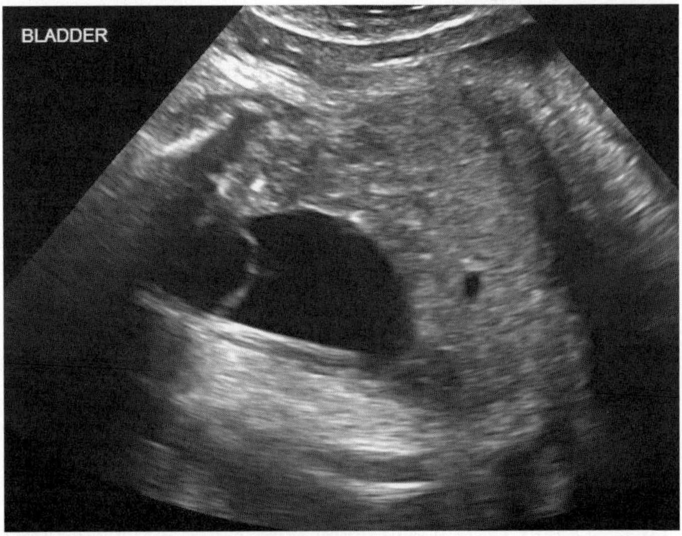

Figure 1-14. Bladder with ureterocele bulging into bladder.

should also be evaluated. Prophylactic antibiotics should be used until reflux has been excluded. The prenatal diagnosis and the use of prophylactic antibiotics from birth has been shown to decrease the incidence of urinary tract infections and secondary operative procedures compared to postnatally diagnosed fetuses.

Posterior Urethral Valves (PUVs)

PUVs are the most common type of bladder outlet obstruction seen in fetuses. The incidence is 1/5000–1/8000. It is limited to males. In the first trimester, a bladder outlet obstruction can be seen as a much dilated bladder; the kidneys may not be well seen and the amniotic fluid is normal, as urine is not yet the main component, though a typical PUV bladder appearance can be seen early in some cases (Figure 1-15). Sometimes, the bladder will rupture and the fetus will present with urinary ascites (Figure 1-16). The characteristic fetal ultrasound appearance

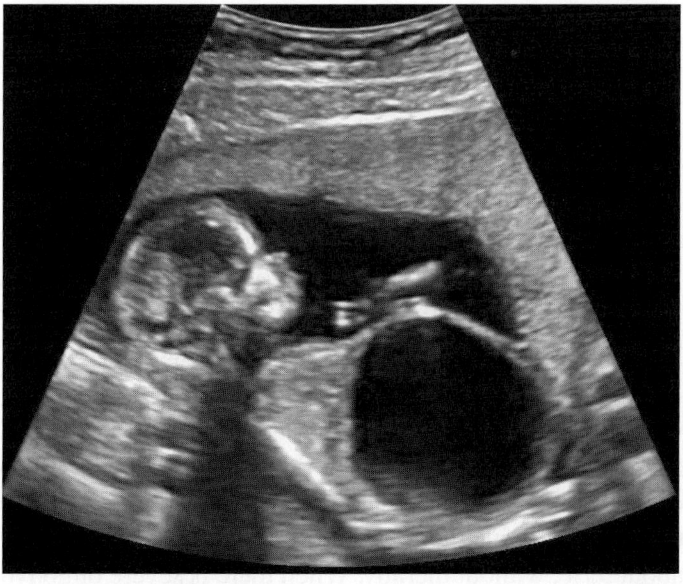

Figure 1-15. Bladder outlet obstruction at 13-week gestation with dilated bladder and normal amniotic fluid.

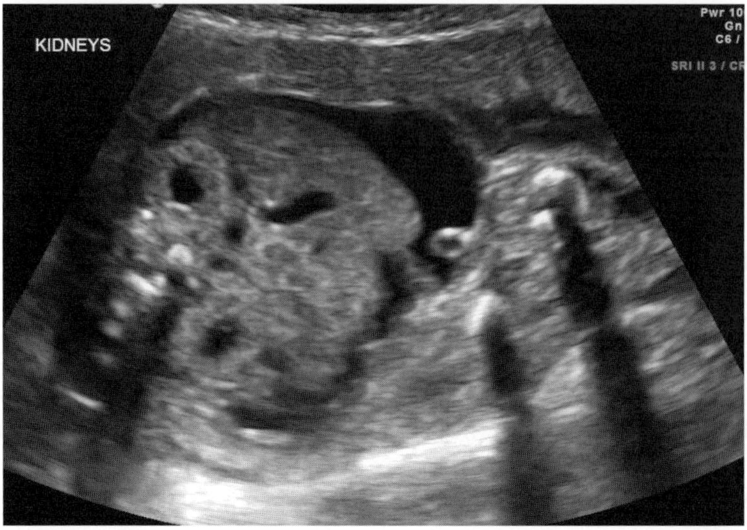

Figure 1-16. Bladder outlet obstruction presenting as a ruptured bladder with urinary ascites, dilated echogenic kidneys with small cortical cysts and no amniotic fluid.

of PUV is a dilated, thick-walled bladder with a dilated proximal urethra, or "key hole" appearance (Figure 1-17), with bilateral dilated ureters and kidneys and oligohydramnios. This appearance, however, can be seen in other forms of bladder outlet obstruction. Not all cases have oligohydramnios. It is important to assess for non-urinary tract abnormalities and this may require an amnioinfusion for better visualization. The incidence of karyotype abnormalities is about 12% and genetic counseling should be provided and genetic testing offered. The differential diagnosis includes other forms of bladder outlet obstruction and megacystis.

PUVs are the result of a membrane (valve) in the posterior urethra blocking the urethra. Since not all cases have severe oligohydramnios, this blockage may not be complete. The prognosis in PUV is variable and may be affected by intrauterine therapy. The overall survival with *in utero* diagnosis is about 55%, without therapy. When there is severe oligohydramnios in the mid-trimester, the mortality is at least 90% and for this group,

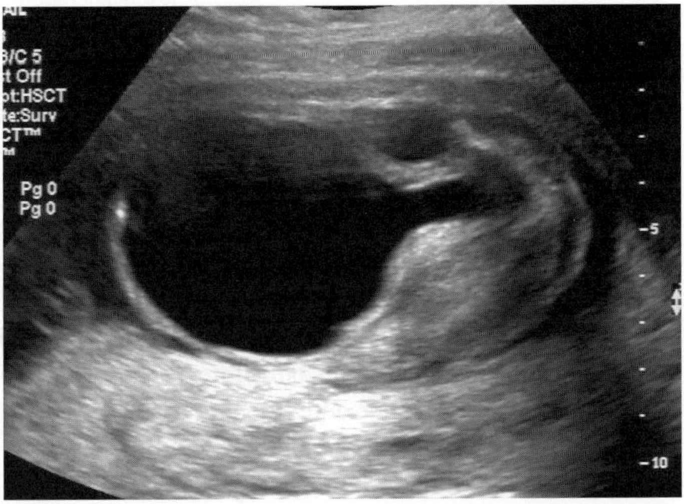

Figure 1-17. Classic appearance of PUV with a dilated, thick walled bladder and dilated proximal urethra (key-hole sign). Normal appearing amniotic fluid is from amniofusion.

termination is an option. Ultrasound markers of poor prognosis are diagnosis prior to 24-week gestation, severe oligohydramnios, echogenic kidneys with cortical cysts (obstructive cystic dysplasia), and non-urinary tract abnormalities or a karyotype abnormality. These fetuses usually succumb to pulmonary hypoplasia. To better differentiate those with a good prognosis, who may benefit from *in utero* intervention, some suggest the serial assessments of urinary electrolytes by vesicocentesis. Good prognosis values would be urinary sodium <90 mmol/L; chloride <80 mmol/L; osmolality <180 mOsm/L; calcium <7 mg/L; total protein <20 md/dL, and beta 2 microglobulin <6 mg/L. Those in the good prognosis group may be candidates for *in utero* intervention with the placement of a vesicoamniotic shunt. In the good prognosis group receiving *in utero* therapy, the survival of 47–91% has been reported with 34–40% of survivors having end-stage renal disease and 44% having persistent respiratory problems. The use and long-term outcomes from this approach are still controversial.

Postnatal evaluation consists of ultrasound, VCUG, and nuclear renogram. Surgery is usually required.

Urethral Atresia

Urethral atresia is the second most common form of fetal bladder outlet obstruction and is the most common in females. It can be detected as early as the first trimester. The typical ultrasound appearance in the second trimester is a massively dilated thin-walled bladder, bilateral hydroureteronephrosis, and severe oligohydramnios (Figure 1-18). Associated anomalies are common and may require an amnioinfusion to visualize. In female fetuses, this may be associated with cloacal anomalies. There is a significant risk for chromosome abnormalities and genetic counseling and testing should be offered. The differential diagnosis is the other causes of bladder outlet obstruction.

Urethral atresia is due to a complete blockage of the urethra or due to the incomplete formation of the urethra. The prognosis is uniformly poor, with most dying soon after birth due to pulmonary hypoplasia. Due to the very poor prognosis, the option of termination should be offered. Some have suggested *in utero* intervention as for PUV, but this is controversial and the experience and success are much less than with PUV.

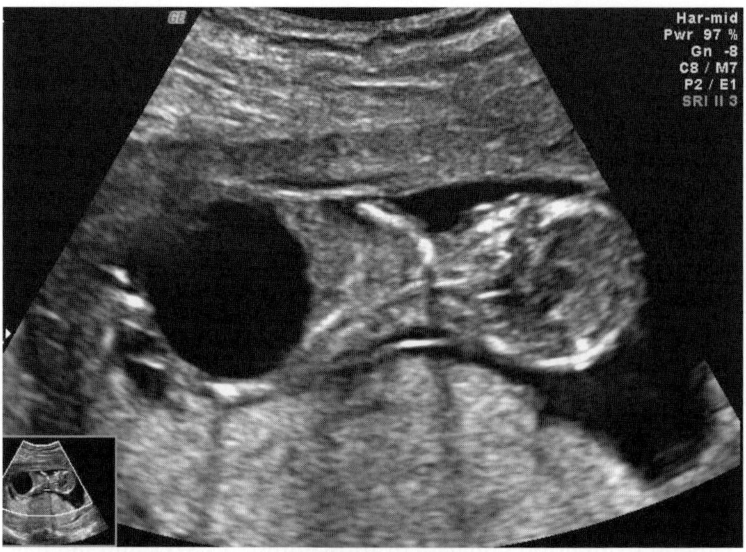

Figure 1-18. Urethral atresia in a female fetus at 16 weeks with a severely dilated thin-walled bladder and no amniotic fluid.

Megacystis Microcolon Intestinal Hypoperistalsis Syndrome (MMIHS)

MMIHS is a rare condition that includes non-obstructed enlarged urinary bladder, bilateral hydronephrosis, microcolon, intestinal malrotation, and functional small bowel obstruction. It is felt to be due to decrease muscle tone of the intestinal and urinary tracts. Ultrasound demonstrates a dilated bladder, bilateral hydronephrosis, and normal amniotic fluid (may be hydramnios in third trimester). Bowel or stomach dilatation can sometimes be seen *in utero*. This is much more common in females.

It has an autosomal recessive inheritance pattern; therefore, the recurrence rate is 25%. Genetic counseling should be offered. The prognosis is very poor, with most infants dying. Postnatal evaluation consists of both urinary tract and gastrointestinal evaluations. No good *in utero* therapeutic options have been developed, though the use of intestinal transplant postnatally has been reported.

Urethral Stenosis

Urethral stenosis is an uncommon form of fetal bladder outlet obstruction. It is due to a narrowing of part or all of the urethra. The obstruction is usually incomplete and there are varying amounts of amniotic fluid noted. On ultrasound, there is often a dilated bladder, usually thin-walled and significant hydroureteronephrosis that tends to worsen over time. The prognosis depends on the degree of pulmonary hypoplasia and renal dysfunction. The postnatal evaluation is similar to that for the other causes of fetal bladder outlet obstruction.

Prune Belly Syndrome (TRIAD Syndrome, Eagle-Barrett Syndrome)

This is an uncommon cause of megacystis and hydroureteronephrosis. The incidence is about 1/50,000 live births. It is almost completely limited to males. The fetal ultrasound appearance is a dilated, thin- or thick-walled bladder, distended abdomen, bilateral hydroureteronephrosis and amniotic fluid volume that ranges from normal to severe oligohydramnios. Non-renal abnormalities are common and should be ruled out. When a vesicocentesis is performed, a laxity in the abdominal wall may be seen.

The syndrome consists of abdominal wall distension, urinary tract obstruction, and cryptorchidism. The abdominal wall musculature is either absent or hypoplastic. There is a very high incidence of vesicoureteral reflux. The differential diagnosis is the other forms of bladder outlet obstruction or megacystis.

The prognosis depends upon the degree of pulmonary hypoplasia, the degree of renal dysfunction, and the amount of abdominal wall laxity. The resultant impaired support of the chest decreases cough and there is an increased risk of respiratory infections. The abdominal wall laxity can cause functional and cosmetic problems. Postnatal evaluation consists of renal ultrasound, VCUG, nuclear renogram, pulmonary evaluation, and plastic surgery consultation.

SUMMARY

Urinary tract abnormalities are some of the most common anomalies noted on antenatal ultrasound. They range from benign simple cysts to lethal bilateral renal agenesis. The evaluation of the urinary tract consists of assessing the kidneys for number, location, size, shape, echogenicity, architecture, and the presence of dilatation; the evaluation of the bladder for presence, location, size, wall thickness, and internal echoes; the visualization of ureters if dilated; and the assessment of amniotic fluid volume. With the presence of any urinary tract abnormality, a detailed anatomic survey of the fetus to look for non-renal anomalies should be performed. Renal dilatation noted in the second trimester should be reassessed in the third trimester and any significant abnormality that remains should be evaluated postnatally. The postnatal evaluation usually consists of some combination of renal ultrasound, VCUG, and nuclear renogram. When the risk of reflux is high, prophylactic antibiotics should be used until it can be excluded. By developing an accurate diagnosis (or differential diagnosis), an appropriate plan for further evaluation and, if necessary, treatment can be made.

COMMENT FROM THE EDITORS

This comprehensive review by Dr. Shlossman shows just the tip of the iceberg of his rich experience in prenatal diagnosis. Although the pediatric urologist must work together with a perinatologist, he/she must be knowledgable about this topic in order to best counsel the expecting parents on the diagnostic measures and possible therapeutic options available to them after the birth of the baby. Regular multidisciplinary meetings to discuss cases prenatally diagnosed anomalies greatly enhance communications and improve patient care. The greatest value of prenatal diagnosis in urology has been a marked decrease in the number of babies with an unsuspected anomaly presenting with sepsis.

FURTHER READING

Atiyeh B, Husmann D, Baum M. Contralateral renal abnormalities in patients with renal agenesis and noncystic renal dysplasia. *Pediatrics* 1993; **91**:812–815.

Blazer S, Zimmer E, Blumenfeld Z, Zelikovic I, Bronshtein Z. Natural history of fetal simple renal cysts detected in early pregnancy. *J Urol* 1999; **162**:812–814.

Bornstein E, Barnhard Y, Donnenfeld A, Ferber A, Divon MY. Fetal pyelectasis: does gender modify the risk of major trisomies? *Obstet Gynecol* 2006; **107**:877–879.

Brophy MM, Austin PF, Yan Y, Coplen DE. Vesicoureteral reflux and clinical outcomes in infants with prenatally detected hydronephrosis. *J Urol* 2002; **168**:1716–1719.

Brun M, Maugey-Laulom B, Eurin D, Didier F, Avni EF. Prenatal sonographic patterns in autosomal dominant polycystic kidney disease: a multicenter study. *Ultrasound Obstet Gynecol* 2004; **24**:55–61.

Decter R. Renal duplication and fusion anomalies. *Pediatr Clin North Am* 1997; **44**:1323–1341.

Feldman DM, DeCambre M, Kong E, Borgida A, Jamil M, McKenna P, Egan JFX. Evaluation and follow-up of fetal hydronephrosis. *J Ultrasound Med* 2001; **20**:1065–1069.

Fernbach SK, Maizels M, Conway JJ. Ultrasound grading of hydronephrosis: introduction to the system used by the Society for Fetal Urology. *Pediatr Radiol* 1993; **23**:478–480.

Gabow PA. Autosomal dominant polycystic kidney disease. *NEJM* 1993; **329**:332–342.

Greenfield SP, Wan J. Vesicoureteral reflux: practical aspects of evaluation and management. *Pediatr Nephrol* 1996; **10**:789–794.

Gunn TR, Dermot MJ, Pease P. Antenatal diagnosis of urinary tract abnormalities by ultrasonography after 28 weeks' gestation: incidence and outcome. *Am J Obstet Gynecol* 1995; **172**:479–486.

Herman TE, Siegel MJ. Prune belly syndrome. *J Perinatol* 2009; **29**:69–71.

Heyman C, Breysem L, Proesmans W. Multicystic kidney dysplasia: a prospective study on the natural history of the affected and the contralateral kidney. *Eur J Pediatr* 1998; **157**:673–675.

Ismaili K, Hall M, Donner C, Thomas D, Vermeylen D, Avni FE. Results of a systematic screening for minor degrees of fetal pelvis dilatation in an unselected population. *Am J Obstet Gynecol* 2003; **188**:242–246.

Karnak I, Woo LL, Shah SN, Sirajuddin A, Kay R, Ross JH. Prenatally detected ureteropelvic junction obstruction: clinical features and associated urologic abnormalities. *Pediatr Surg Int* 2008; **24**:395–402.

Kumar S, Fisk NM. Distal urinary obstruction. *Clin Perinatol* 2003; **30**:507–519.

Levin TL, Soghier L, Blitman NM, Vega-Rich C, Nafday S. Megacystis-microcolon-intestinal hypoperistalsis and prune belly: overlapping syndromes. *Pediatr Radiol* 2004; **34**:995–998.

McLellan DL, Retik AB, Bauer SB, Diamond DA, Atala A, Mandell J, Lebowitz RL, Borer JG, Peters CA. Rate and predictors of spontaneous resolution of prenatally diagnosed primary nonrefluxing megaureter. *J Urol* 2002; **168**:2177–2180.

Nyberg DA, Souter VL, El-Bastawissi A, Young S, Luthhardt F, Luthy DA. Isolated sonographic markers for detection of fetal Down syndrome in the second trimester of pregnancy. *J Ultrasound Med* 2001; **20**:1053–1063.

Obido AO, Raab E, Elovitz M, Merrill JD, Macones GA. Prenatal mild pyelectasis: evaluating the thresholds of renal pelvis diameter associated with normal postnatal renal function. *J Ultrasound Med* 2004; **23**:513–517.

Rabelo EA, Oliveira EA, Diniz JS, Silva JM, Filgueiras MJ, Pezzuti IL, Tatsua ES. Natural history of multicystic kidney conservatively managed: a prospective study. *Pediatr Nephrol* 2004; **19**:1102–1107.

Rossetti S, Harris PC. Genotype-phenotype correlations in autosomal dominant and autosomal recessive polycystic kidney disease. *J Am Soc Nephrol* 2007; **18**:1374–1380.

Sairam S, Al-Habib A, Sasson S, Thilaganathan B. Natural history of fetal hydronephrosis diagnosed on mid-trimester ultrasound. *Ultrasound Obstet Gynecol* 2001; **17**:191–196.

Stock A, Richards D, Frentzen B, Richard G. Correlation of prenatal renal pelvic anteroposterior diameter with outcome in infancy. *J Urol* 1996; **155**:1050–1052.

Upadhyay J, Bolduc S, Braga L, Farhat W, Bagli DJ, McLorie GA, Khoury AE, El-Ghoneimi A. Impact of prenatal diagnosis on the morbidity associated with ureterocele management. *J Urol* 2002; **167**:2560–2565.

Wu S, Johnson MP. Fetal lower urinary tract obstruction. *Clin Perinatol* 2009; **36**:377–390.

Yice J, Wilcox D. Management of fetal hydronephrosis. *Pediatr Nephrol* 2008; **23**:347–353.

Chapter 2

Urinary Tract Infections

Ricardo González and Barbara M. Ludwikowski

Infections of the urinary tract (UTI) may be caused by bacteria, fungi, or viruses. With the exception of the occasional viral cystitis, the majority of infections are bacterial infections. Fungal infections are seen almost exclusively in immuno-suppressed patients or in those with indwelling catheters or complex urinary tract abnormalities after prolonged antibiotic treatment. UTIs are among the most common bacterial infections seen in a pediatric practice. It is estimated that they account for more than one million outpatient visits per year in the USA. The prevalence of UTI in children in the USA is estimated at 5% of the population, being more frequent in girls (8%) than in boys (2%). Except in the first year of life, the UTIs are more prevalent in females than in males. In the first year of life, uncircumcised males have an even greater prevalence of UTIs. Breast-feeding appears to protect infants from UTI.

BACTERIAL INFECTIONS

Bacterial UTIs can be classified as follows:

UPPER TRACT

Acute	Pyelitis
	Pyelonephritis
	Lobar nephronia
	Renal and perirenal abscess
Chronic	Xanthogranulomatous pyelonephritis (XGP)
	Tuberculosis

LOWER TRACT

Acute Cystitis
Urethritis
Epididymitis

Chronic

Although the diagnosis of the different forms of UTI will be discussed in the corresponding sections, some general principles about obtaining and interpreting urine cultures (UC) that apply to all cases are discussed here. Any growth of bacteria, viruses, or fungi in the urine is abnormal. In newborns and infants who require immediate treatment before the results of the culture and antibiotic sensitivities are known, it is imperative to obtain a specimen of bladder urine to avoid errors caused by a contaminated specimen. In girls, a correctly obtained catheterised specimen is sufficient. The same applies to circumcised males. In uncircumcised males in whom the prepuce cannot be retracted, a specimen of bladder urine should be obtained by suprapubic needle aspiration of bladder urine. In older toilet-trained children, a midstream specimen obtained after washing the meatus can be reliable if more 10^5 colonies of a single organism are obtained. For a voided specimen to be reliable in males, the prepuce must be retractable.

Acute Pyelitis, Pyelonephritis, and Lobar Nephronia

Definition

An acute bacterial infection of the renal pelvis and parenchyma. The infection can involve one or more renal lobules. The resulting reaction can cause tissue damage, which may result in loss of renal parenchyma and healing with scar formation. The most common organism is *E. coli*, followed in frequency by *Klebsiella* sp. and *Enterococcus* sp. Gram-positive organisms are occasional offenders. The route of infection is usually ascending. Bacterial adherence factors determined by the intrinsic properties of the bacteria such as the P-fimbriae of *E. coli* and the presence of epithelial receptors in the genital epithelium and the urinary tract facilitate the ascent of bacteria. The presence of vesicoureteral reflux (VUR) facilitates the ascent of less virulent bacteria but the patients with VUR may be more susceptible to permanent scarring.

Urinary tract abnormalities leading to stasis such as upper tract dilatation or incomplete bladder emptying are also predisposing factors. Uncircumcised boys of less than one year of age have an increased risk for UTI (see Chapter 9). Bladder catheterization for diagnostic or therapeutic purposes is the most common cause of iatrogenic UTIs.

In the newborn, renal infections may be hematogenous.

Presentation

The newborns and infants with acute pyelonephritis present with nonspecific symptoms. Listlessness, gastrointestinal symptoms such as vomiting or diarrhea, and fever are common. UTIs account for 7% of febrile infants. Nevertheless, the diagnosis is often overlooked or delayed. Therefore, the urine must be always checked (urinalysis and culture) in all babies with fever greater than 38.5°C. Pyelonephritis must always be included in the differential diagnosis of the septic infant.

Older children usually present with fever and flank or abdominal pain. The symptoms of cystitis may or may not precede the onset of fiber. The differential diagnosis often includes other conditions that may present with abdominal pain and fiber such as ureteral calculi, acute appendicitis, or adnexal inflammation in females.

Diagnosis

The diagnosis is made by the clinical presentation in the presence of an abnormal urinalysis and a positive UC.

Physical examination

Infants and newborns show signs of a generalized infection and the abdomen may be distended. In older children, there is upper quadrant abdominal or flank tenderness. Fever is characteristic in all age groups.

Differential diagnosis includes other causes of sepsis in infants. Ureteral calculus with infection, acute appendicitis, and adnexal infections are in females.

Laboratory findings

The urinalysis is usually abnormal with leukocyturia, with or without blood. The nitrate test is usually positive, as is the test for leukocyte esterase. The UC grows greater than 10^6 colonies of a single organism. In the blood, there is usually leukocytosis and an elevated C-reactive protein level. Blood cultures may be positive. However, the urinalysis may be normal and the culture may be negative if the child has been treated with antibiotics before obtaining the urine specimen. Blood cultures are necessary for patients with temperatures over 38.5°C.

Imaging studies

The confirmation of the diagnosis of acute pyelonephritis requires imaging studies although these are not always obtained or necessary if the diagnosis is clear. A CT scan of the abdomen with intravenous contrast reveals either areas of focal perfusion defects involving one or more renal lobules (Figure 2-1). More rarely, a mass-like lesion is seen. This has been called lobar nephronia or acute focal bacterial nephritis, which seems to be mostly a radiological finding but has no bearing on the treatment or

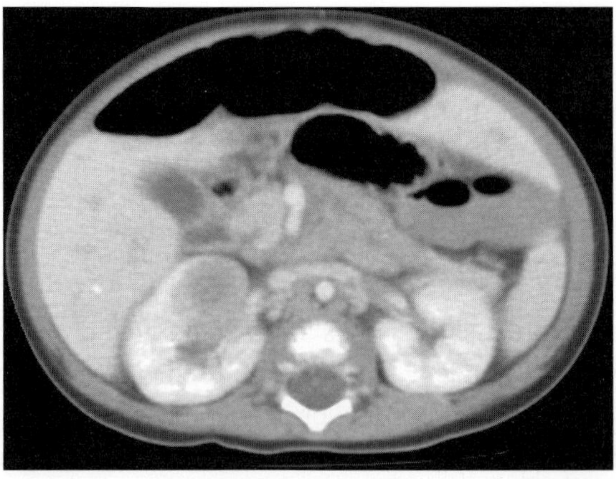

Figure 2-1. Spiral CT of the abdomen with intravenous contrast showing an area of lack of opacification in the right kidney in a child with acute pyelonephritis.

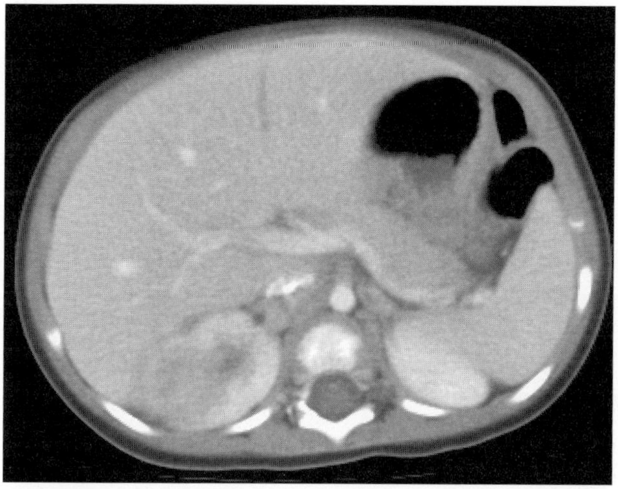

Figure 2-2. Spiral CT of the abdomen with intravenous contrast showing a mass-like lesion in the right kidney in a child with acute pyelonephritis compatible with lobar nephronia.

outcome of the disease (Figure 2-2). The importance of recognizing this imaging manifestation of pyelonephritis, which can also be seen on ultrasound, is that it may lead to the erroneous diagnosis of a renal tumor or abscess. In practice, CT scan is seldom performed unless other intra-abdominal conditions are suspected. A nuclear renal scan using technetium-labeled dimercaptosuccinic acid (DMSA) is also a very sensitive test of renal involvement by an inflammatory process. The characteristic finding in acute pyelonephritis is an area of diminished or absent uptake of the isotope (Figure 2-3). In contrast with CT scanning, with DMSA scanning, it may be difficult to distinguish whether the defect in uptake is caused by an acute process or an established scar, but it has the advantage that radiation exposure is more localized to the kidneys rather than the entire abdomen and that it avoids the adverse effects of contrast medium.

About 50% of children with a febrile UTI, leukocytosis, and an elevated C-reactive protein have normal DMSA scans suggesting the diagnosis of pyelitis, which is a renal infection without parenchymal involvement. Renal involvement increases with the delayed onset of appropriate treatment.

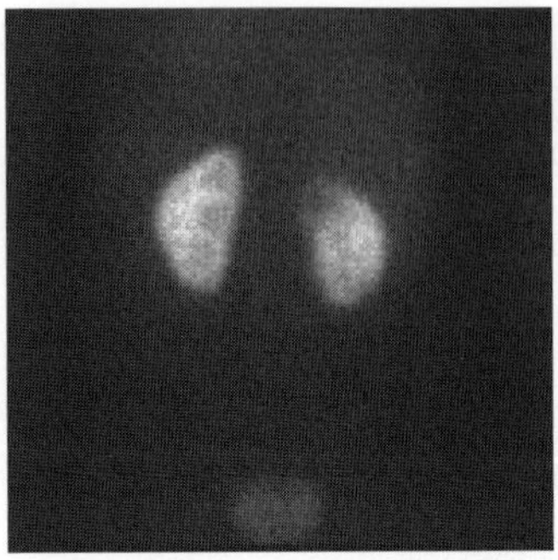

Figure 2-3. DMSA scan showing right upper pole lack of uptake of the isotope typical of acute pyelonephritis.

Since many defects seen during the acute episode healed completely in time, some authors recommend performing only one DMSA scan six to nine months after the acute episode to detect parenchymal scars.

Renal ultrasonography should be done in the acute phase on all children with acute pyelonephritis who have not had previous imaging of the urinary tract. Although ultrasonography is not a sensitive method to diagnose renal infection, it is essential to make sure that there is no urinary tract dilatation which may signal obstruction (Figure 2-4). Supra- or infravesical obstruction is present in 3% of the cases of acute pyelonephritis in children and may require appropriate drainage in addition to antibiotic treatment. In cases of upper tract dilatation, the ultrasound may also reveal the presence of pyonephrosis.

A micturition cystourethrogram (MCUG and VCUG) should be done as soon as convenient to determine whether VUR is present or not (see Chapter 16).

Treatment

Well children may be treated on an ambulatory basis but in practice, most children with acute pyelonephritis are admitted to the hospital to receive intravenous hydration and to initiate antibiotic therapy. Although there appears to be no difference in the outcome of oral versus intravenous antibiotic therapy, in practice, we prefer a short

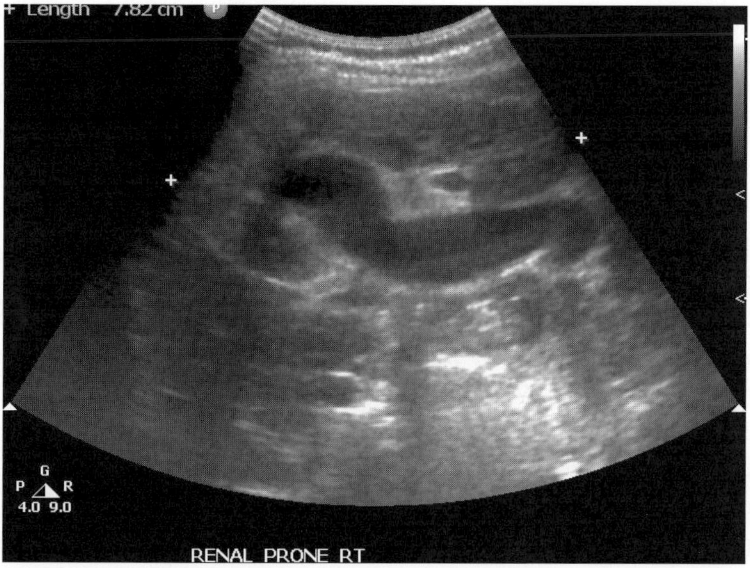

Figure 2-4. Renal ultrasonogram showing the duplication of the right collecting system and the dilatation of the upper pole pelvis and proximal ureter in a child with clinical acute pyelonephritis.

course of intravenous antibiotics followed by the continuation of oral antibiotics at home. Our preference is to start with ceftriaxone 50–75 mg per kg per day once a day or in two divided doses for 48 hours or until the result of the antibiotic sensitivities in the UC become available. In children with normal renal function, aminoglycosides are also effective. For oral antibiotics, cefixime, ceftibuten, and amoxicillin/clavulanic acid are also may effective. The ideal duration of antibiotic therapy has not been determined but most authors recommend 10 to 14 days of antibiotic therapy. Some recommend a three-week treatment course for patients with imaging studies compatible with lobar nephronia.

The treatment of VUR is discussed in Chapter 16. Circumcision should be considered in infants with recurrent infections.

Acute pyelonephritis in the presence of a dilated urinary tract, which does not respond promptly to antibiotics, should be drained either by retrograde placement of a double pigtail stent or by percutaneous nephrostomy.

Renal abscesses are rare and seldom require drainage. Perirenal abscesses are usually hematogenous and caused by Gram-positive organisms.

Prognosis and follow-up

Most patients respond well to treatment. Recurrence of infections is common in infancy. In infants less than six months of age, the recurrence rate is 25% compared to 8% after six months of age. Uncircumcised male infants with a non-retractable prepuce have the highest probability of recurrence. The role of prophylactic low-dose antibiotic therapy in preventing the recurrence of UTI is widely used and probably effective in some cases but currently questioned given the lack of adequate controlled studies. About half of children with abnormal DMSA scans during the acute infection or about 25% of all children with febrile UTIs will develop a permanent scar in the kidney. The presence of VUR increases the likelihood of renal scarring. The presence of bladder dysfunction, although a probable predisposing factor for UTIs, does not increase the risk of renal scarring. Although there is a sense that scar formation is more frequent in young children, they certainly can develop at any age. Renal scars predispose later in the life to microalbuminuria and hypertension. The exact incidence of hypertension with renal scars is uncertain but given sufficiently long follow-up, it may be as high as 10%. Conversely, 21% of children presenting with arterial hypertension have renal scars on DMSA scanning.

Although earlier publications indicated that renal scarring associated with VUR accounted for 5 to 12% of children with end-stage renal insufficiency, the actual numbers may be smaller. Not in all children with renal failure and VUR is the reflux responsible for the renal damage. Congenitally, abnormal renal development also accounts for a proportion of these cases.

Children with known renal scars should have long-term follow-up with urinalysis and blood pressure measurements.

Chronic Pyelonephritis

Formerly, chronic pyelonephritis was the term used to refer to a condition characterized by renal scars and is also referred to as reflux nephropathy. In reality, this represents the result of past infections and not actually a chronic infection and thus the term should be abandoned. There is, however, one condition that can properly be called chronic pyelonephritis and is better known as XGP. Renal tuberculosis is another example of chronic renal infection.

Xanthogranulomatous Pyelonephritis

Definition

It is a chronic bacterial infection of the kidney that causes destruction of the parenchyma. It is characterized by a mass-like lesion, which histologically contains lipid-laden macrophages. Stones and obstruction are the frequent features of the disease.

Presentation

Although more common in adults in whom it is often misdiagnosis as a renal tumor, more than 200 pediatric cases have been reported. Children with XGP present with the generalized symptoms of malaise and poor appetite with or without weight loss. Etiologic agents are in decreasing order of frequency: *Proteus mirabilis*, *E. coli*, *Enterococcus*, and *Pseudomonas* sp. Flank pain and fever are the rule. On examination, a tender flank mass is often present.

Diagnosis

The urinalysis demonstrates pyuria and the UC is positive. On ultrasonography, the kidney is enlarged with dilatation of the intrarenal collecting system and the loss of normal parenchyma. Calcifications are often seen on ultrasonography and always seen on CT scan. Although, in the past, the diagnosis was made after nephrectomy, with modern imaging modalities, a preoperative diagnosis should always be possible. Usually, there is poor function of the involved kidney.

Treatment

Antibiotics and total nephrectomy are the usual recommended treatments although an occasional case treated by partial nephrectomy has been reported. After initial treatment investigation for possible causes of stone formation (see Chapter 21), the prevention of infection and lithiasis are important.

Urinary Tract Tuberculosis

Definition

Renal tuberculosis is a hematogenous infection of the kidney caused by *M. tuberculosis*, which occurs at the time of the primary infection but remains latent for many years. For this reason, it is more common in adults than in children. From the kidney, the infection may spread down to the renal collecting system, ureter, and bladder. Tuberculous epididymitis is considered to be hematogenous. Renal tuberculosis is rare in children but more common in less-developed countries. In adults, urinary tract tuberculosis represents more than 2/3 of the cases of extrapulmonary disease. In review of 385 cases of tuberculosis in children from the UK and Ireland, 15 to 29% were not respiratory in location.

Presentation

In a recent review, the mean age at presentation was 11 years with a mean duration of the symptoms of three to four months. Most patients had lower tract symptoms suggestive of bladder involvement, followed in frequency by constitutional symptoms and hematuria.

Diagnosis

It is important to suspect the diagnosis in order to obtain the necessary laboratory confirmation. Sterile acid pyuria is the classic triad that should lead to suspicion of urinary tract tuberculosis. Cultures for acid fast bacilli should be obtained repeatedly. Because it takes several weeks to get results and the yield is around 30%, urine PCR for *M. tuberculosis* is highly recommended. Sometimes, treatment must be instituted based on a high level of suspicion and the appearance of the kidneys on imaging studies. When bladder involvement is present, cystoscopy shows the evidence of cystitis and a bladder biopsy can be diagnostic. PCR for *M. tuberculosis* should be done on the specimen.

Characteristic findings on imaging studies include calcifications, parenchymal loss, calyceal clubbing, infundibular, pelvic, or ureteral narrowing, and contracted bladder. The chest roentgenogram may be normal.

Treatment

Primary treatment is with antitubercular drugs such as rifampin, isoniazid, and pyrazinamide, which should be undertaken in consultation with the infectious disease specialist. Quadruple therapy may be indicated in some cases. Surgery may be needed to remove non-functioning kidneys in case of poor response to therapy, drainage procedures to relieve obstruction, ureteral replacement, and augmentation cystoplasty for chronically contracted bladders.

Cystitis

Definition

Acute bacterial cystitis is the most common type of UTI seen in childhood. It is more common in girls and *E. coli* is the most frequent infectious agent.

Presentation

Urinary frequency, urgency, and pain with micturition are the characteristic presenting symptoms. Gross hematuria may be present. In some children, the urgency leads to day- or nighttime wetting. Lower abdominal pain and low grade fever may be present.

Diagnosis

The differential diagnosis includes rare cases of viral cystitis, vulvo-vaginits, and bladder dysfunction. In children with chronic symptoms of bladder dysfunction, the symptoms may be misinterpreted. The urinalysis shows pyuria, and the tests for leukocyte esterase and nitrates are usually positive. A UC growing more than 10^5 colonies of a single organism is diagnostic. Imaging studies are not usually recommended.

Treatment

Treatment is usually initiated with a broad spectrum antibiotic before the results of the culture and sensitivities are available. Early treatment may prevent ascending pyelonephritis. Nitrofurantoin which, reaches good urinary concentrations but no tissue levels may be used to treat cystitis. Short courses of the treatment of three to five days are usually sufficient. A UC should be obtained two days after completion of treatment to rule out persistent asymptomatic bacteriuria.

Prognosis

Recurrences are frequent. In cases of recurrent cystitis, predisposing factors should be investigated. Constipation, incomplete bladder emptying, and the other forms of bladder dysfunction such as infrequent voiding should be addressed. In sexually active adolescents, coitus may be a predisposing factor. In cases of frequent recurrent cystitis, a course of antibacterial prophylaxis with trimethoprim or furadantoin may be useful.

Urethritis

Definition

Bacterial urethritis is rare in prepubertal boys. In sexually active males, chlamydial infections are common with a prevalence of two million cases in the USA. Gonococcal infections may occur isolated or in association with chlamydial infections. *Mycoplasma genitalium*, *M. hominis*, and *Ureaplasma* are the other frequent etiologic agents.

Presentation

Painful micturition and urethral discharge.

Diagnosis

Urethral discharge may be confirmed in physical examination. The urinalysis shows pyuria but the UC is usually negative. A urethral swab should be sent for chlamydial and neisserial cultures.

Treatment

Azithromycin and doxycycline appear to be equally effective or chlamydial infections. Azithromycin is preferred for *Mycoplasma*. Infections by *Neisseria gonorrhoea* should be treated with cephalosporins. However, treatment should follow the guidelines of local public health authorities for sexually transmitted diseases (STD). Screening for other STDs, the treatment of sexual contacts, and counseling are beyond the spectrum of this chapter.

Epididymitis

Infections of the epididymis occur in both pre- and postpubertal males and should be discussed separately.

Prepubertal Epididymitis

Definition

Acute inflammatory disease of the epididymis in sexually non-active males is a relatively rare event. As discussed in Chapter 7, many published reports have implicated epididymitis as a frequent cause of scrotal pain and swelling in prepubertal boys. However, it is likely that most of those events are caused by the torsion of Morgagni's hydatid which on scrotal ultrasonography can produce enlargement and hyperemia of the tissues surrounding the testis and of the epididymis itself. In those cases, the urinalysis is normal. True prepubertal epididymitis is invariably infectious and associated with abnormal urinalysis and positive UC. Chronic epididymitis can be caused by *M. tuberculosis* and *Brucella.*

Presentation

The usual presentation is acute painful scrotal swelling usually with fever greater than 38°C. The symptoms of cystitis or urethritis may also be present. Frequently, there is history of a known urological disease such as a urethral stricture, repaired hypospadias, and an enlarged utricle.

Diagnosis

Physical examination reveals a painful swollen scrotum. There may be skin erythema. If a detailed scrotal examination is possible, a retrotesticular mass is palpable. The spermatic cord may be tender and indurated. The urinalysis shows pyuria and the UC is positive. Leukocytosis is frequent. Scrotal ultrasonography reveals an enlarged and hyperemic epididymis with normal blood flow to the testis (Figure 2-5).

Treatment

Broad spectrum antibiotics and analgesics are effective. When the results of the culture are available, antibiotic therapy with the appropriate antibiotic for 10–14 days is recommended.

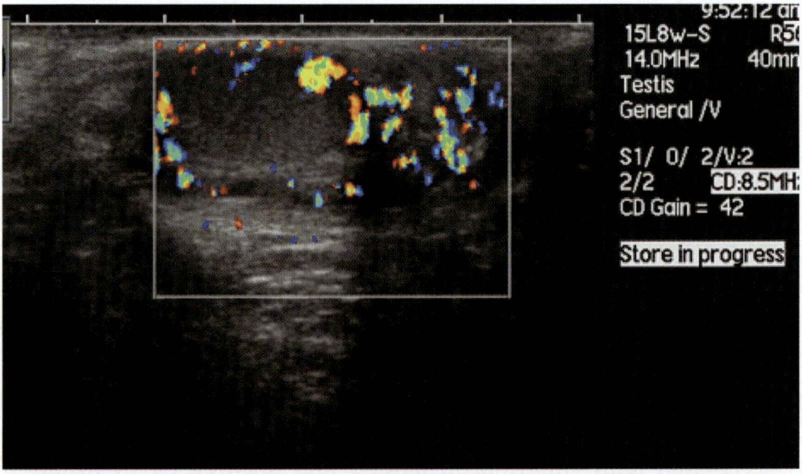

Figure 2-5. Scrotal ultrasonography with color Doppler reveals an enlarged and hyperemic epididymis with normal blood flow to the testis.

Prognosis and follow-up

Infertility is a common consequence of bilateral epididymitis. Evaluation after the acute episode should include a renal and bladder ultrasound and a micturition cystourethrogram. In recurrent cases, the micturition cystourethrogram often shows reflux into the ejaculatory duct or vas deferens. Prevention of recurrence requires the treatment of the underlying problem.

Postpubertal Epididymitis

Definition

In sexually active males, epididymitis usually occurs in the absence of anatomical abnormalities. It is an STD with the same etiologic agents as urethritis.

Presentation

The presentation is acute painful scrotal swelling; fever is unusual. The symptoms of urethritis may precede the onset of scrotal pain.

Treatment and diagnosis

The disease is usually established by physical examination. A tender and enlarged epididymis in a normal location behind the testis can be palpated. The testes may be involved in the inflammatory process. Pyuria is common. Urethral swabs should be obtained and they are tested for the presence of *Neisseria*, *Chlamydia*, and *Mycoplasma*. Differential diagnosis includes the torsion of the spermatic cord and testicular tumors. Ultrasonography of the scrotum is diagnostic.

See treatment of urethritis. Referral to a STD clinic is advisable.

VIRAL INFECTIONS

A variety of viruses can cause urinary tract diseases. In immuno-compromised patients, Polyoma BK virus nephritis has been described. HIV-associated nephritis (HIVAN) is the most common cause of renal failure in HIV-1 seropositive population.

Hemorrhagic cystitis can have a viral etiology. Among immuno-competent children, adenovirus cystitis is most common, but cytomegalovirus cystitis is also reported. The diagnosis of viral hemorrhagic cystitis is made by exclusion when symptoms are present and the bacterial cultures are negative. Serial serum antibody levels may assist in the diagnosis. Viral cultures should be obtained. Bladder ultrasound may reveal a mass-like lesion that may be mistaken for a tumor.

Polyoma BK virus, cytomegalovirus, and adenovirus can also cause hemorrhagic cystitis in immuno-compromised patients; for example, after stem cell transplantation.

Treatment with antiviral agents such as cidofovir may be useful.

PARASITIC INFECTIONS

Schistomiasis

Cystitis caused by *Schistosoma hematobium* is endemic in North Africa but affects mostly adults. Nevertheless, series of pediatric the cases have been reported. Given present migrations, the cases of schistosomiasis can be seen outside the regions where the disease is endemic. Humans are the intermediate hosts in the parasite life cycle. The disease is contracted by contact with contaminated water where the definitive host, a snail, inhabits. The parasites live in the blood vessels of the bladder and cause a granulomatous reaction. Hematuria, often terminal, and painful urination are the common symptoms. Diagnosis is made by isolating the ova in the urine. Serum antibodies can be detected by ELISA test. Associated bacterial infection is common. Treatment with praziquantel is effective. The untreated disease can lead to severe bladder contraction and the development of squamous cell carcinoma. Bladder cancer associated to schistosomiasis has been reported in teenagers.

FURTHER READING

Ahmed MD, *et al*. Dimercaptosuccinic acid (DMSA) renal scan in the evaluation of hypertension in children. *Pediatr Nephrol* 2008; **23**:435–438.

Al-Taheini KA, Pike J, Leonard M. Acute epididymitis in children: the role of radiologic studies. *Urology* 2008; **71**:826–829.

Cendron M. Reflux nephropathy. *J Pediatr Urol* 2008; **4**:414–421.

Cheng CH, Tsau YK, Lin TY. Effective duration of antimicrobial therapy for the treatment of acute labor nephronia. *Pediatrics* 2006; **117**:e84–e89.

Dillon MJ, Goonasekera CDA. Reflux nephropathy. *J Am Soc Nephrol* 1998; **9**:2377–2383.

Dogan D, *et al.* Does early treatment of urinary tract infection prevent renal damage? *Pediatrics* 2007; **120**:e922–e928.

Faust WC, Diaz M, Pohl HG. Incidence of post-pyelonephritic renal scarring: a meta-analysis of the dimercapto-succinic acid literature. *J Urol* 2009; **181**:290–297.

Geisler WM. Management of uncomplicated *Chlamydia* infections in adolescents and adults: evidence reviewed for the 2006 Centers for Disease Control and Prevention sexually transmitted disease guidelines. *Clin Infect Dis* 2007; **44** (Suppl 3):S77–S83.

Hodson EM, Willis NS, Craig JC. Antibiotics for acute pyelonephritis in children. *Cochrane Database Syst Rev* 2007; **17**:CD003772.

MMWR. Update to CDC's sexually transmitted diseases treatment guidelines, 2006: fluoroquinolones no longer recommended for treatment of gonococcal infections. Centers for Disease Control and Prevention (CDC) *Morb Mortal Wkly Rep* 2007; **56**:332–336.

National Kidney and Urologic Disease Clearing House (NKUDIC) website. http://kidney.niddk.nih.gov

Neuhaus TJ, *et al.* Randomised trial of oral versus sequential intravenous cephalosporins in children with pyelonephritis. *Eur J Pediatr* 2008; **167**:1037–1047.

Nerli RB, Kamat GV, Alur SB, Koura A, *et al.* Genitourinary tuberculosis in pediatric urological practice. *J Pediatr Urol* 2008; **4**:299–303.

Paduch DA. Viral lower urinary infections. *Curr Urol Rep* 2007; **8**:324–335.

Teo SS, Riordan A, Alffaham M, *et al.* Tuberculosis in the United Kingdom and Republic of Ireland. *Arch Dis Child* 2009; **94**:263–267.

Shaikh N, Morone NE, Bost JE, Farell MH. Prevalence of urinary tract infection in childhood: a meta-analysis. *Pediatr Infect Dis J* 2008; **27**:302–308.

Sheehan GJ, Sekla L, Harding GK. Urinary schistosomiasis: a report of four cases and a review. *Can Med Assoc J* 1984; **131**:1361–1364.

Shim YH, Lee JW, Lee SJ. Risk factors of recurrent urinary tract infection in infants with normal urinary systems. *Pediatr Nephrol* 2009; **24**:309–312.

Taskinen S, Rintala R. Post-pyelonephritic renal scars are not associated with high voiding pressures. *J Pediatr Urol* 2007; **3**:40–44.

Williams GJ, *et al.* Long-term antibiotics for preventing recurrent urinary tract infections in children. *Cochrane Database Syst Rev* 2006; **3**:CD001534.

Zugor V, Schott GE, Labanaris AP. Xanthogranulomatous pyelonephritis in childhood: a critical analysis of 10 cases and of the literature. *Urology* 2007; **70**:157–160.

Chapter 3

Haematuria

Ahmad H. Bani-Hani

Haematuria is a common finding in paediatric population. It is often encountered during routine screening in urine analysis or during work up for other urological symptoms. Haematuria can be a sign and/or a symptom of underlying renal or bladder disease. Unlike haematuria in adults, most cases of haematuria in children are isolated and benign. The differential diagnosis for haematuria is extensive (Table 3-1); nonetheless, this chapter will focus on the evaluation and management of common causes of haematuria in paediatric practice.

DEFINITION

While macroscopic haematuria is visible to the naked eyes, microscopic haematuria is defined as the presence of more than 5 to 10 red blood cells (RBCs) per high-power field (HPF) of a microscopic examination of a centrifuged urinary sediment in at least two of three urinalyses obtained over two to three weeks. Urine samples should be freshly voided, clean catch, midstream, or catheterised specimens. Morning sample is recommended, as it is unlikely that the urine will be diluted and cause lysis of RBCs. The proper technique for urine microscopy is to centrifuge 10 ml of urine at 2000 rpm for five minutes. Nine milliliter is decanted and the sediment is resuspended in the remaining 1 ml of urine. A drop of this suspended sediment is examined by microscope by HPF that is 400× magnification. Positive dipstick for haeme should always be confirmed by urine microscopy. The causes of false positive test include myoglobinuria,

Table 3-1. Differential diagnosis of haematuria.

A. Glomerular disorders
- Benign familial haematuria.
- PSGN.
- IgA nephropathy.
- Systemic vasculitis (e.g. HSP* and WG).
- Goodpasture's syndrome.
- Alport's syndrome.

B. Renal parenchymal disorders
- Tumours and cysts (e.g. Wilms' s tumour and polycystic renal disease).
- Interstitial nephritis.
- Nephrocalcinosis.
- Papillary necrosis.
- Hypercalciuria.

C. Renal collecting system disorders
- UTIs.
- Trauma.
- Nephrolithiasis.
- Tumours (e.g. rhabdomyosarcoma).
- Haemangiomas and polyps.
- Meatal stenosis.
- Idiopathic urethrorrhagia.
- LPHS.

D. Others
- Exercise.
- Haematological disorders (e.g. sickle cell disease or trait).
- Nutcracker phenomenon.
- Renal artery/vein thrombosis.

* HSP.

haemoglobinuria, povidone/iodine contamination, certain foods (e.g. beets), or low urine specific gravity of less than 1.007 (hypotonic urine can cause the lysis of RBCs). High vitamin C intake can cause the false negative results.

The incidence of macroscopic haematuria is 1.3 per 1000, while the incidence of microscopic haematuria in school children is in the range of 1 to 2%. The American Academy of Pediatrics recommends a screening urine analysis at school entry (4–5 years of age) and a repeat one during adolescence (11–21 years of age) as part of well-child visits.

AETIOLOGY

Haematuria may originate from the urinary tract (i.e. urethra, bladder, ureter, or pelvicalyceal system), glomeruli, renal tubules, or interstitium. The presence of bright-red colour urine, visible clots, or crystals with normal-looking RBCs in microscopic examination suggests bleeding from the urinary tract. In contrast, cola/tea-coloured urine and the presence of RBC casts and/or deformed RBCs (Figure 3-1) in urine microscopy suggest glomerular bleeding. The paediatric population is more prone to have bleeding from the glomeruli than from the urinary tract. Table 3-1 summarises the causes of haematuria in children. For the purposes of diagnostic evaluation, haematuria can be gross, symptomatic microscopic, asymptomatic microscopic with proteinuria, or isolated asymptomatic microscopic. Gross haematuria is relatively unusual, accounting for approximately 1.3 in 1000 visits to a paediatrician. In a series of 342 children with gross haematuria followed over a period of 10 years, only 66% of the patients had an identifiable cause. Boys accounted for 80% of the cohort of which 19% had benign idiopathic urethrorrhaegia, 18% had stones, 14% had trauma, and 14% had urinary tract infection (UTI). Of the

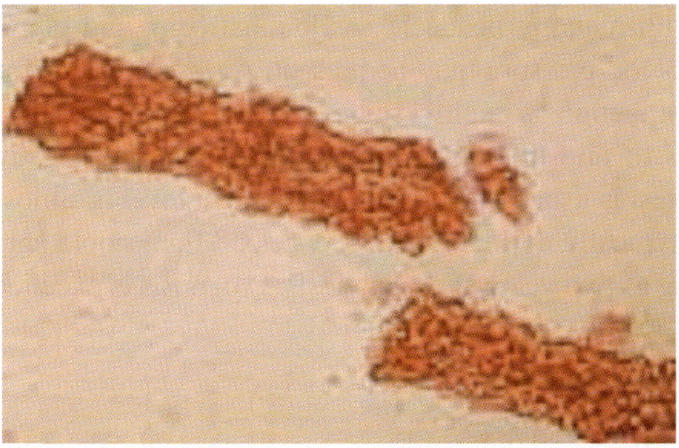

Figure 3-1. RBC cast.

entire cohort, 13% had one or more congenital renal anomaly, 5% had stones, and only 1% had tumours (low-grade transitional cell carcinoma and Wilms' tumour). None of the patients had glomerulonephritis, which is most likely related to author's referral pattern. This series underscores the fact that implications of gross haematuria in children, mostly benign, are different than in adults, especially because genitourinary tumours are rare in children. Moreover, once glomerulonephritis has been excluded, gross haematuria often has a benign underlying cause in children and adolescents. The most commonly encountered aetiologies for the haematuria in children are presented briefly in the following sections.

RENAL GLOMERULAR DISORDERS

Benign Familial Haematuria

The mode of inheritance has not been elucidated. The diagnosis is suspected clinically when more than one member of the family have positive blood in urine analysis in the absence of deafness, ocular manifestation, or progressive renal failure. Diagnosis is made by renal biopsy, which classically demonstrates thin glomerular basement membrane. Prognosis is excellent, as this is a benign disease.

Post-Streptococcal Glomerulonephritis (PSGN)

Patients may be asymptomatic or present acutely with tea-coloured urine associated with malaise, headache, abdominal pain, and oliguria. Oedema and/or high blood pressure may be present. A recent history for pharyngitis and/or skin impetigo is highly suggestive of the diagnosis. Early in the disease, titres of antistreptolysin O antibodies may be negative; however, streptozyme test is usually positive. Complement level is almost always low (C3), which typically normalise in 6–8 weeks. Microscopic haematuria may persist as long as two years after diagnosis. Prognosis is excellent in general.

IgA Nephropathy

IgA nephropathy is probably the most common cause of haematuria in children and is the most common type of glomerulonephropathy worldwide.

The disease is most prevalent in the second and third decades of the life and is rare in infants with male/female ratio of 6:1 in the USA. History alone can highly suggest the diagnosis as the typical presentation is of intermittent and recurrent bouts of gross haematuria following minor infections such as upper respiratory tract infections. Persistent microscopic haematuria is also a common presentation. Diagnosis can be established by obtaining a renal biopsy showing mesangial deposition of IgA. Serum IgA level is elevated in only 50% of patients and its measurement is not clinically useful. Prognosis varies with some children progressing to renal failure after the onset of the disease. Predictors of a poorer outcome include older age at presentation, hypertension, crescentic glomerulonephritis, nephrotic-range proteinuria, and azotemia. Unfortunately, there is no cure for this disease. Children with recurrent bouts of haematuria or with isolated microscopic haematuria who otherwise have minimal (< 1 g/day) or no proteinuria, normal blood pressure, and preserved kidney function should only be monitored periodically to assess disease progression. Children with hypertension and/or mild-to-moderate proteinuria may benefit from angiotensin-converting enzyme (ACE) inhibitors. Nephrotic-range proteinuria and/or severe form of the disease may require steroid and immunosuppressive therapy.

Systemic Vasculitis

Henoch-Schönlein Purpura

Henoch-Schönlein purpura (HSP) is a systemic, small-vessel, and immune complex-mediated leukocytoclastic vasculitis characterised by a triad of purpura, abdominal pain, and arthritis. The disease is mostly seen in the age range of 4 to 15 years. Approximately 50% of children with clinical diagnosis of HSP manifest renal involvement, which may include haematuria, proteinuria, nephrotic syndrome, glomerulonephritis, and acute renal failure. Presumptive aetiology is the exposure to a trigger antigen that causes antibody formation. Antigen triggers include drugs, foods, immunisation, and upper respiratory and other viral illnesses. Diagnosis is usually clinical but skin biopsy of the purpura can be performed showing leukocytoclastic vasculitis. Prognosis is excellent with fewer than 5%

progress to end-stage renal disease (ESRD). For severe cases, steroid therapy can be helpful.

Systemic Lupus Erythematosus

Systemic lupus erythematosus (SLE) is a chronic and multisystemic disease characterised by production of autoantibodies and protean clinical manifestations. It is more commonly seen in females of childbearing age. In children, the peak age at onset is 14 years. Renal manifestations in SLE vary but may include microscopic haematuria, proteinuria, nephrotic syndrome, or acute glomerulonephritis. If the anamnesis is suggestive of the disease, the serological testing with antinuclear antibodies (ANAs) and anti-double-stranded antibodies can be helpful. Primary therapy is dependent on the severity of the disease, most commonly assessed by obtaining renal biopsy, and usually consists of corticosteroids plus additional cytotoxic therapy (e.g. cyclophosphamide and mycophenolate mofetil). Up to 15% of children with lupus nephritis can progress to ESRD.

Wegener Granulomatosis

Wegener granulomatosis (WG) is a multisystem disease generally consisting of a classic triad of: (a) necrotising granulomatous lesions in upper or lower respiratory tract, (b) generalised focal necrotising vasculitis involving both arteries and veins, and (c) focal glomerulonephritis. Similar to SLE, renal involvement includes microscopic haematuria, proteinuria, nephrotic syndrome, and acute glomerulonephritis. C-antineutrophil cytoplasmic antibodies (C-ANCA) or antibodies to proteinase-3 are highly specific for WG but have limited value for following the disease progression or the response to therapy. Treatment is often with combination of corticosteroids and cytotoxic therapy. Overall, the prognosis for WG has dramatically improved in recent decades.

Goodpasture's Syndrome

Goodpasture's syndrome consists of a triad of glomerulonephritis, pulmonary haemorrhage, and antibody to basement membrane antigens.

Documentation of anti-GBM antibody-induced disease may be done by renal biopsy or by establishing the presence of circulating anti-GBM antibodies. Renal involvement can be with acute nephritic picture (hypertension, oedema, haematuria, and reduced renal function). The course of untreated Goodpasture's syndrome is one of progressive renal dysfunctions leading to uremia. Recent studies have shown a marked decrease in mortality to less than 10% related to more rapid diagnosis and treatment. Plasmapheresis to remove circulating anti-GBM antibodies combined with immunosuppressive therapy to prevent new antibody formation is essential steps in management.

Alport's Syndrome

Alport's syndrome is a progressive and classically an X-linked inherited glomerulonephritis accounting for 1 to 2% of patients who develop ESRD. The syndrome is characterised by ocular abnormalities (e.g. anterior lenticonus, yellow-white to silver flecks within the macular, and midperipheral regions of the retina), progressive high-tone sensorineural hearing loss, and hereditary nephritis. The progressive nephritis presents with persistent gross or microscopic haematuria following upper respiratory infections. Low-phosphate, low-protein, and low-salt diets and cyclosporine A are used to manage this condition. Patients who receive a renal allograft have a small risk for developing Alport's disease after renal transplantation.

RENAL PARENCHYMAL DISORDERS

Tumours and Cystic Renal Disease

Tumours and cystic renal disease can present with haematuria. Examples of renal tumours are Wilms' tumour and renal cell carcinoma. Autosomal dominant polycystic kidney disease is an example of cystic renal disease that can present with either gross or microscopic haematuria.

Interstitial Nephritis

Interstitial nephritis can result from administration of analgesics or antibiotics. Discontinuing the offending agent may lead to complete resolution.

Nephrocalcinosis

Nephrocalcinosis refers to calcium deposition within the renal tissue. The most common causes are furosemide therapy in premature neonates, distal renal tubular acidosis, hyperparathyroidism, medullary sponge kidney, hypophosphatemic rickets, sarcoidosis, cortical necrosis, hyperoxaluria, prolonged immobilisation, Cushing syndrome, hyperuricosuria, and renal candidiasis. Diagnosis is usually made by renal ultrasonography. The offending agent must be withdrawn if possible and any underlying disorder must be treated.

Hypercalciuria

Hypercalciuria without signs of renal stones can cause macroscopic or microscopic haematuria. It is assumed that irritation of the urothelium by microcalculi or the microscopic areas of nephrocalcinosis causes bleeding. Symptoms may also include dysuria and/or suprapubic pain. Spot urine calcium to creatinine ratio of more than 0.2 should alert to this possibility.

RENAL COLLECTING SYSTEM DISORDERS

UTIs

UTIs can cause microscopic and gross haematurias. The child often has other concomitant symptoms such as urinary frequency, urgency, and dysuria with or without fever. Urine culture is diagnostic and guides antibiotic therapy. *E. coli* is a frequent aetilogic agent. Infections with *Schistosoma haematobium* are common in some regions and can cause bladder lesions containing eggs and a surrounding granuloma. Adenovirus, a common respiratory virus in children, can cause haemorrhagic cystitis with negative routine urine culture. Viral urine cultures and serial antibody titre determinations may help clarify the diagnosis. On bladder sonography, the bladder wall is thickened and mass effects can be observed. The condition is self-limiting.

Trauma

Trauma is another cause for haematuria in children. As children have higher incidence for pre-existing renal abnormalities (e.g. ureteropelvic junction obstruction and horseshoe kidney) than their counterpart adults, they can be present with a history of haematuria disproportionate to the severity of trauma. Paediatric trauma is usually investigated by CT abdomen and pelvis. Presence of blood at the meatus requires retrograde urethrogram to role out urethral injury.

Nephrolithiasis

Nephrolithiasis is an important cause for both microscopic and gross haematurias in children. Abdominal pain is usually present in this scenario and abdominal ultrasonography is essential in diagnosis.

Tumours

Tumours such as rhabdomyosarcoma of the bladder or prostate can be present with gross and/or microscopic haematuria.

Haemangiomas and Polyps

Haemangiomas and polyps can cause gross haematuria. Klippel-Trenauay and Proteus syndromes are rare hamartomatous disorders that can be associated with gross haematuria. Cystoscopy is diagnostic in these cases.

Meatal Stenosis

Meatal stenosis is a condition that is almost always acquired after neonatal circumcision. Balanitis xerotica obliterans is another cause of meatal stenosis and may lead to urinary retention. The finding of a pinpoint urethral meatus on examination coupled by observing a dorsally deflected urine stream or a forceful and thin stream with great casting distance is diagnostic. Associated symptoms, although may not always attribute to the abnormality, may include dysuria, frequency, terminal haematuria, and incontinence.

Idiopathic Urethrorrhagia

Idiopathic urethrorrhagia is characterised by terminal haematuria and blood spotting on the underwear in prepubertal and pubertal boys.

Diagnosis is mainly clinical by obtaining careful anamnesis. Inflammation of the bulbar urethra has been described at time of cystoscopy but the aetiology remains indeterminate. Radiographic and laboratory evaluations have limited benefit. Cystoscopic examination is not usually indicated. Kaplan and Brock (1982) noted a 20% incidence of stricture in boys with urethrorrhagia who underwent cystoscopy but no stricture in those in whom cystoscopy was not performed. Nevertheless, the process can lead to the formation of bulbar urethral stricture. In almost three-quarters of boys, the condition is self-limiting and resolve within one year, while approximately 8% may have recurrence. Follow-up with serial urine flow until resolution of the symptoms is recommended.

OTHER RARE DISORDERS

1. *Strenuous exercise.*
2. *Haematological disorders* such as sickle cell disease, sickle cell trait, and bleeding disorders.
3. *Nutcracker syndrome* occurs when the left renal vein is compressed between the superior mesenteric artery and aorta, which causes a rise in pressure and development of collateral veins. It can present with left flank pain, unilateral haematuria, and occasionally a varicocele in boys.
4. *Renal artery/vein thrombosis*: in newborns, renal vein thrombosis presents with a palpable abdominal mass and haematuria. Risk factor includes diabetic mother. Doppler ultrasonography is diagnostic.
5. *Loin pain haematuria syndrome* (*LPHS*) was first described in 1967 by Little and colleagues and refers to episodes of unilateral or bilateral lumbar pain accompanied by microscopic or gross haematuria. The diagnosis is made by exclusion. Most patients are females between 20 and 40 years of age; however, the syndrome has been described in children as well. Some authors question the existence of LPHS as symptoms are similar to those found in parents of children with Münchhausen syndrome by proxy. Almost 50% of the patients with LPHS have psychopathological disturbances.

EVALUATION

Evaluation of the child with haematuria begins with a careful history, physical examination, and urine analysis. This will help to determine the level of haematuria (i.e. upper vs. lower urinary tracts) and to determine the urgency of further evaluation based on the likelihood of a particular disease process. Serial urinalyses are helpful in case of microscopic haematuria.

History

Detailed history is an important first step in the evaluation of paediatric haematuria. It will direct the physician in obtaining appropriate and cause-specific laboratory tests to confirm the diagnosis. Key elements in history include:

- *Pain*: abdominal pain can be associated with nephrolithiasis. Associated symptoms of dysuria and/or fever may suggest UTI. Glomerular diseases rarely cause pain except in the conditions such as HSP. In the later case, other symptoms such as diarrhoea, haematochezia, arthralgia, and skin rash may occur at the same time.
- Recent history of pharyngitis or impetigo suggests PSGN.
- Shortness of breath, weight gain, or oedema suggests glomerulonephritis.
- Systemic symptoms such as fever, weight loss, fatigue, mouth ulcers, alopecia, and arthritis may suggest SLE.
- Recurrent painless gross haematuria in association with concurrent respiratory symptoms is highly suggestive of IgA nephropathy.
- Cough or haemoptysis may point towards pulmonary-renal syndrome such as Goodpasture's syndrome or WG.
- An infant with the history of birth asphyxia or the use of umbilical catheters suggests renal vascular thrombosis.
- A newborn of diabetic mother suggests renal vein thrombosis.
- African-American race requires evaluation of a history of sickle cell disease or sickle cell trait.
- Travel history (e.g. exposure to tuberculosis or schistosomiasis).

- Bleeding tendency (e.g. prolonged nosebleeds, heavy menstrual period, or haemarthrosis).
- *Medications*: drug-induced interstitial nephritis can be associated with medications such as antibiotics or anticonvulsants. Non-steroidal anti-inflammatory drugs can lead to papillary necrosis. Cyclophosphamide may cause haemorrhagic cystitis.
- The history of sexual abuse, trauma, foreign body, and menstrual history.
- The family history of ESRD or deafness may suggest Alport syndrome. Benign familial haematuria syndrome can be present with microscopic or macroscopic haematuria.

Physical Examination

Important components of physical examination should address the following:

- Blood pressure measurement to look for hypertension that may indicate glomerulonephritis or renal insufficiency, especially in the presence of oedema.
- *Growth parameters*: failure to thrive (FTT) may indicate chronic renal disease.
- Presence of fever, rash, pallor, and joint involvement suggest systemic disease.
- Abdominal examination for pain, costovertebral angle tenderness or masses.
- External genitalia for the signs of abuse, foreign body, tears, or lacerations.

Laboratory Studies

Detailed history and physical examination will allow targeted investigations to confirm the diagnosis of haematuria (Table 3-2).

- *Urine microscopy*: it should be the first step. This will confirm the presence of RBCs in urine sediment. It will also show whether

Table 3-2. Suggested work-up investigations in select causes of haematuria.

Symptoms	Suspected diagnosis	Laboratory testing
Frequency, urgency, dysuria +/– fever	UTI	Urine culture
Isolated abdominal pain	Nephrolithiasis	Renal ultrasound +/– CT abdomen/pelvis
Pharyngitis and impetigo	PSGN	C3, C4, ASO, and anti-DNAse B
Recurrent painless haematuria	IgA nephropathy	Serum IgA and renal biopsy
Arthralgia, abdominal pain, haematochezia, and skin purpura	HSP	Skin biopsy (leukocytoclastic vasculitis)
Arthritis, malar rash, fever, weight loss, alopecia, oral ulcers, and CNS symptoms	SLE	C3, C4, ANA, anti-double-stranded DNA
Rash, sinusitis, and haemoptysis	WG	ANCA
Fever, haemoptysis, and cough	Goodpasture's syndrome	Anti-GBM antibody
Family history of renal disease and hearing loss	Alport's syndrome	Audiogram and slit lamp examination
African-American race	Sickle cell disease or trait	Sickle cell screen
Medication exposure (NSAIDs, penicillin, etc.)	Interstitial nephritis	Urine eosinophils
Dorsally deflected urine stream	Meatal stenosis	Uroflow

dysmorphic RBCs or RBC casts are present, which indicate glomerular source for haematuria. Absence of RBCs in the urine may indicate pigments (haemoglobin and myoglobin), food substances, drugs, or organic substances.

- *Proteins*: trace amounts of protein in dipstick is normal when evaluating haematuria. This corresponds to excretion of less than

150 mg/24 hours. Anything more than that indicates proteinuria. Nephrotic syndrome typically is associated with excretion of more than 4 gm protein/24 hours.

- *Bacteruria or pyuria* in urine microscopy requires obtaining urine culture to evaluate for UTI (cystitis vs. pyelonephritis).
- *Suspect glomerulonephritis*: obtain CBC and serum creatinine, evaluate also the degree of proteinuria by either obtaining a 24-hour urine collection of protein or spot urine protein: creatinine ration (normal is <0.5 for children less than two years of age and <0.2 for children over two years of age, nephrotic ratio is >3.5). If history is suggestive for recent pharyngitis or impetigo, obtain complement levels (C3 and C4), antistreptolysin O antibody and streptozyme test. For all other immune-mediated GN, obtain ANA and anti-double-stranded DNA antibody.
- *Vasculitis and/or pulmonary-renal syndromes* obtain antineutrophilic cytoplasmic antibody and antiglomerular basement antibody titres.
- *Renal biopsy* may be indicated to establish diagnosis and/or assess the severity of renal involvement.
- *Skin biopsy of purpuric rash* may be needed to establish the diagnosis of HSP.
- *Urine calcium levels*: this can be performed by either 24-hour urine collection for calcium (normal <4 mg/kg/day) or spot urine calcium-creatinine ration (normal <0.2). Hypercalciuria is an important cause of microscopic haematuria in children. It can also lead to macroscopic haematuria believed secondary to adherence of calcium oxalate and phosphate crystals to urothelium.
- *Radiological studies*: renal ultrasound can be utilised to assess structural abnormalities of the collecting renal system e.g. ureteropelvic junction obstruction, look for contour abnormalities such as polycystic renal disease, or investigate kidney stones. CT scan will better assess abdominal and retroperitoneal masses such as rhabdomyosarcoma. CT angiography can also be used to look for rare causes of gross haematuria as in Nutcracker syndrome and arteriovenous fistulas.
- *Other useful studies*: cystoscopy can be helpful in evaluating the urethra and bladder for abnormalities such as polyps, tumours, and haemangioma.

COMMENT FROM THE EDITORS

This chapter represents a comprehensive, yet practical review on the topic of haematuria in children. Patients with microscopic haematuria should be referred to paediatric nephrologists; however, in practice, the urologist receives many of these children and a basic knowledge of the problem is essential to good practice. The most important difference between adult urologic and paediatric practice is that in children cystoscopy plays a minor role in the evaluation of haematuria. The picture should remind us that urologist should learn to look at the spun urinary sediment themselves and learn to recognise the most important findings.

FURTHER READING

Greenfield SP, Williot P, Kaplan D. Gross haematuria in children: a ten-year review. *Urology* 2007; **69**:166–169.

Ingelfinger JR, Davis AE, Grupe WE. Frequency and etiology of gross haematuria in a general pediatric setting. *Pediatrics* 1977; **59**:557–561.

Kaplan GW, Brock WA. Idiopathic urethrorrhagia in boys. *J Urol* 1982; **128**:1001.

Massengill SF. Haematuria. *Pediatr Rev* 2008; **29**:342–347.

Meyers K. Evaluation of haematuria in children. *Urol Clin N Am* 2004; **31**:559–573.

Pan CG. Evaluation of gross haematuria. *Pediatr Clin N Am* 2006; **53**:401–412.

Walker BR, Ellison ED, Snow BW, Cartwright PC. The natural history of idiopathic urethrorrhagia in boys. *J Urol* 2001; **166**:231–232.

Chapter 4

Abdominal, Flank, and Genital Pains and Masses of Genitourinary Origin

Ricardo González and Barbara M. Ludwikowski

PAIN

Definition

Pain is a common presenting complaint for the diseases of the urinary tract. Renal pain may be felt in the flank, abdomen, or both. Bladder pain is usually localized to the lower abdomen but it can be referred to the genitals or perineum. In the first part of this chapter, we discuss urological conditions commonly present with pain.

Conditions Present with Abdominal and Flank Pains

- Ureteral calculi,
- Pyelonephritis,
- Intermittent ureteropelvic junction (UPJ) obstruction, and
- Others.

ABDOMINAL AND FLANK PAINS

Renal pain is the result of tension within the renal capsule. It may result from acute inflammatory processes such as acute pyelonephritis or acute obstruction. Chronic obstruction or chronic inflammation is rarely presents with pain. In young children, the renal pain is often felt in the epigastrium, rather than in the back or flank as is usual in adolescents and adults. The renal pain in older children and adolescents is usually felt in the flank, costovertebral area, and may radiate to the epigastrium, lower abdomen, or genitalia. Vomiting is a frequent consequence of acute ureteral obstruction and is a common feature of ureteral calculi or intermittent hydronephrosis. Dietl's crisis refers to the occurrence of recurrent acute abdominal or flank pain and the vomiting characteristic of intermittent hydronephrosis caused by intermittent UPJ obstruction.

Differential Diagnosis

Acute pyelonephritis presents with fever, pain, and pyuria on the urinalysis. There is usually leukocytosis and an elevated C-reactive protein. The results of the urine culture are generally positive except in case of prior antibiotic administration. In contrast, the pain in acute renal colic from ureteral obstruction is stronger; fever is not common unless the obstruction is complicated by infection. The urinalysis reveals microscopic hematuria but this is not always present. In intermittent obstruction from a UPJ obstruction, the pain is severe; it may be located in the flank or epigastrium and vomiting is the rule. Of course, emesis can also be present in ureteral calculi and acute pyelonephritis.

The differential diagnosis of renal pain in children includes, among many others, acute appendicitis, ovarian torsion, testicular torsion, intestinal invagination, and volvulus. The flank pain of the renal origin needs to be distinguished from that of the musculoskeletal origin. It is beyond the scope of this chapter to discuss the non-renal causes of pain.

Imaging Studies

The initial diagnostic tool is an abdominal ultrasound including the kidneys and bladder. Ultrasonography during the episode of pain is very sensitive to detect dilatation as in the case of intermittent UPJ obstruction but not very sensitive to detect acute pyelonephritis or ureteral calculi. In acute pyelonephritis, the kidney may be enlarged compared to the contralateral side. The presence of renal calcifications may suggest that there is a calculus in the ureter. Ureteral calculi are seen on ultrasonography only when they are at the UPJ or in the retrovesical portion of the ureter.

Examination with a full bladder is necessary. When a ureteral calculus is suspected, but not seen on ultrasonography, a CT of the abdomen without contrast is usually diagnostic. It is better to perform the CT in the prone position to differentiate calculi at the ureterovesical junction (UVJ) from those which have already passed to the bladder. The diagnosis of acute pyelonephritis is usually established on clinical and laboratory grounds. When the urine culture is negative because of prior antibiotic treatment, a DMSA scan of the kidneys or, when not available, a CT of the kidney with intravenous contrast is diagnostic.

Treatment

The treatment depends on the cause (see Chapters 2, 14, and 22).

Conditions Present with Suprapubic, Genital, and Perineal Pains

- Cystitis,
- Urinary retention, and
- Bladder calculi.

BLADDER PAIN

Bladder pain occurs when the bladder is inflamed or over distended. The pain is usually lower abdominal or suprapubic pain. However, bladder pain may be felt in the genital area and the perineum, both in males and in females.

Differential Diagnosis

In addition to pain, acute bladder infections are often present with urinary frequency and urgency and pain during voiding (dysuria). Fever over 38°C is rare. Hematuria and urinary incontinence are sometimes present.

Acute urinary retention causes pain, a palpable lower abdominal mass, and inability to void. Overflow incontinence may be present (see Chapter 6).

Bladder calculi in Western countries are most common in patients with neuropathic bladder and/or bladder augmentation (see Chapter 21). In these cases, pain is rarely the presenting complaint. In the past and in some less developed countries, primary bladder calculi are common. Presentation is usually with pain, stranguria, and hematuria.

The urinalysis helps establish the diagnosis. The specimen obtained should be used for a urine culture that in cases of infection provides the definitive diagnosis and guides the treatment.

Other Diagnostic Studies

A renal and bladder ultrasound and an abdominal ultrasound help to establish the diagnosis when cystitis is not clear-cut.

Further studies and treatment depend on the cause of bladder pain. The treatment for cystitis is discussed in Chapter 2, for stones in Chapter 21, and for urinary retention in Chapter 6.

MASSES

A number of urological diseases in children are present with palpable masses. These include both benign and malignant neoplasms and non-neoplastic conditions.

For painless scrotal swelling and masses, please refer to Chapters 8 and 20.

In the newborn, more than half of the palpable abdominal masses are of genitourinary origin including multicystic dysplastic kidney (MCDK), hydronephrosis, and mesoblastic nephroma.

Abdominal Masses in the Newborn

In the past, many of the conditions listed below were detected during the physical examination of the newborn. At present, in many places where prenatal ultrasonography is performed routinely, the disease is suspected well before the examination.

Physical examination should record the location of the mass, its quality and mobility, and other pertinent features of the general physical examination.

More than half of the palpable masses in the newborn originate in the kidney. Below, we list and briefly describe the most common conditions.

1. MCDK is the most common palpable mass in the newborn abdomen. It is associated with high or low ureteral atresia. The ultrasonographic appearance is characteristic but it is occasionally difficult to differentiate from the massive hydronephrosis or the rare cystic neoplasia of the newborn. On ultrasound, the cystic structures do not communicate with each other or with the often present central cyst, a feature that helps distinguish it from massive hydronephrosis. There may be a variably amount of solid, echogenic components in the mass, representing dysplastic renal tissue. On DMSA or MAG 3 scan function in the involved side is invariably absent.

   Surgery is rarely required. The natural history is one of the gradual spontaneous disappearance resulting from reabsorption of the fluid in the cysts. Rarely, surgery to remove the mass is indicated in the course of follow-up during the first year of life if the mass does not regress or the diagnosis is in doubt.

   Complications are rare. The cases of infection of the MCDK and the arterial hypertension have been reported. The alleged risk of tumor development is extremely rare or null and does not justify routine removal. Bilateral MCDK is incompatible with extrauterine life and it is accompanied by pulmonary hypoplasia, a history of oligo- or anhydramnios and Potter's facies.
2. A large hydronephrotic kidney associated with a high-grade UPJ obstruction is diagnosed by ultrasonography and MAG 3 scan and will usually require early surgical repair (see Chapter 14).
3. Autosomal recessive polycystic kidney disease not detected prenatally (see Chapter 1) presents with large bilateral renal masses. The clinical course is one of the early developments of renal insufficiency. Those children who survive infancy may develop progressive portal hypertension from polycystic liver disease. The diagnosis is made by the family history and ultrasonography. With the early onset of renal failure, peritoneal dialysis may be needed. The lack of space within the peritoneal cavity may necessitate the removal of one of the kidneys. This procedure is attended by high morbidity and mortality.

4. Renal vein thrombosis in the newborn may result from dehydration and a diabetic mother. Proteinuria and hematuria are the rule. Ultrasonography shows an enlarged and hyperechoic kidney and color Doppler detects the lack of flow in the renal vein. The thrombosis may extend into the vena cava. The condition usually resolves with medical management. The loss of renal function is more common on the right side because of the lack of collateral circulation.
5. Posterior urethral valves and other rare causes of urethral obstruction may result in massive bilateral hydronephrosis with palpable kidneys and bladder (see Chapter 17).
6. Mesoblastic nephroma, a benign newborn tumor of the kidney is discussed in Chapter 20. The removal of the tumor in the first few months of the life is recommended to prevent malignant transformation.
7. Neuroblastoma, usually originating in the adrenal gland, represents 10% of palpable masses in the newborn period (Chapter 20).
8. Other neonatal abdominal masses that should be considered in the differential diagnosis include ovarian cysts and tumors, hydrocolpos, choledochal cysts, intestinal duplications, and presacral masses such as teratomas and anterior myelomeningocele.

Careful anamneses including the prenatal history, physical examination, and imaging studies that allow an accurate diagnosis in most cases to direct the appropriate therapy.

Abdominal Masses in Infancy and Childhood

In contrast with masses in the newborn period, which are usually benign, later in infancy and childhood, the abdominal masses commonly are the first manifestation of Wilms' tumors and neuroblastoma (see Chapter 20). However, ovarian masses, a distended bladder and hydrometrocolpos, must also be considered.

Hematocolpos and hematometra present as lower abdominal masses and cyclical abdominal pain after the onset of puberty. The common causes are imperforate hymen, vaginal atresia, transverse vaginal septum, and other causes of vaginal obstruction that escaped detection in infancy. The treatment is surgical correction, which may range from simple hymenotomy to a complex vaginal reconstruction.

Chapter 5

Urinary Incontinence

Julie Franc-Guimond

DEFINITION

Imperfect day- or nighttime control of micturition at an age when this is expected is a common presenting symptom in paediatric urology, which often causes distress to child and family and affects the quality of life.

The function of the urinary bladder is to store urine at low pressure to allow urine produced in the kidneys to continue to enter the bladder between micturitions and the periodic, voluntary, and complete emptying of the accumulated urine. This balanced function requires anatomical integrity of the bladder, internal and external sphincteric mechanisms, and the anatomical and functional integrity of the portions of the peripheral and central nervous systems. Urinary control involves both the somatic and the autonomic nervous systems. It is beyond the scope of this chapter to describe in detail the neurological pathways involved.

To be continent, a child's bladder should have sufficient storing capacity and good compliance and should empty completely at the end of the voiding cycle. In turn, the sphincteric mechanisms should be closed during the filling or storing phase and open during voiding to allow unimpeded and low-pressure emptying.

Hence, urinary incontinence can occur when problems arise during the storage phase, the filling phase, or both but it could also be completely unrelated to the voiding cycle. Aetiologies can be neurological, anatomical, or functional and the pathogenesis can be grouped as failure to

Table 5-1. Classification of urinary incontinence in children.

Failure to store:

- **Neurological**
  (spina bifida, tethered cord, traumatic lesions of the cord or cauda equina, etc.)
- **Non-neurological with normal bladder capacity**
  (urge syndrome, overactive bladder etc.)
- **Non-neurological with reduced bladder capacity**
  (bladder exstrophy, epispadias, bilateral ectopic ureters, etc.)

Failure to empty (overflow incontinence):

- **Neurological**
  (spina bifida, tethered cord, traumatic lesions of the cord or cauda equina, etc.)
- **Non-neurological**
  (myogenic failure such as seen in PBS, PUV, non-neurogenic voiding dysfunction, etc.)

Failure of sphincteric mechanisms:

- **Neurological**
  (spina bifida, tethered cord, traumatic lesions of the cord or cauda equina, etc.)
- **Non-neurological**
  (bladder exstrophy, epispadias, iatrogenic injury to the sphincter, etc.)

Bypass of sphincteric mechanisms:

- Ectopic ureter (in girls)
- Vesicovaginal fistulas

Nocturnal enuresis

store, failure to empty (leading to overflow incontinence), deficiency or bypass of sphincteric mechanisms, or isolated nocturnal enuresis (Table 5-1). In many cases, there are multiple mechanisms involved.

GENERAL CONSIDERATIONS AND INITIAL ASSESSMENT

Voiding happens involuntarily in infants and young children until the age of three to five years, after which it is regulated voluntarily. Even though most children are generally toilet trained by the time they are five years old, the time course for achieving urinary continence varies among them.

Therefore, one should keep in mind that children are growing and maturing individuals and should evaluate them within the context of their developmental age. In general, an appropriate workup includes a thorough history, a physical examination, and non-invasive tests. Invasive studies are reserved for the cases of suspected anatomical or neurological anomaly. While most patients aged five and under normally require no more than a history and a physical examination, some may warrant additional attention if other significant symptoms (urinary tract infections, abnormal stream, haematuria, etc.) are present or anatomical anomalies are suspected.

Anamnesis

The anamnesis should especially inquire the child's voiding habits and past medical history including any antenatal or perinatal particularities that may possibly have a bearing on the present illness. Details that may identify covert neurological or structural anomalies should also be sought. While being born with spinal dysraphism is usually obvious, other pathologies may not be as evident. Delays in learning to walk, frequent falls, gait problems, or faecal incontinence suggest potential occult neurological problems. Obtaining information regarding the family history is also important, as it may reveal medical conditions with genetic predisposition that could play a role in the urological condition. In addition, the medical history should pay attention to the presence of possible psychosocial stressors such as fear of going to the toilet outside of home, eating disorders, emotional stress, and sexual abuse which, although rare, cannot be overlooked.

In order to correctly define the patient's symptoms, the medical terms employed should be clear and free of confusion. Urinary incontinence refers to uncontrollable leakage of urine, which can be continuous or intermittent. It can occur during the daytime, the nighttime, or both. The word daytime is preferred over diurnal, as the latter may imply something that occurs daily over a 24-hour period rather than symptoms that are encountered during the day. Enuresis can be a confusing term since its use varies from one author to the other but should be reserved for nighttime wetting. The onset and the pattern of incontinence need to be established since it will help determine the likely cause. The incontinence can be acute or chronic, congenital or acquired. More specifically, the terms primary vs. secondary urinary incontinences are used to describe patients whom have never been dry for at least six months vs. those who have. The age at which a child became toilet trained will carry some relevance and merits attention but, as mentioned before, it will become more important to acknowledge the patient's symptoms within the context of his or her overall development.

Urinary incontinence may be present during the day, night, or both and can happen occasionally or many times a day. In addition, incontinence may occur at anytime in relation to the voiding cycle or come about just before or after micturition. Urge incontinence occurs when there is an involuntary loss of urine associated to an intense desire to void while leakage of urine in the context of increased intra-abdominal pressure is called stress incontinence. Mixed incontinence is the combination of urge and stress incontinences. Post-void dribbling refers to leakage of urine experienced after voiding usually caused by vaginal reflux in girls. Giggle incontinence or enuresis risoria is a rare type of incontinence, which occurs just prior to or during an episode of intense laughter. Continuous incontinence is when the patient is always wet or damp because of the continuous leakage of urine. This can occur either despite normal voiding cycles or in the absence of voluntary micturition. The former scenario would typically be encountered in a toilet-trained girl who was found to have an ectopic ureter that bypasses the urinary sphincter (paradoxical incontinence). The latter indicates a failure of the sphincteric mechanisms because of structural or neurological pathologies.

Additional lower urinary tract symptoms worth asking include increased or decreased frequency, nocturia, urgency, straining, painful urination or abnormal stream, impression of incomplete emptying, as well as squatting or other holding manoeuvres (standing on tiptoe, crossing legs also referred to as Vincent's curtsy).

It is also imperative to investigate the presence of other symptoms or comorbidities such as haematuria, constipation or encopresis, urinary tract infections, vesicoureteral reflux (VUR), diabetes mellitus (DM), and attention-deficit disorder with or without hyperactivity.

Finally, questioning the patient directly is important since parents often ignore some of their child's symptoms and/or pay very little attention to details that they do not believe to be important. Furthermore, they often devalue symptoms that may prove to be significant or ignore events pertinent to the actual medical problem.

It is also very useful to have the child and parents complete a "Voiding and Stooling Diary" in which during two 24-hour periods each voiding is recorded with time and volume and whether or not there were incontinent episodes in between. Bowel movements are recorded for a week with regards to the characteristics and episodes of encopresis. Ideally, the volume of fluid intake should be recorded as well. Although there is a great variation among individuals, normal micturition frequency is five to eight voids per day, zero to one nocturnal micturition, and three bowel movements per week up to three per day.

Physical Examination

Routine examination should be performed with emphasis on the abdomen, external genitalia, and back. It should also include a neurological examination that focuses on gait, motor skills, reflexes of the lower extremities, and sphincteric integrity. The abdominal inspection should confirm or rule out the presence of a distended bladder or an abdominal mass or it may point to faecal impaction. Examining the genitalia is important, as it could reveal the presence of labial adhesions or signs of local infection or irritation. It may also raise the suspicion of sexual abuse if local tears or signs of sexually transmitted diseases are observed. More importantly, it could reveal abnormalities of the urethral meatus or point to the presence of an ectopic ureter or epispadias in girls. The spine is examined for signs of closed spinal dysraphism (sacral dimple, hair tuft, haemangioma, or lipoma), sacral agenesis, or scoliosis.

Diagnostic Tests

Investigation should begin with non-invasive tests (urine analysis, urine culture, and diary of voiding and bowel habits) to rule out underlying conditions such as a urinary tract infection, DM, and constipation. Non-invasive urodynamic studies consisting of uroflowmetry and sonographic measurement of the post-void residual (PVR) volume are important to

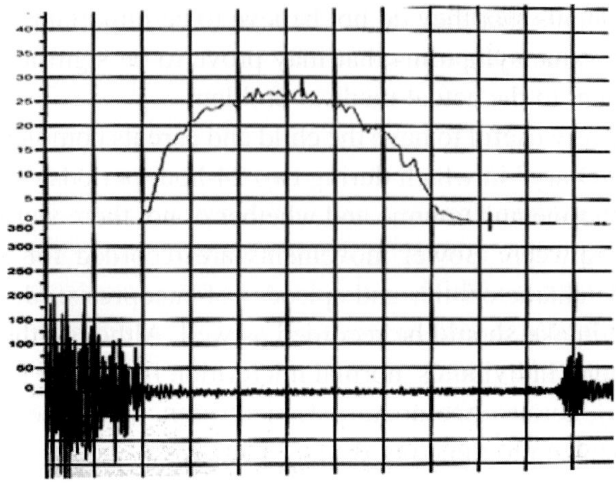

Figure 5-1. Normal uroflowmetry showing a bell-shaped curve and silent EMG.

confirm or rule out normal voiding mechanics. Regarding bladder emptying, a normal uroflowmetry translates into an adequate voided volume, the presence of a bell-shaped curve (Figure 5-1) and a non-significant PVR volume (less than 20 ml is usually considered normal). Many formulas have been proposed to approximate the expected bladder capacity for a particular child such as (age + 1) × 30 in ml. Another way is to calculate the minimal acceptable total bladder capacity for age using 16 (age) + 70 in ml. Of course, these formulas are rough estimates and can only be applied if the patient's body habitus is normal. Another useful rule of thumb is bladder capacity equals body weight × 7.

A plain X-ray of the abdomen may help to ascertain the presence of constipation, pubic diastasis, or gross spinal abnormalities. Additional radiological studies (ultrasound, voiding cystourethrogram, and MRI of the spine) may be needed if there is evidence of previous or current urinary tract infections, or if underlying anatomical or neurological anomalies are suspected. Other abnormal findings such as haematuria should also raise the need for X-rays. Invasive urodynamics (cystomanometry with or without the measurement of intra-abdominal pressure and electrical activity of the pelvic floor) will be performed for voiding dysfunction unresponsive to typical medical treatment or for patients with neurological conditions. The need for any additional imaging and functional studies will be based on the patient's history and physical examination.

Diagnosis

An initial assessment based upon a comprehensive history, examination, and appropriate additional studies should help establish the cause of the incontinence, which can be neurological, anatomical, or functional but should also ensure that serious conditions are not overlooked and that unnecessary tests are not performed. Some causes may give rise to more than one symptom or sign so it may be of assistance, therefore, to consider the various symptoms as a whole in an approach to diagnosis. It can be cautiously suggested that there is less chance for assuming that the urinary incontinence for a particular child is most likely caused by a certain diagnosis. If well diagnosed, the patient's symptoms will improve with the proposed treatment options and if not, more invasive studies can be obtained to better define the patient's medical condition. For example, a child suspected of having detrusor overactivity will benefit from the use of anticholinergics without having to experience an invasive urodynamic study if there is good response to the therapy.

Neurological conditions (closed or open spinal dysraphism, sacral agenesis, spinal cord injury, tethered cord, tumour with neurological impairment, etc.) that may cause urinary incontinence during the childhood are diagnosed based on the history of already known neurological diseases, the history of delay in learning to walk, gait problems, frequent falls, abnormal spinal and/or neurological examination, and well-documented anomalies on urodynamics and specific radiological studies.

Anatomical conditions that may cause urinary incontinence are often present early in life, i.e. before five years of age, because of the history of continuous leakage as well as the absence of voiding cycle in certain cases. The diagnosis is presumed by the history but confirmed by the physical examination and/or additional investigative procedures. Aetiologies include congenital anomalies such as bladder exstrophy, epispadias, ureteral ectopia (in girls) and posterior urethral valves (PUV) (in boys), or acquired anomalies such as meatal stenosis and iatrogenic damage to the external urinary sphincter, etc.

Incontinence caused by all other aetiologies that are not related to the structural or neurological conditions such as voiding dysfunction that presents with urinary incontinence is often referred to as functional incontinence.

As mentioned above, the mechanism for incontinence can be classified regardless of the cause as failure to store, failure to empty (overflow incontinence), deficiency or bypass of sphincteric mechanisms, or isolated nocturnal enuresis (Table 5-1).

Common Conditions

In the following section, some common conditions presenting with urinary incontinence are listed. Figure 5-2 describes an algorithm for the evaluation of the patient with functional daytime wetting.

- In the neurologically normal child without pre-existing conditions (such as epispadias, PUV, pelvic trauma, etc.):

    1. overactive bladder,
    2. dysfunctional voiding,
    3. infrequent voiding,
    4. enuresis nocturna,
    5. vaginal voiding, and
    6. ectopic ureter.

- In the child with known neurological abnormalities (see Chapter 21):

    1. spina bifida,
    2. sacral agenesis,
    3. spinal cord injury, and
    4. cerebral palsy.

- In the child with known urological or pelvic anomalies:

    1. epispadias and exstrophy (see Chapter 23),
    2. posterior urethral valves (see Chapter 17), and
    3. bilateral ectopic ureters.

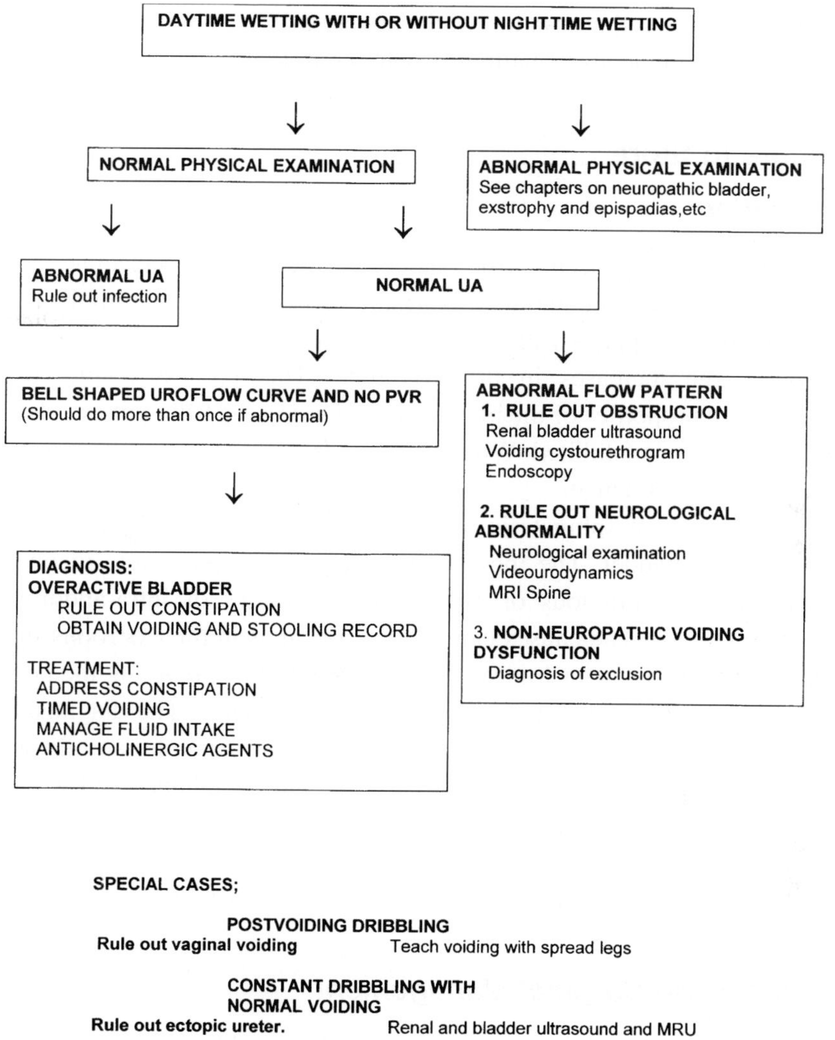

Figure 5-2. Algorithm for the evaluation of the child who presents with daytime wetting.

General Principles of Treatment

Therapeutic modalities vary according to the cause of the incontinence and the concomitant conditions. In general, non-surgical treatment options include behavioural modification, dietary changes, pharmacologic therapy, and/or even self-catheterisation while surgery may be required for children born with anatomic abnormalities or with neurological diseases.

Failure to Store

Definition

Failure to store can occur if the bladder is small; it has inadequate compliance or contract prematurely. Normal bladder compliance implies that bladder filling happens with little or no increase in intravesical pressure, despite large increases in urine volume. This process results from viscoelastic properties of the bladder wall. During the filling phase, detrusor contraction is inhibited. When it is not, detrusor overactivity may lead to urinary incontinence.

The failure of sphincteric mechanisms also leads to failure to store urine in the bladder. The incontinence caused by sphincteric incompetence can be continuous or only during increases of intra-abdominal pressure (stress). The causes can be anatomical as in the exstrophy epispadias complex or neurological. Surgical procedures involving the pelvic floor may lead to iatrogenic sphincteric incompetence. The diagnosis of sphincter failure is often made by exclusion. For example, a child with spina bifida with adequate bladder capacity and compliance and without detrusor overactivity who leaks urine permanently or during efforts has sphincteric incompetence. The presence of a denervated pelvic floor on electromyography supports the diagnosis of sphincter failure.

Medical and Surgical Management

The management of failure to store needs to address the cause (see Chapters 21 and 23). The functional disorders such as overactive bladder and the urge syndrome are treated with behavioural modification (hydration, timed voiding, dietary changes to limit bladder irritants, etc.) anticholinergic agents, and aggressive treatment of comorbid conditions such as urinary infection and constipation.

Likewise, neurological conditions causing failure to store may respond to anticholinergics but surgical bladder augmentation may be needed (Chapter 21). Botulinum toxin has been used to reduce bladder contractility and improve compliance in neuropathic bladder dysfunction but the effect is temporary. The use of botulinum toxin for non-neurological and functional disorders is controversial.

In neurological failure to store, treatments, both medical and surgical, lead to failure to empty and the need to use intermittent catheterisation.

The treatment of sphincteric incompetence is surgical (see Chapters 21 and 23). Non-surgical approaches such as weight reduction, physiotherapy, and the use of alpha-adrenergic medications are rarely used or useful in the paediatric population. Most cases are offered surgical treatment including injection of bulking agents, slings, bladder neck procedures, or implantation of artificial urinary sphincter.

Failure to Empty (Overflow Incontinence)

Definition of the Disease

The reflex of voiding should normally happen under voluntary control. It requires adequate relaxation of the sphincteric outlet structures and complete absence of bladder outlet obstruction with sustained contraction of the bladder until emptying is complete. An infra-vesical obstruction, either functional or anatomical, may cause the bladder to overfill and overflow incontinence.

Aetiologies

Besides storage problems, heterogeneous pathologies such as congenital or acquired spinal anomalies and voiding dysfunction syndromes can also present with an abnormal voiding phase and if emptying is incomplete, incontinence could be the results of an overflow. Therefore, the same neurological and non-neurological medical conditions mentioned in the section above can also present with overflow incontinence. For example, an unstable bladder could trigger the sphincteric guarding reflex and lead to dyscoordination between the sphincter and the detrusor. Such, incoordination may translate into a continuum of abnormal voiding patterns such as the staccato or fractionated patterns with the possibility of incomplete

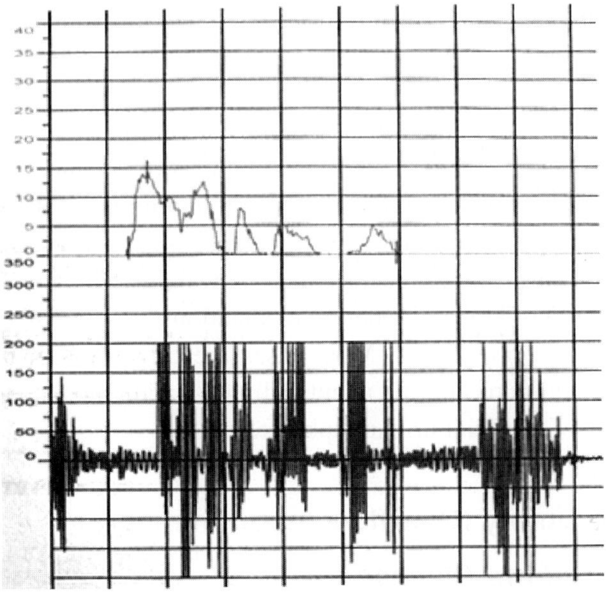

Figure 5-3. Non-invasive urodynamics obtained for a female patient presenting with urinary incontinence reveal that she voids abnormally. Uroflowmetry shows sphincteric dyssynergia resulting in poor bladder emptying and a high PVR.

emptying (Figure 5-3). Eventually, this could result in vesical overdistension with a reduced contraction ability of the detrusor traditionally termed the lazy bladder syndrome.

In addition to the usual neurological and non-neurological disorders, there is, at the critical end of the spectrum, a category of patients with the infrequent Hinman's syndrome, which is also called the non-neurogenic neurogenic bladder or occult neuropathic bladder, who have all the features of a patient with neurogenic detrusor–sphincter dyssynergia but in whom no neurological abnormalities can be found. A related syndrome, the Ochoa syndrome, is similar but the patients also have an abnormal facial expression when laughing.

Other non-neurological entities that may adversely affect bladder emptying and induce overflow incontinence include myogenic failure such as seen in prune belly syndrome (PBS), PUV, congenital urethral atresia, or iatrogenic urethral strictures (see Chapters 17 and 24).

Presentation

Patients with structural or functional pathologies that present with symptoms such as decreased urinary frequency, painful urination, straining to void, and weak or interrupted urinary stream with or without sensation of incomplete emptying most probably have a condition in which there is a dyscoordination between the sphincter and the detrusor, leading to overdistension of the bladder and secondary urinary leakage. They could also present with urinary tract infections or gross haematuria.

Hinman's syndrome or non-neurogenic neurogenic bladder disorder is a diagnosis of exclusion. It is suspected when a child presents with severe wetting accompanied by anatomical and functional changes such as bladder trabeculations, conformational changes of the ureterovesical orifices with or without VUR, and dilatation of the upper tracts along with incomplete emptying in the absence of a proven neurological entity or specific anomaly such as PUV. Renal failure at presentation is often the rule (Figure 5-4).

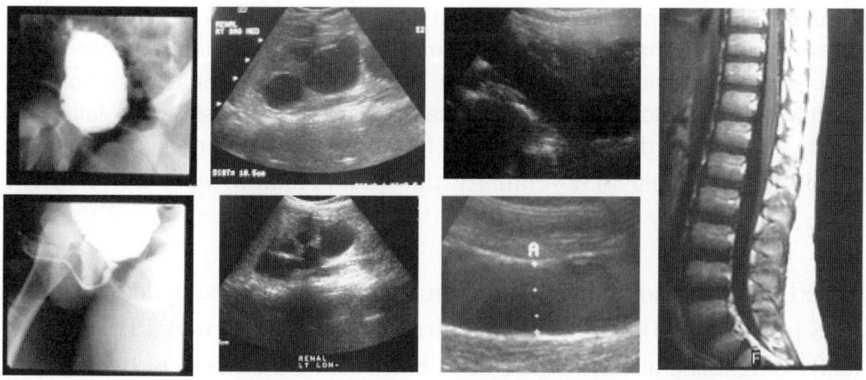

Figure 5-4. VCUG done for an eight-year-old boy who presented with a lifelong history of day- and nighttime incontinences and polydipsia demonstrates a trabeculated bladder without signs of urethral obstruction. In addition, he was found to have a palpable bladder on physical examination, bilateral hydroureteronephrosis on ultrasound and an elevated serum creatinine (5.6 mg/dl) with metabolic acidosis. UDS showed small bladder capacity, poor compliance, and inhibited bladder contraction during the filling phase. Emptying was incomplete with signs of dyssynergia. MRI of the spine was obtained but no anomalies were observed. He is believed to have a non-neurogenic neurogenic bladder otherwise known as Hinman's syndrome.

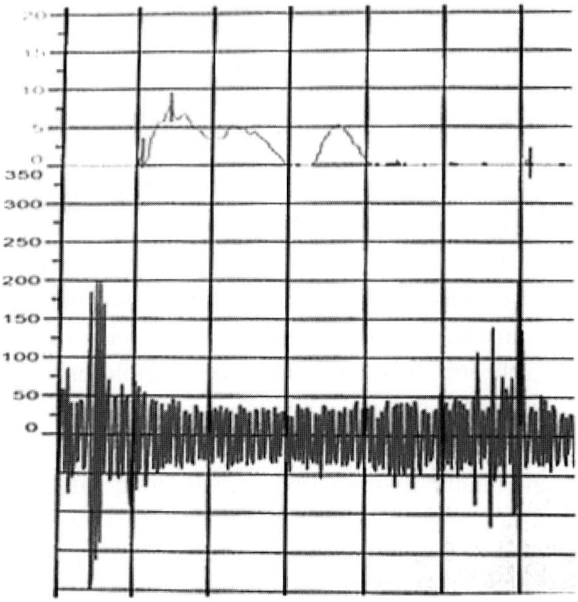

Figure 5-5. Patient born with PUV but diagnosed late in life at 11 years of age presented with urinary incontinence, impression of incomplete emptying, history of two previous urinary tract infections, and renal insufficiency. Uroflowmetry (performed after adequate valve ablation) shows a failure to empty, most likely due to a myogenic failure, with an abnormal flow curve, a silent EMG and a high PVR.

PUV are found in one per 5000 male births while the incidence of the PBS is one in 35,000–50,000 live births. Patients born with PBS are typically diagnosed at birth while boys born with PUV may not be detected early in life. Symptoms of patients known to have PUV, PBS, or other urethral anomalies may vary greatly but all are in relation to a certain degree of obstruction and impairment of bladder emptying (Figure 5-5) (cf. part two in which various chapters discuss these conditions in more details).

Diagnostic Methods

Diagnosing neurological and non-neurological conditions in children whom are believed to have overflow incontinence should begin like described in the preceding section. Additional workup will be obtained if basic tools unveil signs of incomplete bladder emptying such as an abnormal urinary flow with or without activity on the EMG, dilated urinary tracts, a large bladder with or without thickened walls or trabeculations, etc. Frequently used diagnostic methods include serum creatinine measurement to rule out renal failure, renal and bladder ultrasound, VCUG, invasive urodynamics, urethrocystoscopy, nuclear studies, and MRI.

Suspected structural anomalies of the spinal cord are typically confirmed with MRI. Secondary impairment of the urological function is profiled using most diagnostic tools. Children with dysfunctional elimination syndromes that present with overflow incontinence may have irritative symptoms in addition to voiding difficulties. Uroflow, an indirect measure of bladder and sphincter function, is often obtained in conjunction with pelvic-floor electromyography, to evaluate pelvic-floor activity during voiding. It may show normal, staccato, or interrupted patterns with silent or active EMG (Figure 5-3) and significant PVR. VCUG can reveal that patients who fail to open the urethral sphincter during voiding often have an atypical urethral configuration referred to as "spinning top" urethra. Invasive urodynamic studies, reserved for patients with complex forms of functional urinary incontinence, may demonstrate incoordination between the detrusor contraction and the expected relaxation of the urethral sphincter. Abnormalities may also be observed throughout the filling phase.

The diagnosis of non-neurogenic neurogenic syndrome relies on exclusion of obvious neurological pathologies.

PUV and other urethral anomalies are suspected on voiding cystography but confirmed with endoscopy.

Medical and Surgical Management

Adequate management of neurogenic bladder sphincter dysfunction should first acknowledge the patient at risk for upper- and lower-tract deterioration and begin appropriate medical treatment pre-emptively. Clean intermittent catheterisation combined with anticholinergic drugs represents the standard conduct. Early institution of such treatment can prevent secondary bladder-wall changes, hence renal damage thus potentially improving long-term outcomes. Surgery may be required if optimal medical management does not suffice and/or to achieve continence.

Behavioural and pharmacologic therapies are the primary treatments of functional bladder disorders in children. Severe cases may need to perform CIC and/or be offered less conventional therapeutic options such as biofeedback, neuromodulation, and botulinum toxin injections.

Treatment of non-neurogenic neurogenic bladders is complex. Most children will respond well to the traditional combination of anticholinergic agents and CIC while some may continue to have poorly compliant bladders that will require surgical treatment such as bladder augmentation.

PUV are initially managed by stabilisation and valve ablation. Subsequent management is more complex and should be individually based. Timed voiding regimens, prophylactic antibiotics, anticholinergics with CIC, and bladder augmentation are frequently used therapeutic options.

Therapeutic particularities observed in the case of patients born with PBS include early institution of prophylactic antibiotics and close monitoring of renal function especially because limiting instrumentation early in life are often advocated. Urological reconstruction may later be required and is often performed at the same time as orchidopexy and abdominoplasty (for the most severe cases).

Prognosis and Long-Term Complications

Bladders of patient found to have neurogenic bladder sphincter dysfunction and look-alike syndromes can cause severe and irreversible nephropathy years before incontinence arises. The same can be said about the bladder of patients born with PUV or PBS.

As mentioned before, the clinical symptoms of functional urinary dysfunction may vary from mild incontinence to severe disorders with endpoints of irreversible bladder dysfunction with VUR, recurrent urinary tract infections, and resulting renal injuries.

Bypass of Sphincteric Mechanisms

Definition of the Disease

Continuous dribbling of urine with otherwise normal voiding cycles points to a structural anomaly that escapes the sphincteric mechanisms.

Aetiology

Urinary incontinence in girls who have been toilet trained may be due to an ectopic ureter inserting below the urinary sphincter (see Chapter 15). Continuous incontinence in young females or males could also be observed with fistulas that may be congenital or arise after repair of complex genitourinary malformations such as persistent cloaca, anorectal anomalies, or trauma.

Presentation

Patients present with a history of continuous dribbling of urine with otherwise normal voiding cycles in toilet-trained female patients but continuous incontinence is always abnormal even in children whom are not yet toilet trained. Presenting features may also include history of urinary tract infections, abdominal pain, and renal failure. In cases of large fistulas, the incontinence is complete and constant.

Diagnostic Methods

The diagnosis is often delayed, is psychologically stressful, and may be overlooked during physical examination. Findings on ultrasound or VCUG may be subtle. MRI and nuclear scintigraphy may be more helpful than computed tomography but we can only find what we are looking for. Therefore, a very high degree of suspicion is required. Ultimately, most patients will benefit from an examination under anaesthesia with endoscopy performed prior to surgical management.

Surgical Management

The surgical treatment depends on the anatomy and the function of the renal unit or moiety drained by the ectopic ureter. Options include nephroureterectomy for non-functioning kidney, heminephroureterectomy for non-functioning upper pole of duplex kidney with ectopic ureter, ureteropyelostomy, ureteroureterostomy, or ureteral reimplantation.

Prognosis and Long-Term Complications

The surgical outcome in terms of achievement of continence is high if ectopic ureters are part of a duplicated system but not as good if they drain a single system uni- or bilaterally since the integrity of the bladder neck is usually impaired.

Nocturnal Enuresis

Definition

Nighttime incontinence is named monosymptomatic nocturnal enuresis if the symptom of bedwetting occurs in the absence of any other lower urinary tract symptoms. It characterises 80% of all patients presenting with nighttime incontinence. Non-monosymptomatic nocturnal enuresis signifies that other lower urinary tract symptoms (urgency, frequency, daytime incontinence, etc.) are present. The latter points to organic pathologies or to dysfunctional elimination syndromes and differs from primary or secondary monosymptomatic nocturnal enuresis. This section mainly intends to cover monosymptomatic nocturnal enuresis.

Aetiology

Not any reason can explain all the cases of bedwetting. In fact, studies have identified many possible explanations but none applies to all scenarios and many controversies remain. Identified causes include developmental delay, inadequate antidiuretic hormone (ADH) secretion, sleep disorders with or without sleep apnea and upper airway obstructive symptoms, small functional bladder capacity, as well as psychosocial or genetic factors. There is, in fact, a strong family history of bedwetting, suggesting a genetic basis. If one or both parents were bedwetters, a child has a 44 or 77% chance, respectively, of also suffering from enuresis nocturna.

Reports on the genetics of enuresis are available since the 1930s and molecular genetics since 1995, both emphasising the significance of heredity in the aetiology of nocturnal enuresis and many researchers currently focus on the recognition of genes, gene products, and their interaction with environmental factors. Thus far, many findings support the hypothesis of genetic and phenotypical heterogeneities of nocturnal enuresis with linkage to certain markers on chromosomes 12q, 13q, and 22q. Other factors that may contribute to nocturnal enuresis include constipation and diet, in particular, the consumption of mild caffeine drinks with diuretic effects (e.g. cola).

Presentation

Bedwetting is so common that some believe it represents a variant of normal development rather than a disease since the development of bladder control at night is the last to occur. Despite the fact that nighttime incontinence is a symptom that is usually outgrown overtime, incontinence at the normal age of toilet training may cause great distress. It is embarrassing, adversely affects the child's quality of life and can lead to poor self-esteem and unmerited punishment.

Fifteen to 20% of five-year-olds and upto 1–2% of young adults are present with monosymptomatic nocturnal enuresis. Boys tend to be affected slightly more frequently than girls are. Affected children are usually physically and emotionally normal. Without treatment, about 15% of bedwetting children become dry each year. Hence, about 1% of adults remain enuretic.

Diagnostic Methods

Monosymptomatic enuresis nocturna is unlikely related to other diseases. Nevertheless, a thorough questionnaire should aim at making sure that the patient is not minimising daytime symptoms and a complete physical examination needs to be undertaken to assess physical normality. In addition, a calendar should be obtained to keep tract of voiding habits and bowel movements. Important pathologies such as renal failure or DM must be ruled out if there is evidence of increased urine output. Finally, urine analysis and culture help to exclude urinary tract infections. Radiological studies are not necessary if the medical history is typical and the physical examination is normal.

Medical Management

Although it affects many young people, nighttime incontinence at the normal age of toilet training may cause great distress and be embarrassing. Informing and reassuring the patient and her/his parents that many other children are present with the same symptom and that it is no one's fault is of the outmost importance. Hence, no punishment should take place in any way, shape, or form. On the contrary, they will need a lot of understanding and patience. Treatment should only be considered in patients older than five years and if and only if they wish to do something about it, since monosymptomatic nocturnal enuresis is not dangerous if left untreated and because it usually disappears naturally over time.

Pharmacological, psychological/behavioural, and a diversity of less conventional interventions (psychotherapy, acupuncture, or homeopathy) are used in the management of bedwetters. Only the most commonly used interventions will be addressed in this chapter. In general, therapeutic options aim at modifying the possible factors that are believed to play a role in the pathophysiology of nighttime incontinence. However, none of the techniques or pharmaceutical alternatives mentioned below insures success. In fact, most proposed options offer a 70% success rate at best.

Pharmacological agents useful in the treatment include desmopressin acetate or DDAVP and imipramine, a tricyclic antidepressor. Desmopressin acetate is a synthetic analogue of the natural pituitary hormone 8-arginine vasopressin, an ADH affecting renal water conservation. In theory, it mimics the native compound causing the kidneys to produce less urine at night, roughly the same as a non-bedwetting child. In turn, bedwetting is less likely to occur. Good response is therefore more likely to be observed in patients with nocturnal polyuria and low nocturnal urine osmolality. DDAVP has been approved for children but it is important to use it as prescribed and to limit beverages before bedtime in order to maximise the effectiveness of the medication and prevent complications, i.e. to avoid the possible risk of water intoxication.

Although initially intended for short-term use or on special occasions, using it nightly for longer periods may be appropriate for some children. Currently, only oral administration is recommended. It is given one hour prior to bedtime with its effects lasting for upto twelve hours. Desmopressin has been shown to reduce effectively the number of wet nights suffered by bedwetting children but this effect is not sustained after treatment stops. However, since spontaneous resolution is expected at some point, it has been suggested that treatment should be withdrawn for at least one week every three months, pending reassessment.

More recently, combination therapy with desmopressin plus oxybutynin for the treatment of paediatric nocturnal enuresis has been suggested but published results show that the success of that pharmaceutical combination is greatest when enuresis is combined with daytime incontinence.

Imipramine, a tricyclic antidepressant, has a proven efficiency in enuretic patients, but due to its known possible side effects, it is often reserved for therapy-resistant cases. Tricyclics act on the central nervous system by blocking the synaptic alpha-receptors' re-uptake of noradrenaline and serotonin into the neurones and they have anticholinergic and/or anti-spasmodic effects. More interestingly, they also have local anaesthetic properties and affect the sleep centre. If used, it is very important to give imipramine to a child as prescribed and to keep it out of the reach between doses, as too much can lead to a fatal overdose.

Although tricyclics and desmopressin are effective in reducing the number of wet nights, most children relapse after discontinuation of active treatment.

Common non-pharmaceutical ways of tackling bedwetting include limiting nighttime fluid consumption, voiding before going to bed, and developing routines for waking up. Also, parents of bedwetters often bring into play a reward system but withholding a recompense for wet nights can look like a punishment and be a hindrance to a child's self-esteem. In fact, some studies suggested that penalties for wet beds appeared to be counter-productive. Such approaches are therefore not encouraged. Another way to induce behaviour modification is to suggest the use of a moisture alarm. Of the various treatment options, enuresis alarm has been widely advocated as being effective for treating nocturnal enuresis, but its use can be demanding since this approach requires a substantial degree of effort and motivation on the part of the child as well as the parents. In fact, if one or both parents are already bothered by a child's nighttime incontinence, alarms have been shown to intensify the annoyance. Reported success rates vary widely and are difficult to assess since the quality of many trials is poor. According to a recent review, about two-thirds of children became dry during alarm use compared to patients without treatment, but it can take weeks or even months to observe results. In the meantime, the child will usually continue to wet the bed. Moreover, relapse rates are high since using an alarm system on its own to condition children to wake before they wet the bed appears effective for only half of them after treatment stops.

Combining various behavioural interventions with pharmacotherapy is more effective than each component alone. Pharmacotherapy can insure relief of enuresis beforehand, while behavioural therapy may lead to greater long-term results. The positive effect of attaining nighttime dryness with pharmacotherapy can persuade the child to continue behavioural therapy.

Prognosis

Although it is not a life-threatening condition, monosymptomatic nocturnal enuresis is a socially disturbing and stressful state that affects the quality of life of the patients and their families. Luckily, the prognosis is good for most since the spontaneous resolution rate approximates 15% per year, i.e. nighttime incontinence persists in adulthood for only 1% of young bedwetters.

In the meantime, pharmacotherapy and behavioural therapy alone or in combination may help with the symptoms and offer, perhaps, a remedy.

CONCLUSION

Having a good understanding of the anatomy and the physiology of the lower urinary tract and disease mechanisms is critical. A detailed medical history, a good physical examination, and requesting appropriate diagnostic modalities are necessary to insure suitable strategies for attaining continence.

COMMENT FROM THE EDITORS

The child who wets is commonplace in the practice of a paediatric urologist. This topic is often daunting to the beginner. This chapter presents the perfect introduction to the topic. Although most cases of wetting are rather easily treated and do not present a major threat to the child's physical health, one must be alert to detect those children with similar presentation who are at risk to develop serious complications, including renal insufficiency.

FURTHER READING

Afshar K, Mirbagheri A, Scott H, MacNeily AE. Development of a symptom score for dysfunctional elimination syndrome. *J Urol* 2009; **182**(4 Suppl): 1939–1943.

Bernard-Bonnin A-C, Franc-Guimond J, Clermont MJ. Dictionnaire de thérapeutique pédiatrique Weber, 2e édition, Énurésie, 2007; **90**:511–514.

Bloom DA, *et al.* Toilet habits and continence in children: an opportunity sampling in search of normal parameters. *J Urol* 1993; **149**:1087–1090.

Curran MJ, *et al.* The overactive bladder in childhood: long-term results with conservative management. *J Urol* 2000; **163**:574–547.

Glazener CM, Evans JH, Peto RE. Alarm interventions for nocturnal enuresis in children. *Cochrane Database Syst Rev* 2005; (2):CD002911 (Review).

Glazener CM, Evans JH. Desmopressin for nocturnal enuresis in children. *Cochrane Database Syst Rev* 2002; (3):CD002112 (Review).

Hinman F Jr. Nonneurogenic neurogenic bladder (the Hinman's syndrome) — 15 years later. *J Urol* 1986; **136**(4):769–777.

Holmdahl G, *et al.* Does treatment with clean intermittent catheterization in boys with posterior urethral valves affect bladder and renal function? *J Urol* 2003; **170**(4 Pt 2):1681–1685.

Houle AM, *et al.* What volume can a child normally store in the bladder at a safe pressure? *J Urol* 1993; **149**(3):561–564.

Joinson C, Heron J, von Gontard A. Psychological problems in children with daytime wetting. *Pediatrics* 2006; **118**(5):1985–1993.

Loening-Baucke V. Urinary incontinence and urinary tract infection and their resolution with treatment of chronic constipation of childhood. *Pediatrics* 1997; **100**:228–232.

Loeys B, *et al.* Does monosymptomatic enuresis exist? A molecular genetic exploration of 32 families with enuresis/incontinence. *BJU Int* 2002; **90**(1):76–83

Nijman RJ. Role of antimuscarinics in the treatment of nonneurogenic daytime urinary incontinence in children. *Urology* 2004; **63**:45–50.

Nevéus T, *et al.* The standardization of terminology of lower urinary tract function in children and adolescents: report from the Standardisation Committee of the International Children's Continence Society. *J Urol* 2006; **176**(1):314–324.

Oakley GP Jr. The scientific basis for eliminating folic acid-preventable spina bifida: a modern miracle from epidemiology. *Ann Epidemiol* 2009; **19**(4):226–230 (Review).

Pohl HG, *et al.* The outcome of voiding dysfunction managed with clean intermittent catheterization in neurologically and anatomically normal children. *BJU Int* 2002; **89**:923–937.

Porena M, *et al.* Biofeedback successfully cures detrusor-sphincter dyssynergia in pediatric patients. *J Urol* 2000; **163**:1927–1931.

Roy Choudhury S, *et al.* Spectrum of ectopic ureters in children. *Pediatr Surg Int* 2008; **24**(7):819–823.

Spindel MR, *et al.* The changing neurourologic lesion in myelodysplasia. *JAMA* 1987; **258**(12):1630–1633.

von Gontard A, *et al.* The genetics of enuresis: a review. *J Urol* 2001; **166**(6): 2438–2443.

Chapter 6

Urinary Retention

Ricardo González

Incomplete bladder emptying or inability to empty the bladder (urinary retention) may be acute or chronic and it is a frequently present complaint in pediatric urology and it may indicate a serious organic or functional disorder. Bladder emptying after normal voiding is usually complete with no more than 10% of the voided volume remaining in the bladder. In this chapter, the main causes of acute and chronic retentions are presented. In most instances, the specific disease processes and treatments are discussed in other chapters.

DEFINITIONS

Acute retention is the inability to void occurring in a patient who was until then voiding normally. Chronic retention is the chronic inability to empty the bladder completely. The patient may simple void incompletely in an apparently normal fashion or simply dribble urine constantly (overflow incontinence).

PRESENTATION

Acute retention in a patient with normal sensation presents with suprapubic pain, extreme urgency to void, and lower abdominal distention. In children with impaired sensation, the only manifestation may be the lack of urination and the presence of a lower abdominal mass.

Chronic urinary retention may present with overflow incontinence, urinary tract infections, or lower abdominal pain.

DIAGNOSIS

The diagnosis of acute retention is usually obvious. Anamnesis, physical examination, and abdominal ultrasound will confirm the presence of a full bladder in the absence of voiding. If an ultrasound is performed, the kidneys should be inspected as well as ureteral and upper tract dilatation may be present.

Chronic retention may be more subtle. A urinary flow examination followed by a pelvic ultrasound to measure residual urine volume should be done in all patients with lower urinary tract symptoms. If the flow pattern or values are abnormal (see Chapter 5) or if the residual urine volume exceeds 10% of the voided volume, the studies should be repeated to rule out the possibility of artifact.

CLASSIFICATION AND ETIOLOGIES

Obstructive

Urethral obstruction can cause acute or chronic urinary retention. In *urethral stricture*, the urinary flow pattern is flat, voiding time is prolonged, and the maximum flow rate is significantly reduced. The bladder may empty completely for a long time until the detrusor decompensates.

Posterior urethral valves are usually detected prenatally or in the neonatal period (see Chapter 16); however, occasionally children may present with episodes of acute urinary retention, precipitated by urinary tract infection.

The other causes of urethral obstruction are partly discussed in Chapter 16. Rarely, an ectopic ureterocele will present with acute urinary retention. Bladder calculi obstructing the bladder neck and those impacted in the urethra may also be present in this manner.

Particularly serious is the acute urinary retention that causes by an obstructing tumor of the prostate, usually a rhabdomyosarcoma (see Chapter 20). A rectal examination is important in all boys presenting with acute retention.

Diagnostic tests for obstruction include retrograde urethrography, micturion cystourethrogram, and endoscopy.

Neuropathic

The neurological mechanisms of urinary retention, acute or chronic, include paralysis of the detrusor or incoordinated contraction of the pelvic floor. These conditions are discussed in Chapters 5 and 21. Occult neurologic processes, such as a tethered cord, demyelinizing diseases, and tumors of the spinal cord, should be ruled out by MRI when the other causes of urinary retention have been excluded.

Myopathic

Detrusor hypo- or acontractility can occur in patients with an intact central and peripheral nervous system. Primary or secondary failure of the detrusor can be seen in the later stages of patients with chronic bladder outlet obstruction (see Chapter 16) and in the Prune Belly Syndrome (Chapter 24). There is no pharmacological treatment for this condition. Intermittent catheterization is needed.

Postoperative

Urinary retention can be seen after any operation under general, epidural, or caudal anesthesias. Since sensation may be altered in the early postoperative period, the surgeon must be alert to this potential complication to avoid bladder overdistention that may lead to temporary myogenic failure.

Associated with Constipation

Children with chronic constipation and chronically dilated rectal ampoules can develop acute or chronic urinary retention in the absence of neurological abnormalities (see Chapter 5).

Idiopathic and Psychogenic

Young women can develop acute urinary retention in the absence of any other abnormalities. In a neurologically normal female with a normal ultrasound of the pelvis, once constipation and sexual abuse have been ruled out, one is often left with the diagnosis of idiopathic urinary retention. This condition may require periods of catheterization but is usually self-limiting and can be recurrent. Some debate exists in the literature as to whether this is a psychogenic process or it represents some form of voiding dysfunction.

Drug Induced

Anticholinergic agents, alpha adrenergic agents, opiates, and many psychotropic medications cause urinary retention as a side effect. A complete anamnesis will help disclose the cause. Some of these agents contribute to postoperative urinary retention.

Chapter 7

Acute Scrotal Pain

Ricardo González and Barbara M. Ludwikowski

Acute scrotal pain and swelling are common symptoms that often prompt an emergency consultation. The differential diagnoses include:

1. torsion of the spermatic cord,
2. torsion of a testicular appendage,
3. scrotal involvement in Schönlein–Henoch purpura and idiopathic scrotal edema,
4. acute epididymitis,
5. incarcerated hernia,
6. scrotal trauma, and
7. varicocele.

In a series of 100 consecutive patients under 15 years of age who presented with "acute scrotum", Melekos *et al.* (1988) reported that 42% had torsion of the spermatic cord and 32% had torsion of the testicular appendage. Table 7-1 summarises the main diagnostic features of the most common causes of acute scrotal pain. The remaining patients had a variety of diagnosis including idiopathic scrotal edema, acute epididymitis, hernia, or varicocele.

TORSION OF THE SPERMATIC CORD

Definition

Torsion of the spermatic cord is a condition that requires prompt diagnosis and management since it often leads to ischemic testicular necrosis. The

Table 7-1. Differential diagnosis.

Condition	Pre- or post-pubertal	Emesis or nausea	Cremasteric reflex	Urinalysis	Sexual activity	Ultrasound
Torsion of spermatic cord	Usually post pubertal	Yes	No	Normal	Maybe	No flow or abnormal waveform
Torsion of hydatid of Morgagni (testicular appendage)	Usually pre pubertal	No	Yes	Normal	Usually no	Normal arterial flow; enlarged epididymis, may be hyperemic; appendage may be visible; hydrocele may be present
Epididymitis	Usually post pubertal	No/yes	Yes	Pyuria	Yes	—

torsion of the spermatic cord can be intra- or extravaginal. Intravaginal testicular torsion (IVT) can only occur when the testes hang inside the tunica vaginalis like the clapper of a bell (bell-clapper deformity) (Figure 7-1). This variation of the reflection of the tunica vaginalis is present in 12% of the males, but only 1 in 4000 males less than 25 years of age will develop torsion. It is important to recognize that the malformation is usually bilateral and therefore both sides may be at risk. The immediate causes of torsion are not known. IVT can occur at any age but it is most common in young postpubertal adolescents. Extravaginal torsion occurs pre- or post-natally in the newborn period; it presents with a scrotal mass and is discussed in Part 1 of Chapter 8.

For IVT, the presentation is with acute onset of pain, sometimes during the night. Nausea and vomiting are present in 40% of the cases. The pain is usually scrotal, but can be felt also in the inguinal area, thigh, or abdomen. The pain is intense but subsides with time. On physical examination, the patient is in acute distress. The involved hemi-scrotum is swollen. The testis

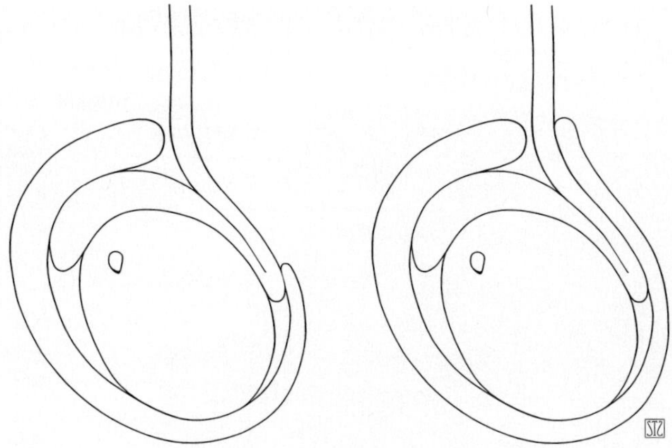

Figure 7-1. Bell clapper deformity of the tunica vaginalis.

and epididymis may ride high in the scrotum. There may be skin erythema and edema. On palpation, there is exquisite tenderness in the scrotum and often in the groin. The testes cannot be differentiated from the epididymis. The cremasteric reflex (elevation of the testes in response to scratching the inner aspect of the ipsilateral thigh) is typically absent.

The torsion of the spermatic cord can resolve spontaneously and recur later. Intermittent testicular torsion should be suspected in patients with the symptoms of recurrent and severe scrotal pain and normal examination between episodes of pain is recommended.

Diagnosis

In typical cases, the diagnosis can be established by the history and physical examination and prompt surgical therapy can be instituted. The confirmation of the diagnosis can be obtained by color Doppler ultrasound. At the onset, the testes may be enlarged; with time, the parenchymal architecture suffers changes and becomes heterogeneous. The arterial blood flow is typically absent but in 180° torsion, the blood flow may be present. In these cases, it is important to measure the amplitude of the pulse wave and compare it to the normal side (Figure 7-2). The performance of an ultrasound should not delay surgical exploration.

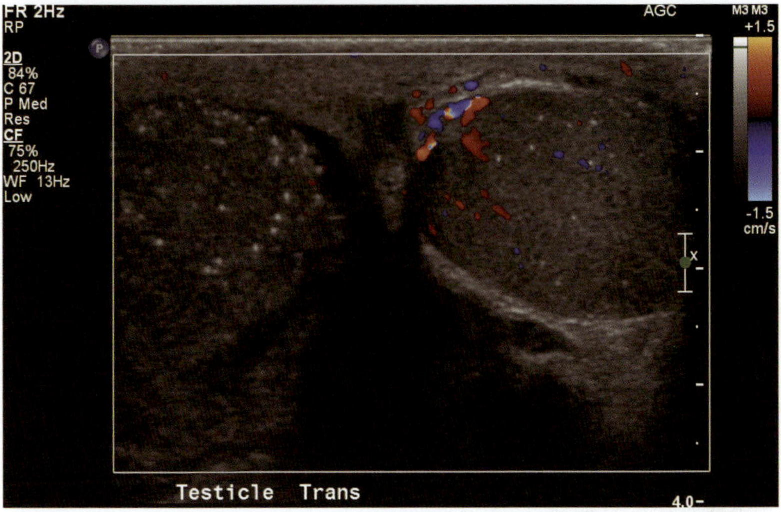

(A)

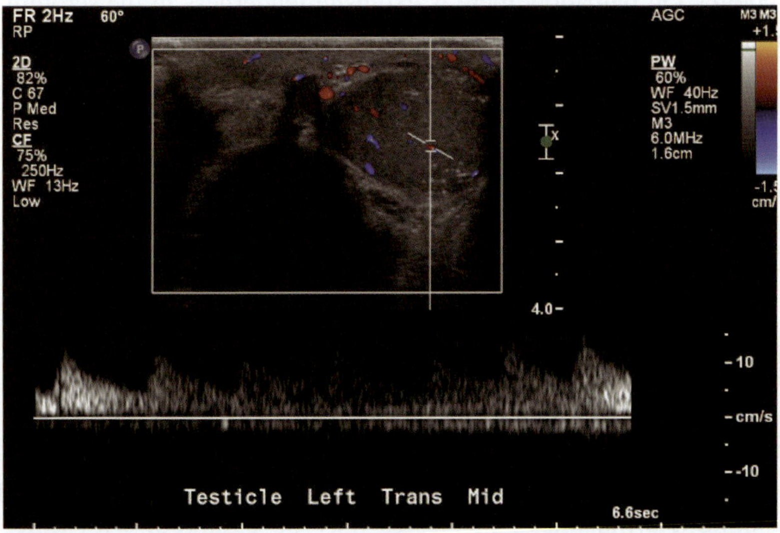

(B)

Figure 7-2. (A)–(C) Ultrasonogram of the scrotum with color Doppler showing normal blood flow in the left testis and absent in the right.

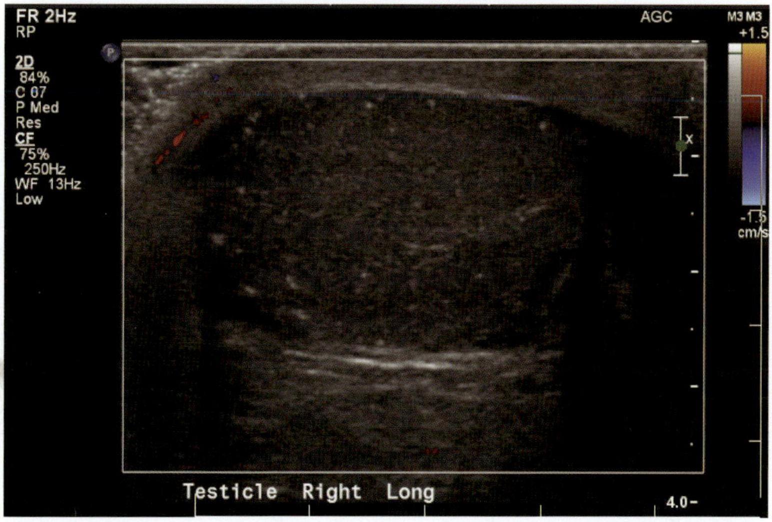

(C)

Figure 7–2. (*Continued*)

Treatment

Although manual detorsion can be attempted in order to shorten the ischemia time, it should be done only by experienced surgeons and only while operating room is prepared. We discourage it as a routine measure. Surgical exploration is typically done through the scrotum (Figure 7-3). The involved side is explored, the cord is untwisted, and the testes wrapped with compresses soaked in warm saline solution. The contralateral side is explored and the testes fixed in place to prevent future torsion. Attention is redirected to the side of the torsion. If the testis has recovered, its normal color it can be fixated to the scrotal wall and the wounds are closed. In cases of doubtful recovery of blood flow, a Doppler probe can be used to determine if there is arterial flow at the mediastinum testis. Alternatively, a small incision can be made in the tunica albuginea to see if it bleeds. Obviously, necrotic testes should be removed. The predictors of no-recovery are history longer than 10 hours, no flow on color Doppler and no bleeding when a small incision is made in the tunica albuginea after detorsion.

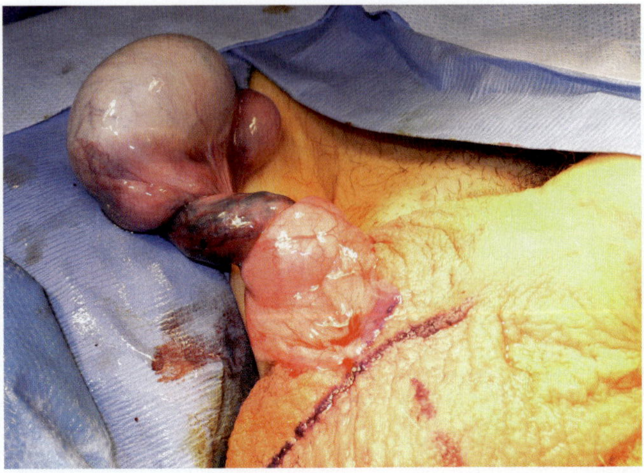

Figure 7-3. Intraoperative finding in right testicular torsion.

Some surgeons perform the exploration through a midline scrotal incision and attach the testes to the scrotum by placing three non-absorbable sutures between the tunica albuginea and the scrotal wall. We prefer to perform separate transverse incision and to place the testes in epidartal pouches. This method of fixation avoids placing sutures in the testes, which may be detrimental to function.

Outcomes and Prognosis

The reported salvage rate with conventional management of IVT is around 50%. The factors that contribute to this rather low salvage rate include: Delay in seeking medical treatment. Many adolescents suffer pain and are too embarrassed to tell their parents. Information about testicular torsion should be included in the sex education curriculum in schools. In general, almost no testis can be salvaged when the twist is 360° and the duration of symptoms is more than 10 hours. Delayed or missed diagnosis in patients that seek consultation in a timely fashion. Torsion can be missed in patients presenting with abdominal pain in which the genitals are not examined. A misdiagnosis is more likely in prepubertal boys in whom the torsion of an appendage is much more likely than IVT. Color Doppler scrotal ultrasound is particularly useful in this group of patients. When the diagnosis is in doubt, a surgical exploration is the safest course of action. However, with careful examination and color Doppler scrotal ultrasound done competently, the number of negative explorations and missed torsions can be kept to a minimum. In situations where emergency ultrasonography is not available, the number of unnecessary explorations and missed torsions are higher.

TORSION OF A TESTICULAR APPENDAGE

Definition

Torsion of a testicular appendage is the most common cause of acute scrotal pain before puberty. There are five vestigial structures described adjacent to the testes and epididymis. From the clinical point of view the most important is the appendix testes of hydatid of Morgagni. Acute pain and inflammation caused by an enlarged hydatid are thought to be an ischemic phenomenon caused by the torsion of the structure. However, histologically there is evidence of acute inflammation in the absence of infectious microorganisms. The typical age of presentation is in the late childhood before the onset of puberty. The torsion of the hydatid may present with symptoms similar to those of the torsion of the spermatic cord, but usually the pain is less severe and children typically present to the emergency department longer after the onset of pain.

On examination, the involved hemiscrotum may be red and tender because of the underlying inflammatory process. The cremasteric reflex is usually present. If the palpation of the scrotal contents is possible, the tenderness can be localized to the upper part of the testis or caput epididymis. A tender and supra-testicular mass may be palpable in about one-third of the cases. The "blue dot" sign is seen in about 20% of the children. This is a dark spot seen by trans-illumination in the upper part of the scrotum. Care must be taken not to confuse these findings with the mass created by the twist of the cord in cases of IVT. In some children, the tenderness is so intense or the inflammatory process so marked that detailed palpation is not possible.

Diagnosis

The urinalysis is normal. Properly interpreted, color Doppler ultrasound is useful to help differentiate this condition from the testicular torsion. Typically, there is significant hyperemia of the para-testicular structures including the epididymis. The testicular blood flow is normal and symmetrical. A supra-testicular mass without blood flow may be identified representing the twisted hydatid (Figure 7-4A–7-4C). The presence of hyperemia and sometimes the enlargement of the epididymis is frequently interpreted by the radiologist as epididymitis. This misinterpretation may lead to unnecessary antibiotic therapy or further investigations. It should be remembered that an acute epididymitis in the prepubertal age in the presence of a normal urinalysis or known genitourinary malformations or diseases is extremely rare.

Treatment

The treatment is symptomatic with decreased physical activity and anti-inflammatory agents. Rarely, when the diagnosis is in doubt, the surgical exploration and removal of the offending appendage is necessary. The other side does not need to be explored. With conservative management the discomfort subsides after four or five days but may recur if the child becomes very active.

Outcome and Prognosis

The recurrence of the symptoms or asynchronous involvement of the other side is occasionally seen. The prognosis is otherwise excellent.

SCROTAL INVOLVEMENT IN SCHÖNLEIN–HENOCH PURPURA AND IDIOPATHIC SCROTAL EDEMA

Schönlein–Henoch purpura is a systemic vasculitis, which is associated with scrotal swelling and discoloration in 13–20% of the cases. For the urological consultant, it is important to recognize the systemic nature of

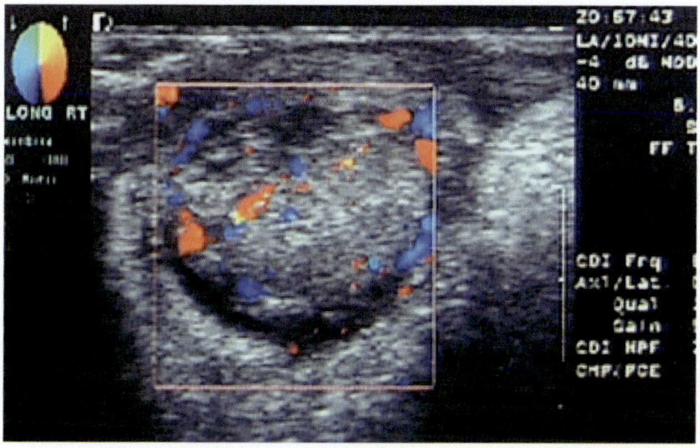

(A)

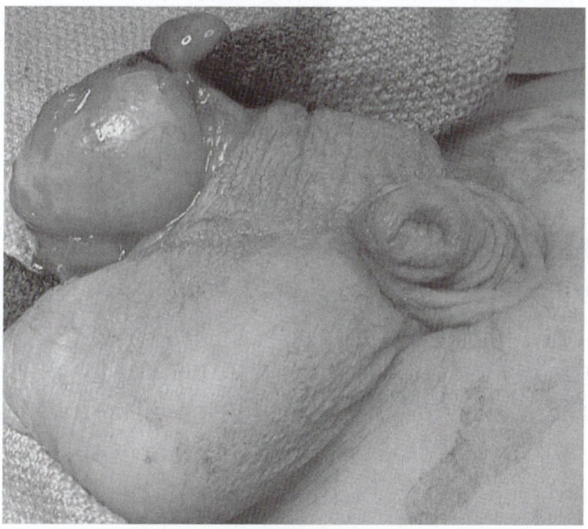

(B)

Figure 7-4. **(A)–(B)** Torsion of right hydatid of Morgagni. **(A)** Normal blood flow to the testis, and **(B)** intraoperative finding in a child explored because of equivocal clinical findings.

the disease to avoid unnecessary surgical exploration for suspected testicular torsion.

Idiopathic scrotal edema is a rare condition presenting in early puberty with pain, edema, and erythema in one hemiscrotum without the history of trauma. In some cases, the regional lymph nodes are enlarged. Scrotal ultrasound shows thickening of the scrotal skin, hyperemia, and a normal underlying testes.

ACUTE EPIDIDYMITIS

Definition

Epididymitis is an inflammatory process of the testes that may also occasionally involve the testis (orchioepididymitis). It is most commonly seen in sexually active males and the most common etiology is an ascending infection caused by *Chlamydia trachomatis* or *Neisseria gonorrhoeae*. Mycobacterial infections are seen in areas with high prevalence of tuberculosis. In prepubertal children, using strict criteria of diagnosis, acute epididymitis is rare and is almost always associated with Gram-negative bacteria and an underlying genitourinary abnormality.

Diagnosis

In prepubertal and non-sexually active males presenting with acute scrotal pain, the differential diagnosis should include testicular torsion and the torsion of the hydatid of Morgagni. The presence of an enlarged or hyperemic epididymis on color Doppler ultrasonography is not sufficient to establish the diagnosis. Additional diagnostic criteria should include two or more of the following: fiber >38.5°C, leukocytosis, pyuria, or positive urine culture (Al-Taheini *et al.*, 2008). If such criteria are met, the treatment with antibiotics is indicated and the subsequent evaluation of the urinary tract should be undertaken.

In sexually active males, the diagnosis is usually made by physical examination confirmed by color Doppler ultrasonography. Swabs of the urethra should be obtained and the appropriate workup and treatment protocol for sexually transmitted diseases are applied.

Treatment

In prepubertal males, wide spectrum antibiotics should be administered till cultures and sensitivities are reported. Thereafter, the treatment with the appropriate antibiotics should be administered for at least two weeks. Surgery is exceptionally needed in cases of non-response to antibiotics or abscess formation.

Postpubertal males referred to a clinic for sexually transmitted diseases are recommended to institute the currently recommended treatment and to track down and treat sexual contacts.

Outcome and Prognosis

Bilateral epididymitis can lead to infertility. Untreated epididymitis can progress to orchioepididymitis and abscess formation requiring surgical drainage and sometimes orchiectomy.

INCARCERATED HERNIA

Definition

Indirect inguinal hernias have a prevalence of 10–20 per 1000 live births or about one in 75 boys. Incarceration occurs when abdominal contents (usually ileum) get trapped in the hernia sac and do not reduce spontaneously. The risk of incarceration is greater in the first two years of life and it may be as high as 30% in the first two months of life. Nevertheless, incarceration can take place at any age.

Diagnosis

Infants usually present with pain and vomiting and a palpable and non-reducible inguinal or scrotal mass is present. In older children, scrotal, inguinal, or abdominal pain, usually accompanied with nausea and vomiting, is the usual presentation. Examination reveals a tender and non-reducible mass in the groin, commonly extending to the scrotum. If the testis is not palpable, an ultrasound may be useful to establish its location before the repair.

Treatment

Manual reduction under analgesia or sedation should be attempted first. If successful, the child is admitted for observation and the hernia is repaired within two weeks of the occurrence. If reduction is not possible, surgical exploration should be undertaken. The risks of the delayed treatment of a non-reducible hernia are compromised blood supply to the intestinal wall or the testis.

At the time of exploration, the compromised bowel is covered with warm and wet compresses until its color improves. The need for bowel resection is rare. Testis with compromised blood supply should be left in the scrotum and the parents counseled about possible atrophy.

Outcome and Prognosis

Testicular atrophy is a potential complication of incarceration. The recurrence rate after repair is less than 1%.

SCROTAL TRAUMA

Traumatic lesions of the scrotal contents and their management are discussed in section "scrotal trauma" of Chapter 12. Sometimes, patients with other conditions, such as IVT or the torsion of the hydatid, may give a history of trauma. The examination and evaluation usually make the differential diagnosis and appropriate management possible.

VARICOCELE

Varicocele is discussed in Part 1 of Chapter 8. Primary varicocele is common in early adolescence but symptoms are rare. Spontaneous or traumatic rupture of a known or previously undiagnosed varicocele presents as a painful scrotal mass. Examination may detect a varicocele or the swelling may be such that a scrotal color Doppler ultrasound is necessary to establish the diagnosis. The treatment should be symptomatic and spontaneous resolution of the hematoma is the rule. The surgical management of the varicocele, if indicated, should wait till the resolution of the acute episode.

FURTHER READING

Al-Taheini KM, Pike J, Leonard M. Acute epididymitis in children: the role of radiologic studies. *Urology* 2008; **71**:826–829.

Melekos M, Asbach H, Markou S. Etiology of acute scrotum with regard to age distribution. *J Urol* 1988; **139**:1023–1025.

Caesar RE, Kaplan GW. Incidence of the bell-clapper deformity in an autopsy series. *Urology* 1994; **44**(1):114–116.

Cimador M, DiPace MR, Castagnetti M, DeGrazia E. Predictors of testicular viability in testicular torsion. *J Pediatr Urol* 2007; **3**(5):387–389.

Cuckow PM, Frank JD. Torsion of the testis. *BJU Int* 2000; **86**:349–353.

Hayn MH, *et al.* Intermittent torsion of the spermatic cord portends an increased risk of acute testicular infarction. *J Urol* 2008; **180**(4 Suppl):1729–1732.

Pepe P, *et al.* Does color Doppler sonography improve the clinical assessment of patients with acute scrotum? *Eur J Radiol* 2006; **60**(1):120–124.

Rabinowitz R. The importance of the cremasteric reflex in acute scrotal swelling in children. *J Urol* 1984; **132**(1):89–90.

Rakha E, Puls F, Saidul I, Furness P. Torsion of the testicular appendix: importance of associated acute inflammation. *J Clin Pathol* 2006; **59**:831–834.

Rushton HG. Editorial comment. *J Urol* 2004; **171**:391–394.

Chapter 8

Painless Scrotal Swelling

Ricardo González and Barbara M. Ludwikowski

In this chapter, we shall discuss the common conditions that present with painless scrotal swelling from newborn period to adolescence that include:

- hydrocele and inguinal hernia,
- varicocele,
- tumors,
- neonatal torsion, and
- other conditions.

HYDROCELE AND HERNIA

Definition

Inguinal hernias are among the most common malformations in boys (one in 75 live births) and are more prevalent in preterm born babies in whom the risk of incarceration is greater. A hydrocele is the presence of fluid in the virtual space of the tunica vaginalis. When there is a patent processus vaginalis, the origin of the fluid is peritoneal. In postpubertal males with a closed processus, it is a posttraumatic or postinflammatory exudate. A childhood inguinal hernia is also a manifestation of a patent processus vaginalis with abdominal contents (omentum or intestine, or ovary) present in the scrotum. Thus, the vast majority of childhood hernias are indirect. Direct and femoral hernias are less common and do not present with painless scrotal swelling and they are beyond the scope of this chapter.

Classification

One can distinguish newborn and infantile, childhood, and adolescent types of hydroceles and hernias. This distinction is important because of the different pathogenesis, natural history, and therapy. Hernias are more frequent on the right side and about 10% are bilateral except in premature babies in whom the incidence of bilaterality is as high as 30%. Metachronous development of a contralateral hernia occurs in about 5% of the cases. Data from laparoscopy or routine contralateral exploration suggests that the incidence of a contralateral patent processus is about 30%, but it is clear that only a small percentage of those will develop a clinical hernia, making routine contralateral exploration unjustified. The risk of incarceration is about 10% and more common in the first few months of life. Incarcerated hernia is discussed in Chapter 7.

A funicular hydrocele (hydrocele of the cord) is one that does not involve the tunica vaginalis. A special type of hydrocele is the abdominoscrotal hydrocele in which the palpable mass extends in the lower abdomen. In these cases, the processus is usually not patent; however, they are usually tense masses and the testes cannot be palpated (Figure 8-1).

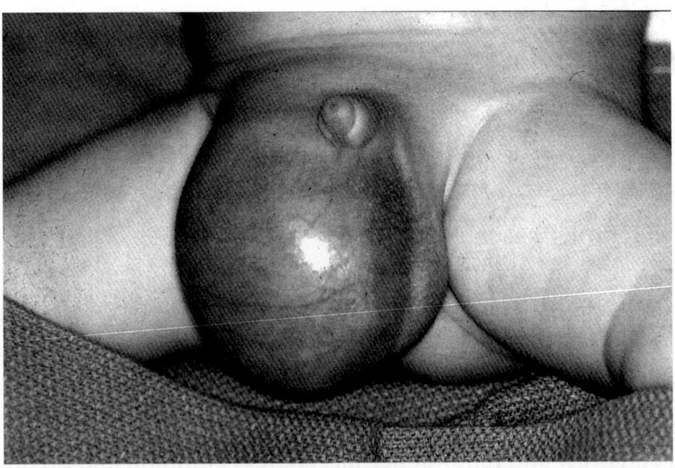

Figure 8-1. Right-sided abdomino-scrotal hydrocele.

Newborn and Childhood

Presentation

Painless scrotal swelling which may be constant or vary in degree with time, increasing or decreasing in size.

Diagnosis

On physical examination, there is obvious scrotal enlargement. Transillumination (i.e. the transmission of light across the mass) is positive when the content of the tunica vaginalis is fluid and negative if there is omentum or intestine. The swelling may be obvious only during crying or straining. When the content of the scrotum is fluid and the size of the mass is variable, we are dealing with a communicating hydrocele, which means the communication across the patent processus is rather large. If the size of the fluid-filled mass is constant, the communication across the processus is likely to be small. Only rather large diameter patent processus allows the passage of omentum or intestine into the scrotum.

Older children may present with a history of recurrent groin or scrotal swelling provided by the caretakers but the physical examination fails to confirm the diagnosis. The child must be routinely examined in the supine and upright positions. The palpation of a thickened spermatic cord (silk glove sign) is suggestive of a hernia. Some rely on ultrasound findings to confirm the diagnosis in questionable cases. Occasionally, the indication to treat a hernia has to be based exclusively on the anamnesis.

Imaging studies

A scrotal ultrasound is useful when the testes in the involved side cannot be palpated. Otherwise, the diagnosis is mostly based on the anamnesis and the physical examination. The usefulness of ultrasonography of the spermatic cord is highly operator dependent but may be useful in case in which a hernia is suspected but not confirmed on examination.

Management

Non-communicating hydroceles, which is those with rather constant size over time, tend to resolve spontaneously in the first year of life and only need surgery when they persist beyond two or three years of age. Communicating hydroceles should be repaired electively in the first year of life when anesthesia is safe. A new onset of a hydrocele beyond the neonatal period is usually a manifestation of a hernia. Obvious hernias containing intestine, omentum, or ovary require prompt surgical correction to prevent incarceration in premature babies; the hernia should be repair prior to discharge from the hospital. Both hydroceles and hernias are approached through a small inguinal incision, which allows high ligation of the processus vaginalis (hernia sac). The repair of the posterior wall of the inguinal canal is not necessary in infants. When a hydrocele with a small communication is present and the fluid does not drain spontaneously through the groin, the cephalad portion of the hydrocele sac is delivered through the inguinal incision by gentle pressure on the lower scrotum and it is the open widely taking care not to injure the cord or epididymis. Recently, laparoscopic repair has been preferred in some centers. Arguments in favor of a laparoscopic approach to the closure of the patent processus include the ability to visualize the other side, minimal risk of injury to the vas deferens, and the ability to detect other defects such as direct or femoral hernias; however, controlled studies comparing open with laparoscopic repairs are not available.

Exploration of the contralateral side, frequently performed in the past, is not justified. The risk of metachronous hernia is about 5% and mostly occurs within one year of the repair. Occasionally, a hydrocele persists despite the correct ligation of the processus; observation till resolution and rarely a transscrotal operation are needed.

Results and complications

Recurrence is reported in about 1% of the cases. Increased intra-abdominal pressure, ventriculo-peritoneal shunts, peritoneal dialysis, and abnormal abdominal wall anatomy (as in bladder exstrophy) predispose to recurrence. Injury to the vas deferens, testicular atrophy, and the malposition of the testes should be exceptional but the exact frequency of occurrence is not clear.

Adolescence

In this age group, the distinction between a hydrocele and a hernia is usually clear in the anamnesis and physical examination. All the diagnostic considerations regarding inguinal hernias in childhood apply for the adolescent. From the treatment viewpoint, a large and long-standing inguinal hernia in an adolescent or teenager may require not only high ligation of the sac but also a repair of the posterior wall of the inguinal canal using the Bassini or Mac Vay techniques.

Adolescent hydroceles often result from scrotal trauma or inflammation (epididymitis). The testis should be evaluated by ultrasonography prior to the repair to avoid missing a tumor or other underlying lesions. When the testis is normal, a scrotal approach using a plication or inversion of the parietal tunica vaginal is usually effective.

VARICOCELE

Definition

Varicocele is an abnormal dilatation of the tributaries of the internal spermatic vein in the scrotum (pampiniform plexus) with venous stasis and reverse flow with increased abdominal pressure. Varicocele is more common on the left side and is sometimes associated with testicular atrophy and male subfertility.

Classification

Primary or idiopathic varicocele is due to venous insufficiency (see below). Secondary varicocele is caused by the obstruction of the spermatic vein by a retroperitoneal mass or the thrombosis of the left renal vein or vena cava.

Pathogenesis

There are normally valves in the cephalad third of the spermatic veins that prevent retrograde blood flow. When the valves are absent or insufficient, retrograde blood flow occurs in the upright position or with increased intra-abdominal pressure. The reasons given to explain the greater prevalence of varicocele on the left side include the fact that the left spermatic vein enters the left renal vein at a right angle, whereas the right vein enters the vena cava at acute angle, allegedly preventing reflux. The "nutcracker phenomenon" is a more attractive theory. The left spermatic vein enters the left renal vein to the left of the aorta. The left renal vein then passes between the aorta and the superior mesenteric artery. When the angle between the two arteries is very acute; the left renal vein is partially compressed, causing reverse spermatic venous flow. This is particularly seen when there is little retroperitoneal fat, which may also explain why left varicoceles occur almost always in males with low body mass index (BMI). It is not clear why varicocele usually present around the onset of puberty.

When varicocele is associated with male subfertility, the sperm analysis usually reveals the so-called "stress pattern" with normal sperm concentration but decreased motility and increased abnormal forms. About 20% or more of males presenting with subfertility have a varicocele. On the other hand, 17% of males requesting vasectomy were found to have a clinical varicocele.

Also unclear is by what mechanism might varicocele affect spermatogenesis. We will mention here only the most plausible theories. (a) The venous stasis increases scrotal temperature, which is a factor well known to interfere with spermatogenesis. (b) The reflux of adrenal catecholamines from the left spermatic vein, which affects spermatogenesis. Since most varicoceles are left-sided and there are no vascular connections between the right and left spermatic venous systems, how a unilateral process might affect both testis is also unclear. The pathogenesis of secondary varicocele is self-explanatory.

Presentation

Varicoceles are usually found on routine physical examinations in early pubertal stages; rarely, they are discovered before the onset of puberty.

Occasionally, the patient himself discovers them or there is a complaint of dull scrotal pain or discomfort during physical exercise. The rare presentation with acute pain because of bleeding is discussed in Chapter 7. Three grades of varicocele are described: Grade I is a subclinical varicocele when reverse venous flow is detected on a Doppler ultrasound examination; Grade II is a varicocele palpable only during the Valsalva maneuvre; and Grade III is a varicocele that is both palpable and visible during examination in the upright position (Figure 8-2).

Diagnosis

The diagnosis of varicocele is established by physical examination. The examination must be conducted both in the upright and supine positions. In primary varicocele, the distended veins collapse when the patient is supine and relaxed. When the venous distension remains unchanged in the supine position, an abdominal ultrasound is necessary to rule out a

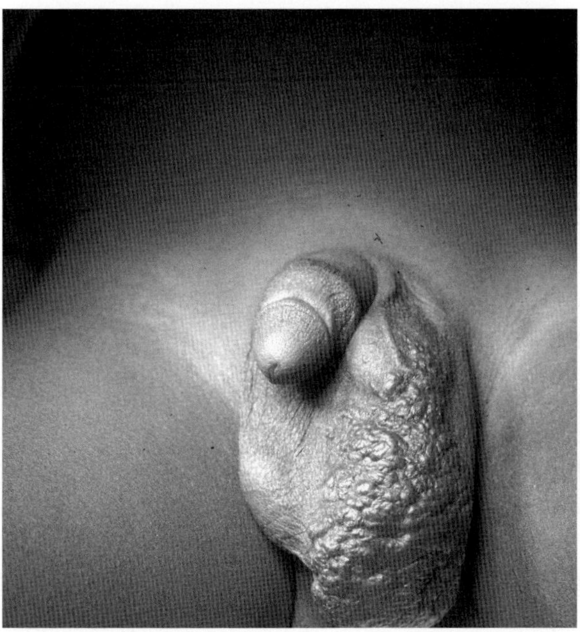

Figure 8-2. Grade 3 varicocele, left.

compressing mass of venous thrombosis. The stage of puberty and the size of the testes measured with the Prader orchidometer should be recorded.

Imaging Studies

Besides the above-mentioned cases in which an abdominal ultrasound is indicated, a scrotal ultrasound confirms the diagnosis and may also be helpful to determine testicular volume. In our experience, the physical examination volume tends to be greater than that recorded by ultrasound; however, what is important is to compare one side against the other. Absolute volume may also be important since some authors have reported that both sides may be smaller than expected for Tanner stage.

Sperm Analysis

Except in symptomatic cases, the treatment of adolescent varicocele aims at preserving fertility. The role of sperm counts is doubted by many. On the one hand, there are no standards for normal values for males who are younger than 18 years and on the other hand, some argue that the testicular lesion caused by varicocele is progressive; therefore, a normal sperm count at one point in time should not preclude treatment.

Management

The management of asymptomatic adolescent varicocele is controversial. There is general agreement that when the left testis is smaller than the right toward the end of pubertal development (Tanner stages IV and V), surgical treatment is indicated. There is no evidence that this approach improves or preserves future fertility.

The surgical treatment of varicocele consists mainly on occlusion of the internal spermatic vein to impede the retrograde reflux of blood, which can be done in a variety of ways that is open, laparoscopic or transvascular. There is no evidence favoring of one approach over another.

Open Procedures

Ligation of the spermatic vain can be approached inguinally or suprainguinally. Suprainguinal approaches have the advantage of not risking damage to the deferential artery, which provides the main blood supply to the testis in case of injury to the internal spermatic artery. Suprainguinal approaches may aim at the retroperitoneal ligation of the internal spermatic vein only (Ivanissevich) or deliberately ligate both artery and vein (Palomo). Recognition that the latter procedure carries a significant risk of hydrocele formation has led some authors to recommend sparing the lymphatic vessels that run along the spermatic vessels.

Some favor inguinal ligation (Bernardi) based on the assumption that it has a greater success rate. The inguinal approach is more cumbersome because at this level, one may encounter several tributaries of the main vein and it carries the risk of damaging other structures and the spermatic cord. The use of an operating microscope is recommended for this approach.

Laparoscopically, it is possible to ligate the vein (Ivanissevich), the vein and the artery together, and also to preserve the lymphatics.

Endovascular procedures consist of embolization of the internal spermatic vein via a transfemoral or transjugular access. Embolizing material and sclerosing substances have been used. This approach has not gained popularity in the pediatric population.

Results

In cases of left testicular atrophy, the Palomo procedure has been reported to cause enlargement of the left testes. Other procedures have also been reported to induce catch-up growth of the testes. Whether this enlargement is due to a beneficial effect of the ligation or interstitial edema caused by interfering with venous and lymphatic returns remains unclear. Unfortunately, there are no long-term studies addressing later fertility after varicocele surgery in adolescence.

TUMORS

Definition

Testicular and paratesticular neoplasias are found during routine physical examination or they present as a painless scrotal mass detected by the child or the parents (Figure 8-3). Scrotal ultrasound is diagnostic. This topic is discussed in detail in Chapter 20.

NEONATAL TESTICULAR TORSION

Definition

Perinatal torsion of the spermatic cord leads to ischemia and necrosis of the testis. It can occur prenatally, during labor, or postnatally. It is seen in 1 of 7500 newborn males. As opposed to torsion in childhood and adolescence, which is intravaginal and requires the presence of an abnormal reflection of the tunica vaginalis (see Chapter 7), the perinatal torsion is said to be extravaginal and is caused by the lax fixation of the parietal layer of the vaginalis to the scrotal wall (Figure 8-4).

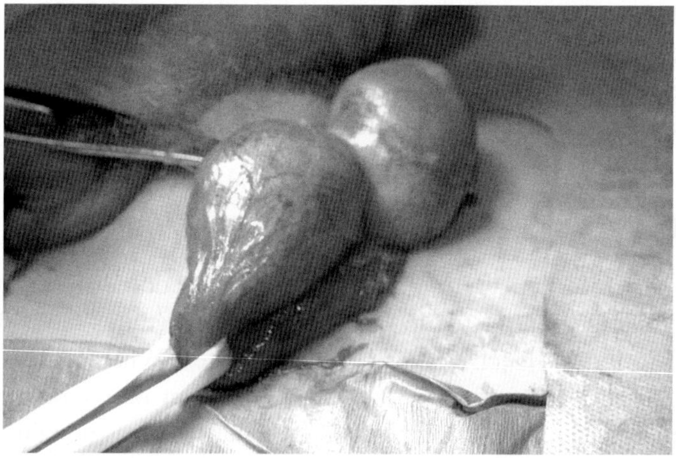

Figure 8-3. Dermoid tumor of the spermatic cord, presenting as a painless scrotal mass.

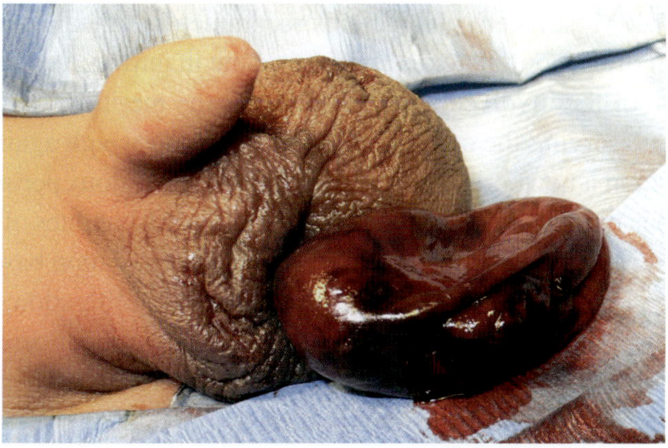

Figure 8-4. Neonatal extravaginal torsion of the spermatic cord presenting as an asymptomatic mass on newborn examination.

Presentation

Scrotal swelling in a newborn.

Differential Diagnosis

The causes of unilateral scrotal swelling in a newborn are — in decreasing order of frequency — hydrocele, inguinal hernia (see above), perinatal torsion, tumors, and in some cases, the swelling is a manifestation of an intra-abdominal process, which in the presence of a patent processus, extends in the scrotum (acute appendicitis and meconium peritonitis).

Diagnosis

Diagnosis is suspected on physical examination in which a hard scrotal mass is easily palpated. An ultrasound examination of the scrotum confirms the absence of a tumor and also serves to evaluate the contralateral side.

Treatment

Salvage of a testis affected by perinatal torsion is exceptional. When diagnosed several hours or days may have gone by, the treatment is, therefore, controversial. Most recent publications recommend immediate exploration and fixation of the contralateral testes as is done in intravaginal torsion. The salvage rate of the involved side is about 3%; the merits of this approach, directed at preserving the contralateral testis, need to weigh against the risk of anesthesia in a newborn. The exact risk of metachronous perinatal testicular torsion is not known and many think that it is rare but rates of up to 22% have been reported. Often, the advocates of early exploration base their recommendation on anecdotal cases that have resulted in litigation.

When a surgical exploration is conducted and the diagnosis of torsion is certain, the scrotal approach is preferred. When the diagnosis is in doubt, the inguinal approach should be used.

As in the case of intravaginal torsion (see Chapter 7) if ultrasonography is not available or not reliable in a given institution, the number of surgical exploration will be higher.

Left untreated the involved testis undergoes gradual atrophy. When a non-operative approach is chosen, it is not clear if at a later day fixation of the contralateral testis is beneficial.

OTHER CONDITIONS

Other causes of painless scrotal swelling are rare and they include, among others, the sebaceous cysts of the scrotum, hemagiomas, lipomas, neurofibromas, etc.

FURTHER READING

Ahmed SJ, Kaplan GW, DeCambre ME. Perinatal testicular torsion: preoperative radiological findings and the argument for urgent surgical exploration. *J Pediatr Surg* 2008; **43**(8):1563–1565.

Barroso U Jr, *et al.* Surgical treatment of varicocele in children with open and laparoscopic Palomo technique: a systematic review of the literature. *J Urol* 2009; **181**(6):2724–2728.

Brisson P, Patel H, Feins N. Cremasteric muscle hypertrophy accompanies inguinal hernias in children. *J Pediatr Surg* 1999; **34**(9):1320–1321.

Carmignani L, *et al.* Sclerotherapy of the pampiniform plexus with modified Marmar technique in children and adolescents. *Urol Int* 2009; **82**(2):187–190.

Diamond DA, *et al.* Varicocele surgery: a decade's experience at a children's hospital. *BJU Int* 2009; **104**(2):246–249.

Cozzi DA, *et al.* Infantile abdominoscrotal hydrocele: a not so benign condition. *J Urol* 2008; **180**(6):2611–2615.

Depasquale R, Landes C, Doyle G. Audit of ultrasound and decision to operate in groin pain of unknown aetiology with ultrasound technique explained. *Clin Radiol* 2009; **64**(6):608–614.

Ein SH, Njere I, Ein A. Six thousand three hundred sixty-one pediatric inguinal hernias: a 35-year review. *J Pediatr Surg* 2006; **41**(5):980–986.

Giseke S, *et al.* A true laparoscopic herniotomy in children: evaluation of long-term outcome. *J Laparoendosc Adv Surg Tech A* 2010; **20**(2):191–194.

Guerra LA, *et al.* Management of neonatal testicular torsion: which way to turn? *Can Urol Assoc J* 2008; **2**(4):376–379.

Kyriazis ID, *et al.* Extravaginal testicular torsion: a clinical entity with unspecified surgical anatomy. *Int Braz J Urol* 2008; **34**(5):617–623.

Kursh ED. What is the incidence of varicocele in a fertile population? *Fertil Steril* 1987; **48**(3):510–511.

Luo CC, Chao HC. Prevention of unnecessary contralateral exploration using the silk glove sign (SGS) in pediatric patients with unilateral inguinal hernia. *Eur J Pediatr* 2007; **166**(7):667–669.

Maddox MM, Smith DP. A long-term prospective analysis of pediatric unilateral inguinal hernias: should laparoscopy or anything else influence the management of the contralateral side? *J Pediatr Urol* 2008; **4**(2):141–145.

Tsao CW, *et al.* The relationship between varicoceles and obesity in a young adult population. *Int J Androl* 2009; **32**(4):385–390.

Uemura S, *et al.* Early repair of inguinal hernia in premature babies. *Pediatr Surg Int* 1999; **15**(1):36–39.

Wilson JM, *et al.* Hydrocele in the pediatric patient: inguinal or scrotal approach? *J Urol* 2008; **180**(4 Suppl):1724–1727.

Zampieri N, *et al.* Testicular catch-up growth after varicocelectomy: does surgical technique make a difference? *Urology* 2009; **73**(2):289–292.

Chapter 9

Male Genital Anomalies and Diseases

Ricardo González and Barbara M. Ludwikowski

The male external genitalia are one of the most frequent sites for congenital malformations from undescended testis seen in 2% of newborn males to hypospadias, which occurs in 1:300 newborn males. Circumcision is the most frequently performed surgical procedure and in certain cultures, it is often requested by the parents upon the birth of a male. Although most male genital anomalies seldom require treatment in the newborn period, they are a source of anxiety for the parents. Early consultation with a pediatric urologist serves to educate the parents and to outline a plan of treatment for the child, thus reducing parental anxiety. Scrotal swelling and scrotal pain are discussed in greater detail in Chapters 7 and 8. For ambiguous genitalia, see Chapter 11. Undescended testis is discussed in Chapter 18, hypospadias is discussed in Chapter 19, and epispadias is discussed in Chapter 23.

PENIS

- Phimosis and circumcision,
- Paraphimosis,
- Concealed penis,
- Meatal stenosis,
- Balanitis and balanoposthitis,
- Warts,
- Micropenis,

- Penile agenesis,
- Hypospadias,
- Epispadias,
- Penile curvature and torsion, and
- Priapism.

SCROTUM (EXCLUDING PAIN AND SWELLING)

- Empty scrotum,
- Bifid scrotum,
- Scrotal transposition, and
- Necrotizing fascitis.

Phimosis and Circumcision

The prepuce is the skin that covers the glans. It consists of an inner layer and an outer layer. The inner layer is devoid of hair follicles or sweat glands. At birth, the inner layer of the prepuce and the skin of the glans form one layer. During infancy and childhood, the layers become separated allowing the prepuce to be retracted exposing the glans during sexual intercourse. The prepuce serves as a protective sheath for the glans, whose skin is normally thin, lightly keratinized, and sensitive. The circumcised glans is covered by thickly keratinized skin analogous to the rest of the penis. In this section, we shall deal with the care of the uncircumcised penis, phimosis and its treatment, and the current indications for circumcision in the absence of phimosis, including neonatal circumcision.

Care of the Uncircumcised Penis

Retraction of the prepuce may be possible in infancy but typically it may take until puberty till the skin layers are completely separated. The forceful retraction of the prepuce or the disruption of the normal adhesions is to be avoided, as it leads to injury and scar formation and may lead to the development of secondary phimosis. As a boy becomes more aware of his body, he will most likely discover how to retract his own foreskin. But foreskin retraction should never be forced. Until the foreskin layers fully separate, one should not attempt to pull it back. Forcing the foreskin to retract before it is ready can cause severe pain, bleeding, and tears in the skin. The appearance of small lumps of white material representing desquamated cells that eventually work their way out of the preputial cavity is normal but often mistaken for infection. Washing under the prepuce is not necessary until it becomes spontaneously retractable. When the prepuce becomes retractable, it is important to instruct the boy to always bring it forward after retraction for hygiene, micturition, or sexual activity. Failure to do so may result in paraphimosis (see below).

Phimosis

Definition

Phimosis is the inability to retract the prepuce after puberty due to a narrow preputial opening. Although the diagnosis of phimosis is often made in childhood, in most cases, it is just an excuse to justify circumcision. True phimosis in infancy and childhood is rare, however, and can lead to retention of urine within the prepuce. Commonly misdiagnosed as phimosis is the inability to retract the prepuce seen in prepubertal children due to incomplete separation of the skin layers of the glans and inner prepuce. This is a normal phenomenon, which does not require treatment. The incidence of true phimosis in an English study was 0.4 cases per 100 boys per year or 0.6 boys affected before their 16th birthday. Secondary phimosis refers to a phimosis that develops after the prepuce has become completely retractable. Premature forced retraction of the prepuce is a common cause in areas where forced retraction of the prepuce is a common pediatric practice. Another cause of secondary phimosis is lichen sclerosus (LS) also known in its penile location as Balanitis xerotica obliterans or BXO. LS is a chronic inflammatory skin disease that is responsible for approximately half of all cases of acquired phimosis, the cause is unknown.

Diagnosis

Examination of the penis should be done gently to avoid hurting the child. Forceful retraction of the prepuce in childhood amounts to abuse. If the

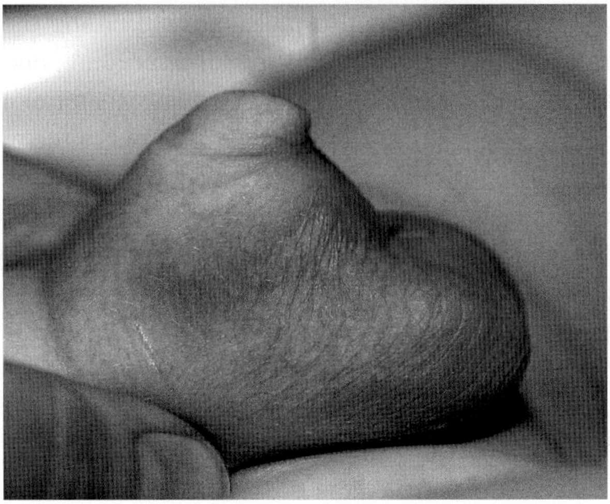

Figure 9-1. Marked phimosis in a newborn with obstruction to urine flow resulting in ballooning of the preputial space.

patient cannot easily retract the prepuce after the onset of puberty, the diagnosis of phimosis should be entertained and treatment considered. A variant of a narrow preputial opening leading to a megaprepuce is shown (Figure 9-1). In these cases, the penis is concealed by a very tight phimotic ring and voiding into the preputial cavity is obvious on examination. LS is characterized by patches of white and dry skin that can be seen in the prepuce and glans. Occasionally, the disease may extend into the urethra.

Treatment

The initial line of treatment of primary phimosis should be topical treatment with steroids and daily gentle preputial retraction. A variety of topical steroid preparations have been reported to be effective including fluticasone propionate and betamethasone. In general, twice-a-day application with gentle and non-traumatic retraction of the prepuce for a period of four weeks has proven better than a placebo cream. The treatment is successful in 70–90% of cases and the results seem to be long-lasting. This treatment can also be effective in cases of LS *per se* or as a complement to excision of the affected skin.

When medical treatment fails, circumcision is the treatment of choice for phimosis with or without LS. Topical tacrolimus has been successfully used to treat LS. LS is considered a precursor of penile cancer. Beyond the neonatal period, pediatric circumcision requires general anesthesia, but can usually be done on ambulatory basis. A routine circumcision in cases of megaprepuce leads to unsatisfactory results.

Other Uses of Circumcision

In addition to the treatment of phimosis, ritual removal of the prepuce has been performed since antiquity in many cultures. It is not within the scope of this chapter to discuss this topic. Suffice it to say that the pediatric urologist is often called to perform circumcision without medical indication and face the difficult ethical dilemma of performing a medically unnecessary operation on a child that cannot give consent.

Ritual and cultural

Circumcision is used in many religions, most notably among Jews and Moslems. Minimal or no medical intervention takes place among Jewish ritual circumcision, which is performed by mohels on the eighth day of life. Many Moslems groups, however, prefer to circumcise their boys later in childhood or at the onset of puberty. When these groups settle in medically advanced cultures, they usually resort to surgeons to perform the operation. Each society has a unique way to pay for the cost of this practice, whether or not the state or private insurance providers pay for it. It should be up to the individual surgeon to decide whether or not to participate in this practice.

Cultural

In some developed countries, notably the United States of America (USA) and South Korea among others, families wish their newborn males circumcised for cultural reasons. Hygiene and to “look like the father” are among the most commonly given reasons. Some American States and insurance companies pay for the procedure while others do not. Neonatal circumcisions are performed by a variety of pediatric, surgical, or obstetric specialists before the baby is discharged from the hospital. A variety of devices are used for this purpose to avoid having to suture the skin edges and to aid in hemostasis. The use of local blocks or no anesthesia varies regionally. The rate of newborn circumcision in the USA is 55 to 80% according to region and ethnic background.

UTI

There is evidence that febrile urinary tract infections (UTI) in the first three months of life are more prevalent in uncircumcised than in circumcised males. Although some authors claim that routine neonatal circumcision would be a cost-effective measure to prevent UTI, other factors including race, congenital anomalies of the urinary tract, and breastfeeding have to be taken into account. Before an invasive procedure, such as circumcision is recommended as a public health measure to prevent UTI, a prospective randomized study of a given population taking into account other risk factors would be necessary.

If accepted by the parents, it may be reasonable to recommend neonatal circumcision for male at high risk for developing UTI in infancy such as those with prenatally detected hydroureteronephrosis or vesicoureteral reflux. Evidence that in this population, circumcision is more protective, safer, or more cost-effective than antibiotic prophylaxis is lacking. In at least one study, ritual circumcision increased the risk of UTI in the first few weeks of life.

HIV

In parts of Africa where the prevalence of heterosexually transmitted HIV infection is high, circumcised males have a lower risk of becoming infected through vaginal intercourse. At least one study in the USA supports this view. Other African studies have cast some doubt on these findings, probably because many circumcisions were performed after initiation of sexual activity. However, programs aimed at implementing easily available circumcision services have met with high complication rates. There is no evidence that circumcision protects men who have sex with men.

Penile cancer

Penile carcinoma is more common in uncircumcised males. However, penile cancer also occurs in circumcised males. Factors other than the presence of the prepuce, including phimosis, poor hygiene, LS, human papillomavirus infections, and lower socio-economic level are also risk factors. Although neonatal circumcision is protective, the influence of other factors is evidenced by the fact that the prevalence of penile cancer is the same in Japan than in the USA, which are the two populations with widely different rates of neonatal circumcision. The widespread use of neonatal circumcision does not seem justified in parts of the world with a low prevalence of the disease. The problem in areas with high prevalence of penile cancer, such as parts of Africa and Brazil, is the difficulty providing safe access to neonatal circumcision to the population with the lowest socio-economic level, which is the most affected by the disease.

Complications of Circumcision

Although circumcision is a simple procedure, it is not free of complications. In cultures in which the procedure is performed as a ritual outside medical setting, the incidence of complications appears to be higher. Infection, bleeding, partial amputation of the glans, and urethral fistulas are among the most serious adverse events associated with circumcision. Neonatal circumcision can lead to the development of urethral meatal stenosis, which usually requires surgical treatment later in the life (see below). Persistent adhesions between the remaining collar of inner preputial skin and the glans are frequent but are resolved spontaneously at puberty. Dense skin bridges that develop between the denuded glans and the circumcision scar require division, which can often be done with local anesthesia. Parental dissatisfaction with the appearance of the child's penis often leads to cosmetic revisions. Another very disturbing complication of neonatal circumcision is the healing of the circumcision scar in front of the glans causing the penis to be buried and invisible. The problem is usually the result of excessive removal of outer preputial skin including penile shaft skin, leaving in place too much inner preputial skin. Urinary obstruction can result from this condition. If detected early, the treatment with topical steroids and the gentle retraction of the skin may be effective. Surgical reconstruction is often necessary. Another serious problem is the removal of too much skin leading to a wide separation of the skin margins. This is best allowed to heal by second intention. Skin grafts are rarely needed. Some of these complications such as meatal stenosis and undesirable appearance of the penis are common and add to the hidden cost of neonatal circumcision and are often not taken into account in cost-benefit analysis.

Paraphimosis

Definition

Paraphimosis is the entrapment of the prepuce in a retracted position, which can happen when the opening of the prepuce is still narrow (some degree of phimosis) or if the prepuce remains retracted for a prolonged period. Edema of the prepuce produces further constriction of the preputial ring behind the corona making the reduction of the paraphimosis difficult.

Diagnosis

On examination, there is tenderness and marked edema of the prepuce, which forms a tight collar around the glans. In cases of short duration, the glans is edematous but the blood supply is not compromised. In cases of long duration, the blood supply of the prepuce and glans may be impaired. The cases of gangrene associated with paraphimosis have been reported.

Treatment

Paraphimosis should be considered as emergency. In most cases, the child is in pain and sedation or anesthesia may be required for the treatment. The reduction of the edema by applying pressure to the swollen prepuce and glans is usually all that is required to reduce the paraphimosis. When this is not sufficient, the application of ice or granulated sugar may help reduce the edema and facilitate reduction. In long-standing cases when conservative methods fail, a dorsal incision of the prepuce (dorsal slit) may be needed.

Prevention

For prevention of paraphimosis, see Section "Care of the uncircumcised penis" above. Once a patient has had an episode of paraphimosis, the situation needs to be reassessed two to three weeks later; during this period, the retraction of the prepuce should be avoided. If there is clear evidence of phimosis, treatment should be instituted as described in Section "Phimosis". For most patients who have had a dorsal slit for the treatment of the acute episode, circumcision may be required for cosmetic reasons.

Concealed Penis

Definition

When the penis is concealed from view in the normal course of inspection. Three different types are recognized.

Classification and Treatment

The most common cause is a prominent prepubic fat pad with loose attachments between the skin and Scarpa's fascia at the base of the penis. Often children are also obese. Although operations have been described to improve the appearance of the genitalia and they are performed at many centers, the most reasonable course of action is reassurance and to request the primary physician to address weight management. In non-obese children, the condition is rare.

The second kind has been described in Section "Phimosis and circumcision" and is illustrated in Figure 9-1. Surgical correction is required.

The third variety is a complication of neonatal circumcision and it has been addressed earlier in this chapter in Section "Complications of circumcision".

Meatal Stenosis

Definition

Narrowing of the urethral meatus is usually acquired and may cause the symptoms of painful micturition, the deviation of the urinary stream, spraying or the need to strain to urinate. The main causes of meatal stenosis are neonatal circumcision (see previous section) and LS. The latter occurs mostly in uncircumcised males. Other skin diseases such as epidermolysis bullosa have been reported as the causes of meatal stenosis.

Diagnosis and Treatment

The diagnosis is established by the physical examination. Most patients with the postneonatal circumcision variety present after toilet training because of the dorsal deflection of the urinary stream that makes it difficult to urinate standing up. On examination, the urethral meatus is narrow with the loss of the slit-like appearance. The stenosis occurs in the ventral aspect of the meatus. Observation of the stream during micturition is diagnostic. Treatment is surgical meatoplasty, with the incision of the meatus toward the fraenulum and the suturing of the skin to urethral mucosa with fine absorbable sutures. Postoperative home dilatation is unnecessary. Treatment by simple meatotomy or dilatation has a high recurrence rate.

Meatal stenosis associated with LS causes obstructive symptoms with pain or straining during micturition. On examination, the prepuce or just the glans surrounding the meatus appears white and thickened. In older patients, the disease may extend into the urethra. Uroflow examination is helpful in these cases. The typical flow pattern is flattened as in all urethral stenosis. Treatment is done by circumcision and meatoplasty. The meatoplasty may be ventral or dorsal according to the configuration of the meatus. If urethral involvement is suspected, cystoscopy should be performed at the time of the circumcision.

Balanitis and Balanoposthitis

Definition

Balanitis is an inflammation of the glans penis; it is referred to as balanoposthitis when it involves the prepuce. We have already discussed balanitis xerotica obliterans or LS in the sections of phimosis and meatal stenosis. More common, particularly, in uncircumcised males is the development of bacterial or fungal infections of the glans and prepuce.

Diagnosis and Treatment

Presenting complain is pain in the penis. Micturition may be painful as well. On examination, the prepuce is erythematous, swollen, and tender to palpation. There may be purulent discharge, which should be cultured. Inguinal lymphadenopathy may be present. The most common etiologic agents are staphylococci and *E. coli*. Treatment with wide spectrum antibiotics leads to prompt resolution of the inflammation. After resolution of the infection, the evaluation of the prepuce and the eventual treatment of phimosis are necessary (see Section "Phimosis").

Penile Warts

Genital warts caused by human papilloma virus (HPV) (types 6 and 1) also called condyloma acuminata in children can be acquired during birth from an infected mother, through hand contact from the parents or through sexual abuse. The vulva is a more frequent site than the penis and it will be discussed in the pertinent section. In newborns, spontaneous regression is the rule. In older children, local destruction can be done but it will not control the viral infection; therefore, recurrences are common.

Another type of warts in children is molluscum contagiosum, which is a viral infection of the skin and mucous membranes that is caused by the molluscum contagiosum virus. It can be acquired by skin-to-skin contact, which may occur during play, in a swimming pool, or through sexual contact. In postpubertal males, viral infections through sexual contact are common.

Micropenis

By the 13th week of gestation in the male embryo under the influence testosterone produced by the fetal Leydig cells, the structural development of the penis is complete. In the following months of gestation, the penis continues to grow to reach the normal newborn size at term. Thus, the initial presence of the testes is essential for the formation of the organ. Subsequent growth requires the presence of functioning testes until term.

The failure of testosterone production by the fetal testes after the 13th week of gestation will cause a normally formed penis to be small.

Definition

When a normally developed penis is less than two standard deviations below the mean length and width for age. For a term newborn of average size, the mean size of the stretched penis from the pubic symphysis to the tip of the glans is 3.5 cm. Below 2.4 cm, it is considered to be small, or micropenis. The commonest cause of micropenis is fetal hypogonadism, which may be primary (testicular failure), hypogonadotropic, or idiopathic.

Diagnosis and Management

The penile size should be recorded and interpreted in relation to a child's age. Premature infants have smaller penises than full-term newborns. A normal urethral meatus and prepuce indicate that testosterone-producing tissue was present in the first 12 weeks of gestation. The presence or absence of gonads in the scrotum should be noted. Additional abnormalities that may indicate syndromic micropenis should be sought. If testes are present, their volume should be recorded. A karyotype is usually done and reveals 46XY. A pediatric endocrinology consult is essential.

Primary or secondary hypogonadism is the usual underlying reason for the micropenis. The measurement of testosterone, luteinizing hormone, and follicle-stimulating hormone should be performed. This should be done in the newborn period and repeated in the first two or three months of life to take advantage of the normal testosterone surge.

In infancy, testicular function and penile response can be evaluated by the human gonadotropin (HGC) stimulation test. Serum testosterone is measured before and after three or four injections. When there is little or no testosterone rise, as in the case of primary hypogonadism, the parenteral injection of testosterone can be used to assess penile response to stimulation.

If the testes are not palpable, an ultrasound of the groin and abdomen may be helpful. Eventually, laparoscopy is necessary to rule out the possibility of intra-abdominal testes or to establish that the patient has vanished testes (see Chapter 18).

Eventually, the treatment will be done by an endocrinologist with testosterone replacement. In most instances, there will be a good response to exogenous testosterone. There seem to be no advantage to testosterone stimulation before the age at which the onset of puberty is desirable except to test future response. In extreme cases, for psychological reasons, prepubertal testosterone may be advisable but care must be taken not to interfere with somatic growth.

Penile Agenesis

Definition

It is the congenital absence of the penis. The urethra enters the anterior rectal wall or anal verge. The scrotum and testes are normal. Associated renal anomalies are common and the condition, which is rare, often results in intrauterine fetal or newborn death.

Diagnosis and Management

The diagnosis may be suspected prenatally when the penis is not visible by the 30th week in an XY fetus. In these cases, the scrotum is usually visible whereas in complete androgen insensitivity of gonadal dysgenesis, it is not.

The management of urinary tract anomalies is essential for survival. In the past early removal of the testes and female gender assignment with subsequent feminizing, genitoplasty used to be the rule. Male gender assignment with postpubertal phalloplasty is another option. The problem with female gender assignment is the risk of subsequent wish to reverse to the male gender. The problem with male gender assignment is growing up without a penis and the less than satisfactory results of phalloplasty. Neonatal decision should be done with a team approach involving surgeons, pediatricians, endocrinologists, and psychologists with informed active participation of the parents.

Hypospadias

Definition

It is a congenital anomaly of the penis characterized by a ventral and proximal position of the urethral meatus. In addition, the prepuce is usually not developed on the ventral side forming a hood rather than a sleeve around the glans (Figure 9-2). Ventral curvature of the penis (chordee) of various degrees is common as well as axial rotations (Figure 9-3). In severe cases, particularly when the urethral meatus is very proximal, the scrotum may be bifid or extend cephalad to the base of the penis (partial scrotal transposition) (Figure 9-4). Hypospadias is usually an isolated anomaly, but when the penis is small or the testes undescended, the disorder of sexual differentiation or endocrinopathies should be suspected. For a detailed discussion of hypospadias, see Chapter 19.

Epispadias

Definition and Classification

It is a congenital anomaly of the penis, which is the milder end of the spectrum of the bladder exstrophy/epispadias complex. A common feature

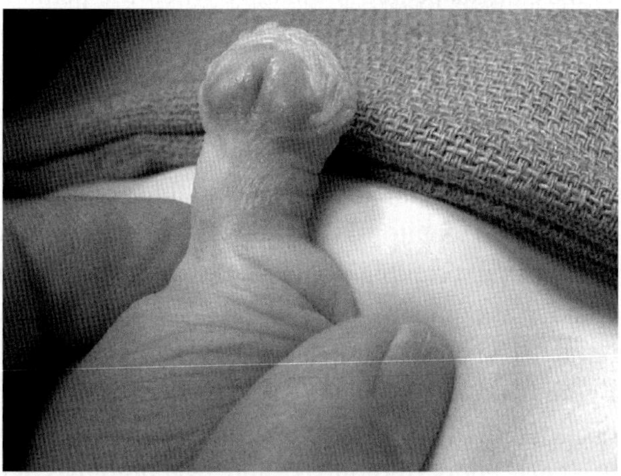

Figure 9-2. Distal hypospadias with a straight shaft, meatus at the coronal sulcus, and a ventrally deficient prepuce (hooded prepuce).

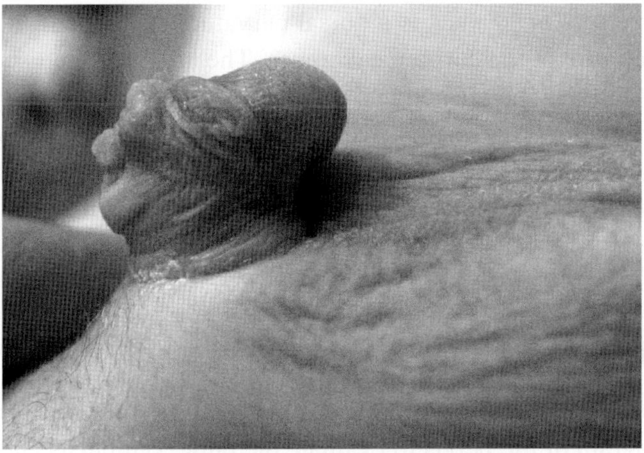

Figure 9-3. Mid-shaft hypospadias with ventral curvature of the shaft, deficient ventral skin, and hooded prepuce.

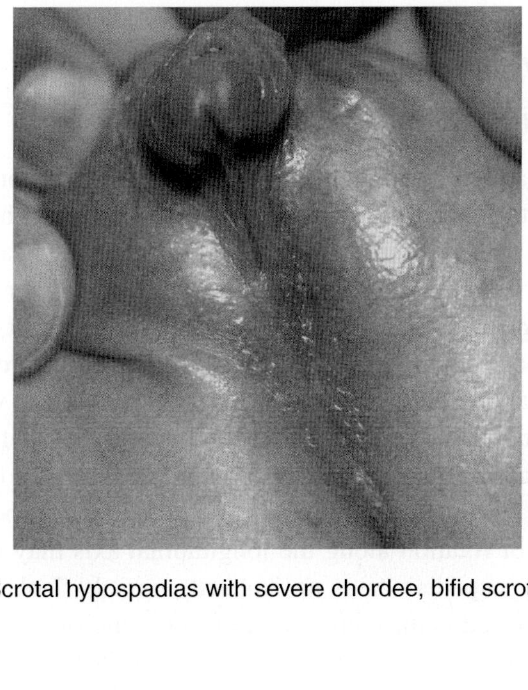

Figure 9-4. Scrotal hypospadias with severe chordee, bifid scrotum, and incomplete prepuce.

of all degrees of epispadias is a dorsal curvature of the penis determined by the curvature of the corpora cavernosa. The urethral meatus is dorsally displaced and may be located in the dorsum of the glans, the penile shaft, or just below the pubic symphisis. The penis tends to be short and wide. In the more severe cases, the pubic symphisis is separated as in bladder exstrophy and the bladder neck and the proximal urethra are wide and urinary incontinence is common.

Evaluation and Management

In addition to the physical examination, evaluation should include a plain roentgenogram of the pelvis to evaluate the pubic symphisis and, in proximal cases, a micturition cystourethrogram to evaluate bladder capacity and to rule out vesico-ureteric reflux. In distal cases, reconstructive surgery can be done before the second birthday. For treatment of proximal cases, please refer to Chapter 23.

Penile Curvature and Torsion

Definition and Classification

A ventral curvature of the penis during erection is commonly referred to as chordee. Although, in most cases, it is associated with hypospadias, it can also occur in the presence of a normally positioned meatus. The penis may be otherwise normally developed or it may have other features associated with hypospadias such as hooded prepuce, deficient ventral penile skin, or a hypoplastic ventral urethral wall. The curvature may also be lateral or dorsal. These curvatures are usually associated with a normal prepuce and urethra. They are caused by an intrinsic deformity of the corpora cavernosa. Ventral penile curvature may be due exclusively to deficient ventral skin or to an intrinsic deformity of the corpora cavernosa. Penile torsion or rotation along the longitudinal axis may be seen in the presence of hypospadias or as an isolated anomaly. Isolated rotation is usually only noticed in the course or after a circumcision and has no functional consequences.

Treatment

When isolated, the decision to treat any of these anomalies should be based on the estimation of potential adverse effect on sexual function and not only for cosmetic consideration. When a ventral curvature is due to a skin problem alone, it can usually be corrected by re-arranging the penile skin, usually in the course of a circumcision. Intrinsic deformities of the corpora require coropal plications with or without grafting the opposite side of the curvature.

Priapism

Definition

Priapism is an abnormal prolonged penile erection without sexual desire and failure to subside despite orgasm. Two types are recognized; first, low-flow priapism is painful and can lead to irreversible ischemic damage of the erectile tissue. It is often associated with predisposing factors, the most common of which is sickle cell anemia followed by leukemia and other hematological disorders. Spinal cord injury and spinal cord degenerative process as well as a variety of pharmacological agents have also been implicated in the etiology of priapism. Second, high-flow priapism is secondary to perineal blunt trauma and the formation of an arterio-venous fistula in the proximal corpus cavernosum. This form of priapism is not associated with ischemic changes and is not painful.

Diagnosis

The diagnosis is established based on a history of a prolonged erection confirmed on physical examination. The corpora are rigid but the glans is not. A history of concurrent predisposing factors such as perineal trauma or sickle cell disease should be sought. However, in some conditions such as leukemia or sickle cell disease, priapism may be the initial manifestation of the disease. In addition to the history and the presence or absence of pain, cavernous blood gas analysis and color Doppler ultrasonography of the corpora help establish the differential diagnosis. A typical picture of post-traumatic high-flow priapism in a prepubertal boy is shown in

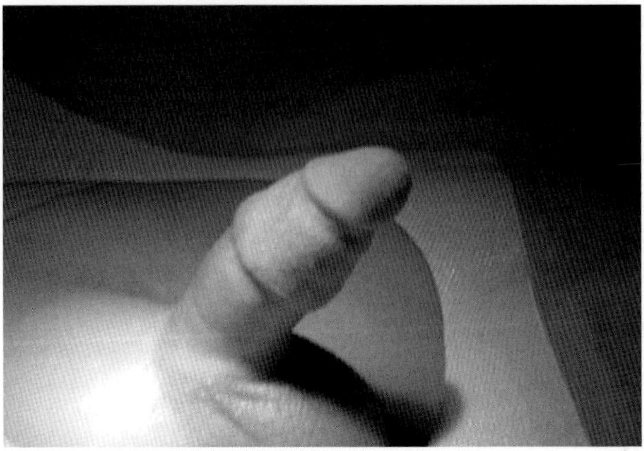

Figure 9-5. Erect penis with post-traumatic high-flow priapism.

Figure 9-5. Figure 9-6 shows the color Doppler ultrasound appearance of the post-traumatic arterio-venous fistula on the right corpus, which was responsible for the priapism.

Management

The management of low-flow priapism should start with the treatment of the underlying cause. There is some urgency in relieving the erection, not only for pain control but also to prevent irreversible ischemic damage to the erectile tissue. Corporal irrigation and intra-corporeal alpha adrenergics can be useful. When more conservative measures fail, the creation of a shunt between the corpora cavernosa and the spongiosum, which is not involved in the process, may be indicated. This can be done at the level of the glans (winter shunt) or surgically in the perineum.

High-flow priapism is best treated by super selective embolization of the fistula in the course of pelvic angiography. In the early stages, the external compression of the fistula has been reported to be effective.

Empty Scrotum

Absence of the testes in the scrotum in a full-term newborn requires immediate investigation. In the presence of a normal penis, the differential

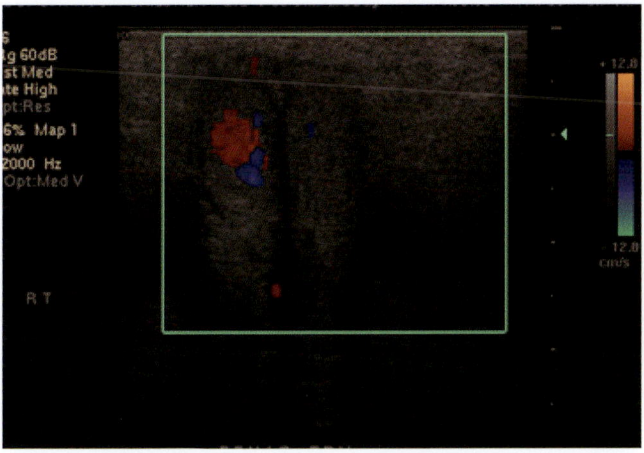

Figure 9-6. Ultrasonographic image of the perineum with color Doppler showing an arterio-venous fistula on the right corpus cavernosum.

diagnosis includes bilateral undescended testes or bilateral vanished testes. If the penis is small (less than two standard deviations below the mean), an empty scrotum may reflect the deficient production of gonadotropins. If the phallus is hypospadiac, an immediate investigation for possible female with 21-hydroxylase deficiency, a potential life-threatening condition, must be undertaken. These topics are discussed in detail in the Chapters 11 and 17 dealing with cryptorchidism and disorders of sexual development.

Bifid Scrotum

During the development under the influence of testosterone, the genital folds fuse to form the scrotum. Therefore, a bifid scrotum is a manifestation of incomplete virilization and is usually associated with hypospadias (Figure 9-4) (see Chapter 18).

Scrotal Transposition

Scrotal transposition occurs when a part or the entire scrotum is located cranial to the base of the penis (Figure 9-7). The anomaly is associated with hypospadias in 80% of the cases (see Chapter 18) but it may occur

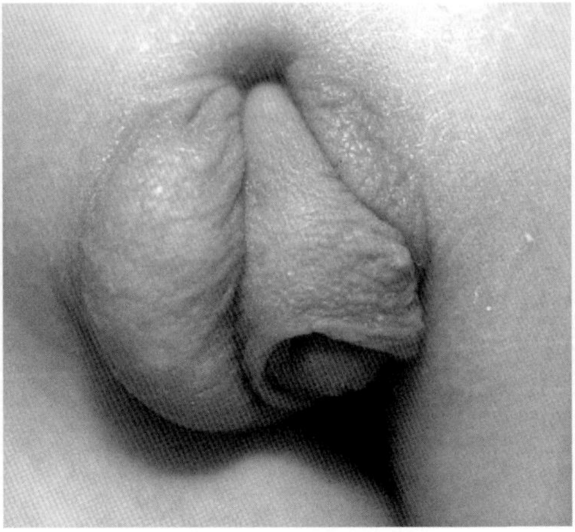

Figure 9-7. Partial penoscrotal transposition (or shawl scrotum).

in the presence of a normal penis. It has also been reported to be genetic and associated with anomalies in other organ systems.

Necrotizing Fascitis

Genital necrotizing fascitis also known as Fournier's gangrene is uncommon in children. It has been reported to follow skin infections, circumcision, or anorectal trauma. Affected patients commonly have debilitating conditions such as malignancy or other systemic diseases. In childhood, Gram-positive organisms are usually responsible. Treatment should be promptly instituted with antibiotics and judicious surgical debridement.

FURTHER READING

Bailey RC, Egesah O, Rosenberg S. Male circumcision for HIV prevention: a prospective study of complications in clinical and traditional settings in Bungoma, Kenya. *Bull World Health Organ* 2008; **86**:669–677.

Byakika-Tusilime J. Circumcision and HIV infection: assessment of causality. *AIDS Behav* 2008; **12**:835–841.

Ceylan K, *et al*. Severe complications of circumcision: analysis of 48 cases. *J Pediatr Urol* 2007; **3**:32–35.

Connolly CA, *et al*. Male circumcision and its relationship to HIV infection in South Africa: results from a national survey in 2002. *S Afr Med J* 2008; **98**:789–794.

De Castro R, *et al*. Phalloplasty and urethroplasty in children with penile agenesis: preliminary report. *J Urol* 2007; **177**:1112–1116.

Esposito C, *et al*. Topical steroid application versus circumcision in pediatric patients with phimosis: a prospective randomized placebo controlled clinical trial. *World J Urol* 2008; **26**:187–190.

Favorito LA, *et al*. Epidemiologic study on penile cancer in Brazil. *Int Braz J Urol* 2008; **34**:587–591; discussion 591–593.

Ghysel C, *et al*. Long-term efficiency of skin stretching and a topical corticoid cream application for unretractable foreskin and phimosis in prepubertal boys. *Urol Int* 2009; **82**:81–88.

Gollaher DL. *Circumcision*. New York: Basic Books, 2000. ISBN 0-465-04397-6.

Ha TS, Lee JS. Scrotal involvement in childhood Henoch-Schönlein purpura. *Acta Paediatr* 2007; **96**:552–555.

Hendren WH. The genetic male with absent penis and urethrorectal communication: experience with 5 patients. *J Urol* 1997; **157**:1469–1474.

Hsieh TF, Chang CH, Chang SS. Foreskin development before adolescence in 2149 schoolboys. *Int J Urol* 2006; **13**:968–970.

Jesus LE, Dekermacher S. Priapism in children: a review of the pathophysiology and treatment. *J Pediatr (Rio J)* 2009; **85**:194–200.

Leibowitz AA, Desmond K, Belin T. Determinants and policy implications of male circumcision in the United States. *Am J Public Health* 2009; **99**:138–145.

Mackway-Jones K, Teece S. Best evidence topic reports. Ice, pins, or sugar to reduce paraphimosis. *Emerg Med J* 2004; **21**:77–78.

Mårild S, *et al*. Protective effect of breastfeeding against urinary tract infection. *Acta Paediatr* 2004; **93**:164–168.

Meyer-Bahlburg HF. Gender identity outcome in female-raised 46,XY persons with penile agenesis, cloacal exstrophy of the bladder, or penile ablation. *Arch Sex Behav* 2005; **34**:423–438.

Millet GA, *et al*. Circumcision status and risk of HIV and sexually transmitted infections among men who have sex with men: a meta-analysis. *JAMA* 2008; **300**:1674–1684.

Pinke LA, *et al.* Penoscrotal transposition: review of 53 patients. *J Urol* 2001; **166**:1865–1868.

Prais D, Shoov-Furman R, Amir J. Is ritual circumcision a risk factor for urinary tract infections? *Arch Dis Child* 2009; **94**:191–194.

Roussey-Kesler G, *et al.* Antibiotic prophylaxis for the prevention of recurrent urinary tract infection in children with low grade vesicoureteral reflux: results from a prospective randomized study. *J Urol* 2008; **179**:674–679.

Sandler G, *et al.* Pediatric high-flow priapism and super-selective angiography — an Australian perspective. *J Pediatr Surg* 2008; **43**:1898–1901.

Shaik N, *et al.* Prevalence of urinary tract infection in childhood: a meta-analysis. *Pediatr Infec Dis J* 2008; **27**:302–308.

Shankar KR, Rickwood AM. Incidence of phimosis in boys. *BJU Int* 1999; **84**:101–102.

Schoen EJ, Colby CJ, Ray GT. Newborn circumcision decreases incidence and costs of urinary tract infections during the first year of life. *Pediatrics* 2000; **195**:789–793.

Van Howe RS. Effect of confounding in the association between circumcision and urinary tract infection. *J Infect* 2005; **51**:59–68.

Volgger H, Pfefferkorn S, Hobisch A. Posttraumatic high-flow priapism in children: noninvasive treatment by color Doppler ultrasound-guided perineal compression. *Urology* 2007; **70**:590. e3–5.

Warner L, *et al.* Male circumcision and the risk of HIV infection among heterosexual African American men attending Baltimore sexually transmitted disease clinics. *J Infect Dis* 2009; **199**:59–65.

Zavras N, *et al.* Conservative treatment of phimosis with fluticasone propionate 0.05%: a clinical study in 1185 boys. *J Pediatr Urol* 2009; **5**(3):181–185.

Chapter 10

Genital Anomalies and Diseases in Girls

Ricardo González and Barbara M. Ludwikowski

This chapter describes the most common genital anomalies and diseases seen in females excluding disorders of sexual development, which is discussed in Chapter 11.

CONGENITAL ANOMALIES

- Persistent urogenital sinus with and without rectal atresia.
- Epispadias.
- Clitoral and labial hypertrophies.
- Interlabial masses (Skene's glans cysts, imperforate hymen, and prolapsing ureterocele).
- Müllerian anomalies.

ACQUIRED DISEASES

- Interlabial masses (urethral prolapse and tumors).
- Vulvovaginitis.
- Condyloma.
- Foreign bodies.
- Fusion of the labia minora.

PERSISTENT UROGENITAL SINUS WITH AND WITHOUT RECTAL ATRESIA

Definition

In the course of normal development, the process of exstrophy and the eversion of the distal part of the urogenital sinus give rise to the development of the vestibule and separate openings for the urethra and vagina. When the process of separation is incomplete, the vagina and urethra fuse to open through a common channel (persistent urogenital sinus).

Classification

Three types of persistent urogenital sinus are recognized: (i) isolated, not associated to endocrine abnormalities and with a normal anus and rectum, (ii) associated with fetal virilization, most common in cases of congenital adrenal hyperplasia due to 21-hydroxylase deficiency, and (iii) associated with anal or rectal atresias as in persistent cloaca.

Primary Urogenital Sinus

Presentation and Diagnosis

A primary urogenital sinus may remain unrecognized until the onset of sexual activity (Figure 10-1). Routine examination of the external genitalia during well-baby examinations should allow recognition in early infancy. It is important that the examination be done in a gentle and non-intimidating manner, preferably by a female physician or in the presence of a nurse. In children over three years of age, proper preparation and explanation should precede the examination. The vulva is best examined by gentle downward traction of the labia majora, which allows the best visualization of the urethral meatus and vaginal introitus. When the anatomy does not appear normal during an office visit, examination under sedation is indicated. At times, the junction of the vagina to the sinus is narrow and causes retention of mucus and secretions stimulated by maternal estrogens. Occasionally, urine may be trapped in the vagina. This condition is called hydro- or mucocolpos and may be detected prenatally on fetal ultrasonography as a

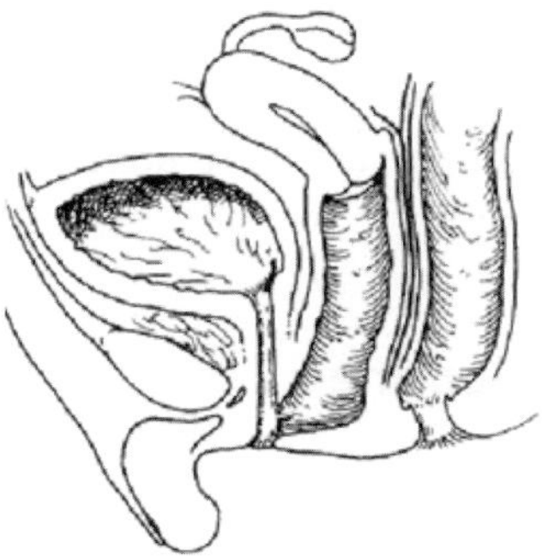

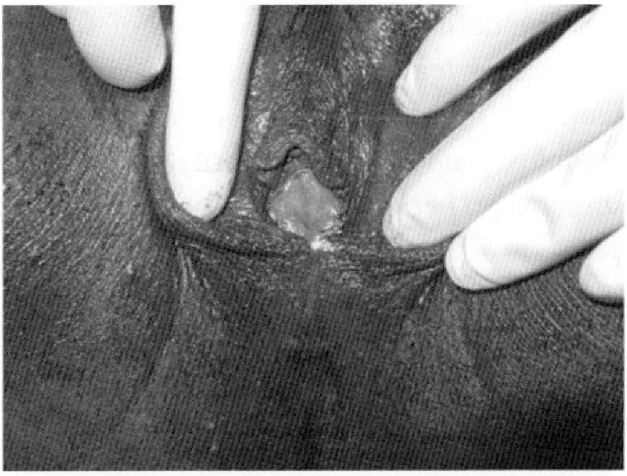

Figure 10-1. Left: Artistic representation of urogenital sinus with normal anus and rectum and low confluence of the urethra and vagina. Right: Urogenital sinus in an African female with untreated congenital adrenal hyperplasia. Notice the absent vaginal introitus and the uncharacteristic lack of clitoral hypertrophy.

pelvic mass in the third trimester of gestation. When a hydromucocolpos exists, it requires immediate postnatal attention since it may cause ureteral or urethral obstruction. A primary urogenital sinus may also be associated with a short urethra and urinary incontinence. Urinary tract infections can also be the presenting manifestation of this condition.

The evaluation consists of defining the internal genital anatomy as well as the urinary tract anatomy by means of pelvic and renal ultrasonography, a retrograde contrast study through the sinus external opening. Magnetic resonance imaging may be useful but may require heavy sedation or anesthesia to obtain adequate images. Eventually, urethroscopy, cystoscopy, and vaginoscopy are needed to determine the exact anatomy and to plan the surgical repair. Laparoscopy may be useful when the internal genital anatomy has not been well defined with the imaging studies.

Treatment

The treatment of the newborn with hydromucocolpos requires decompression. This can often be accomplished endoscopically; however, occasionally, percutaneous drainage of the distended vagina may be needed.

The definitive repair consists of surgery to separate the urethra from the vagina leaving two separate vestibular openings. It is beyond the scope of this handbook to describe the surgical options, which can be complex, and given the rarity of the malformation are best done by surgeons experienced in this type of repairs.

Urogenital Sinus Associated with Endocrine Abnormalities

Definition

Under the influence of virilizing substances in an XX fetus, the distal urogenital sinus persists and the urethra acquires male characteristics. In very severe cases, the urethra will end up in a phallic position. The same virilizing factors lead to clitoral hypertrophy (Figure 10-2) and this is the

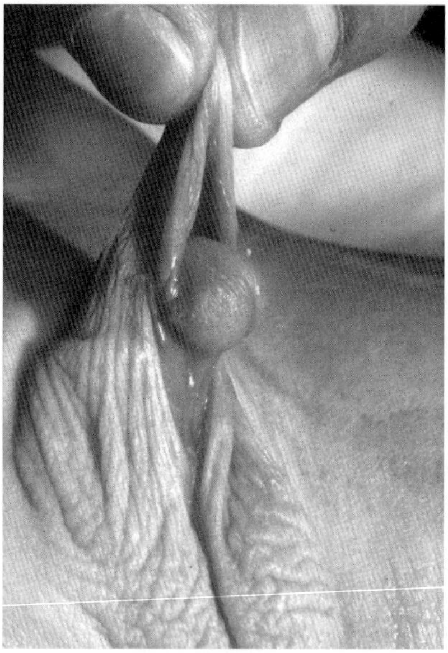

Figure 10-2. Genitalia of an XX female with congenital adrenal hyperplasia and Prader IV virilization. Notice the enlarged clitoris and scrotalized labia resembling a proximal hypospadias. The lack of palpable gonads in such a case should prompt an immediate neonatal evaluation.

salient feature of these newborns, which leads to a diagnostic investigation. This topic is discussed in greater detail in Chapter 11.

Causes

Virilization of a female fetus is most commonly caused by 21-hydroxylase deficiency that prevents cortisone synthesis; precursors with the androgenic activity accumulate leading to virilization. This is a life-threatening disorder in the newborn and is discussed in detail in Chapter 11. Less common causes of virilization of a female fetus are the exposure to exogenous androgens, placental aromatase deficiency and maternal androgen producing tumours.

Evaluation and Treatment

The evaluation and treatment of the virilized female is discussed in Chapter 11.

Urogenital Sinus Associated with Anal or Rectal Atresia (Persistent Cloaca)

Definition

This is the most severe form of imperforate anus and rectal atresia in females. The rectum, vagina (often duplicated), and urethra converge into a common channel or cloaca, which typically opens behind the clitoris (Figure 10-3). A variant, called posterior cloaca (Figure 10-4), in which the opening is on the anterior anal margin is not a true cloaca; in that the rectum is normal. It simply represents a urogenital sinus with a posterior opening.

Presentation and Diagnosis and Evaluation

The diagnosis may be suspected prenatally or established during the newborn examination. As illustrated in Figure 10-3, there is a single opening in the perineum, behind the clitoris. In some girls, the labia minora are often displaced anteriorly and occasionally; these girls are believed to have a disorder of sexual differentiation.

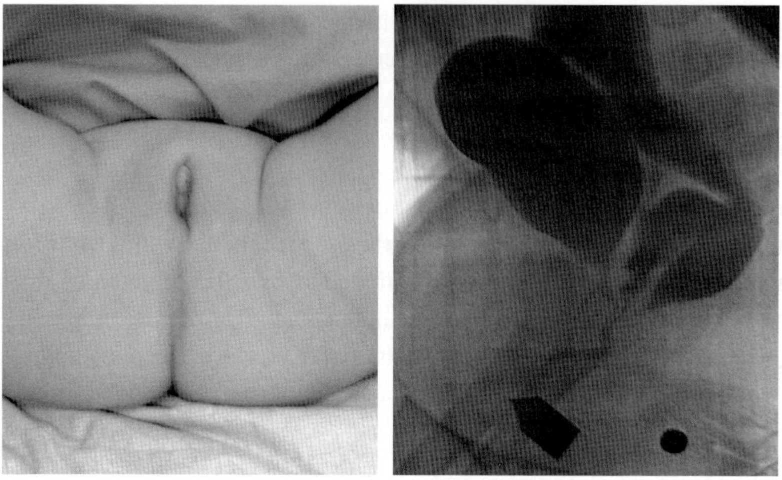

Figure 10-3. Left: The view of the perineum of a girl with the persistence of the cloaca. There is only one perineal opening. Right: Contrast image showing the convergence of the rectum, vagina, and urethra in the same patient.

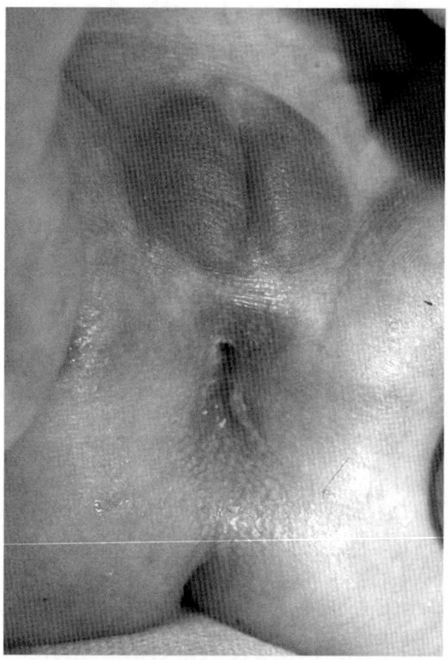

Figure 10-4. The posterior opening of a persistent urogenital sinus with normal anus (misnomer posterior cloaca). Notice the opening of the urogenital sinus just in front of the anus.

The evaluation should include the spine, the genital and urinary tracts, and the cardiovascular system. Urologic anomalies including vesicoureteral reflux, renal agenesis, and hydronephrosis are common. The vagina may be single, duplicated, or absent, as can be the uterus. Spinal anomalies, particularly of the lumbosacral spine, are present in about half of the cases and are important for the prognosis regarding rectal and urinary continences. A spinal ultrasound and eventually an MRI or the lumbosacral spine are important.

Treatment

The pediatric anorectal and genitourinary surgeons should manage these cases jointly. Initially, a totally diverting high sigmoid or transverse colostomy is done. At the time of the colostomy, an endoscopic examination of the cloacal channel will determine its length and will help planning the future reconstruction. If there is a hydrocolpos, the entrance to the vagina into the cloaca can be dilated to drain it and if necessary to do intermittent catheterization. Hydrocolpos can be responsible for hydronephrosis. A vaginostomy is seldom necessary and complicates the subsequent reconstruction.

These girls may need cardiological and neurosurgical consultations to address associated anomalies.

FEMALE EPISPADIAS

Definition

This rare anomaly is a part of the exstrophy/epispadias complex discussed in Chapter 23. In its most severe form, the urethra is short and wide, the clitoris is bifid, and the pubic rami do not meet in the midline (diastasis of the symphysis pubis) (Figure 10-5).

Presentation

Ideally, epispadias should be detected in the newborn examination or during the well-baby examinations in infancy. However, when it occurs

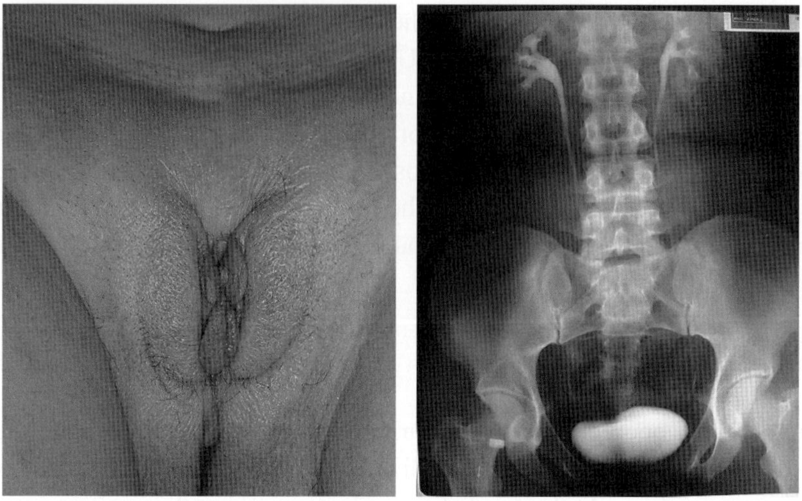

Figure 10-5. Left: Female epispadias exhibiting the bifid clitoris. Right: Excretory urogram showing a wide pubic diastasis. The anomaly in this incontinent female was not recognized until after puberty.

without bladder exstrophy in females may go unrecognized for years until the child presents with urinary incontinence. The importance of correct genital examinations cannot be overemphasized.

Evaluation

In addition to the external genital anatomy, the length of the urethra, the skeletal anatomy of the pelvis, and the bladder capacity should be evaluated. Because of the lack of outlet resistance in severe cases, the bladder may be small. Vesicoureteral reflux may be present.

Treatment

The treatment of the malformation and attending urinary incontinence are discussed along with bladder exstrophy in Chapter 22. In cases of pure epispadias, some authors favor the implantation of an artificial urinary sphincter to treat urinary incontinence.

CLITORAL AND LABIAL HYPERTROPHY

Clitoral enlargement is most commonly seen in the cases of prenatal virilization but it may occur in isolation. If treatment is deemed necessary, it is better to wait till after puberty to obtain informed consent from the patient since loss of sensation may occur. Every girl with clitoral hypertrophy should be evaluated for the possible causes of virilization, which can be prenatal (see Section "Urogenital sinus associated with endocrine abnormalities" of this chapter and Chapter 11) or postnatally acquired as may be the case of ovarian or adrenal tumors.

Adolescents may present with hypertrophy of the labia minora, which usually requires more reassurance than cosmetic corrective surgery.

CONGENITAL INTERLABIAL MASSES

Definition, Presentation, and Treatment

Masses present in the labia minora in newborn girls may represent one of the several conditions including Skene's glans cysts, imperforate hymen, or a prolapsing ureterocele.

Skene's glans or paraurethral glans can be obstructed and full of secretions in the newborn. These cysts can be uni- or bilateral. They are easily recognized because they arise lateral to the urethral meatus. A simple puncture usually solves the problem.

Imperforate hymen leads to the accumulation of mucus from vaginal secretions stimulated by maternal estrogens (Figure 10-6). On examination, there is a thin membrane bulging where the introitus should be. The urethral meatus is in front and normal. An ultrasound of the pelvis may reveal a vagina distended with secretions. Incision under sedation solves the problem.

A *prolapsing ureterocele* is the most serious on congenital interlabial masses. The cystic mass protrudes within the urethral meatus. The evaluation of the entire urinary tract is necessary and immediate treatment instituted (see Chapter 15).

MÜLLERIAN ANOMALIES

The Fallopian tubes, uterus, and upper vagina arise from the ducts of Müller, which in males involute under the influence of Müllerian inhibiting

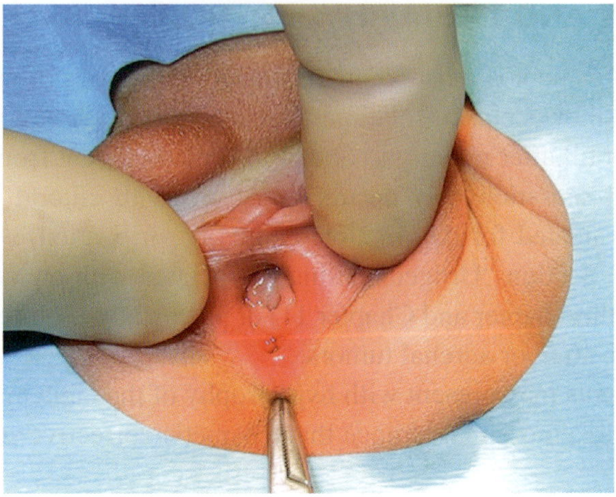

Figure 10-6. Vaginal duplication with obstruction of the right hemivagina (notice the bulging hymen), an open left hemivagina and an anterior anus. The hemostat indicates the normal location of the anus (Herlyn-Werner-Wunderlich syndrome with perinal fistula).

substance secreted by the Sertoli cells of the testis. The development of the Müllerian structures is intimately related to the development of the Wolffian ducts from which the ureters and internal male genital ducts originate. Several anomalies of the Müllerian system are of significance to the pediatric urologists.

Transverse vaginal septa, vaginal atresia and absent vagina can all have associated renal anomalies. Diagnosis may be made in the course of a routine childhood examination (Figure 10-7) or girls may present at puberty with amenorrhea or cyclical abdominal pain.

Mayer-Rokitansky-Kuster-Hauser (MRKH) Syndrome

Definition

The absence of uterus and upper vagina associated with renal anomalies, principally unilateral agenesis or renal ectopia. It is rarely associated with skeletal anomalies or rectal malformations. Its prevalence is 1:5000 female births.

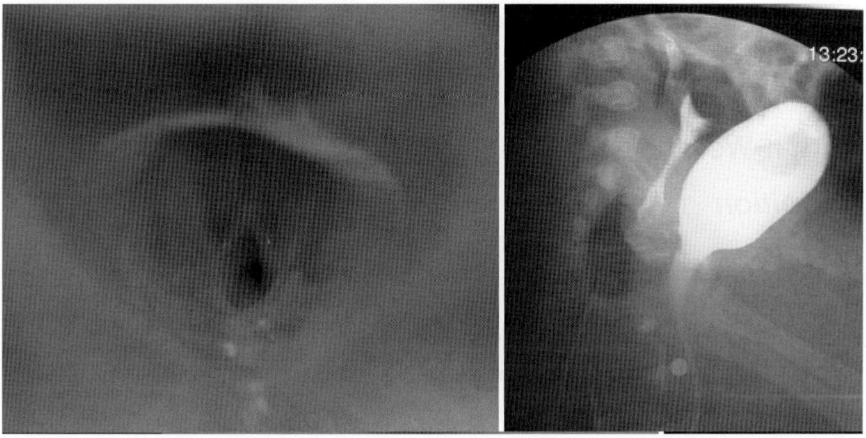

Figure 10-7. Left: Distal vaginal atresia or septum. The opening seen is the urethral meatus. Right: Contrast study through the urethra and existing vaginostomy, showing the lack of communication of the vagina with the perineum or the urethra. This girl presented at birth with a large pelvic mass causing ureteral obstruction (courtesy of Dr. Katharina Roth, Aarau, Switzerland).

Presentation

MRKH syndrome can be suspected prenatally in girls with renal agenesis or it may be an incidental finding during the course of a urologic evaluation for other causes. Females who reach puberty undetected present with primary amenorrhea of which, MRKH syndrome is the second most frequent cause.

Diagnosis

Pelvic and renal ultrasound as well as MRI are useful to define the internal genital anatomy. Laparoscopy is sometimes needed.

Treatment

Uncomplicated renal agenesis or ectopia requires no treatment. The treatment of the absent vagina is controversial. Since a distal shallow vaginal pouch is often present some recommend dilatation starting after the onset of puberty. Some authors favor vaginal replacement with an intestinal segment.

Herlyn-Werner-Wunderlich (HWW) Syndrome

Definition

HWW syndrome is a rare Müllerian anomaly consisting of uterine didelphys, vaginal septum, and ipsilateral renal agenesis. There is vaginal duplication with an obstructed septum in one of the sides. Renal agenesis on the side of the Müllerian obstruction is common.

Presentation

As with MRKH syndrome, HWW syndrome can be suspected prenatally in girls with renal agenesis or it may be incidentally discovered during the course of imaging studies (Figure 10-6). Presentation is otherwise after menarche with cyclic abdominal pain despite normal menstruation.

Treatment

Uncomplicated renal agenesis or ectopia requires no treatment. The vaginal septum can usually be incised through the open vagina to drain the obstructed duplicated vagina.

INTERLABIAL MASSES OUTSIDE THE NEWBORN PERIOD

Definition

Interlabial masses detected outside the newborn period may represent a urethral prolapse or neoplasias.

Urethral Prolapse

Urethral prolapse is more common in black girls than in Caucasian or Asian (Figure 10-8). Presenting symptoms include vulvar bleeding or

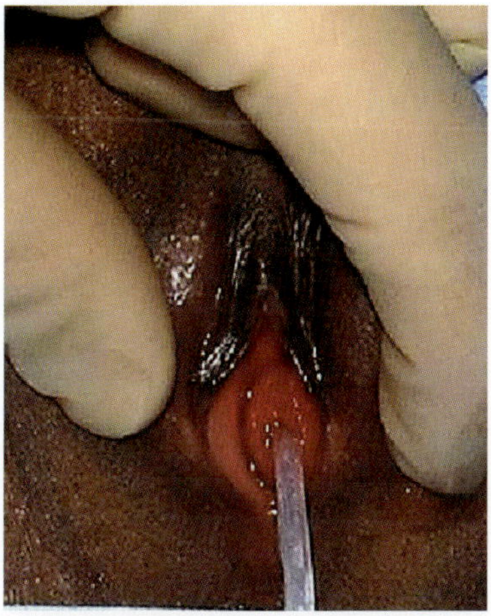

Figure 10-8. Urethral prolapse in African–American female. The urethral meatus (catheter) is in the center of the prolapsed mass.

rarely urinary retention. Treatment may begin with topical estrogens for a limited period followed by surgical excision when there is no response. Antibiotics may be needed in the cases complicated with infection.

Neoplasias

Benign neoplasias such as hemangioma (Figure 10-9) can be treated by local excision. The most common malignant neoplasia of the vagina in children is embryonal rhabdomyosarcoma that can present as an interlabial mass, which may resemble a bunch of grapes (sarcoma botryoides). Malignant tumors are discussed in Chapter 20.

VULVOVAGINITIS

Various types of inflammation of the vulva can be seen in girls. The commonly occurring symptoms are pruritus, pain, or dysuria with or without discharge. These include contact dermatitis, lichen sclerosus, psoriasis, and bacterial and mycotic infections. Frequent pathogens are *Staphylococcus aureus* and *S. pyogenes.* Vulvar lesions or infections caused by other organisms should arise the suspicion of sexual abuse.

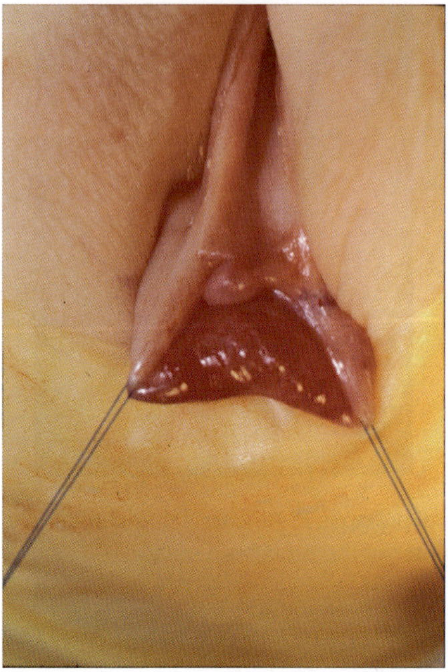

Figure 10-9. Clitoral hemangioma.

CONDYLOMA

Genital warts caused by human papilloma virus (HPV types 6 and 1) also called condyloma acuminata in children can be acquired during birth from an infected mother, through hand contact from the parents, or by sexual abuse. The vulva is usually affected. In newborns, spontaneous regression is the rule. In older children, local destruction can be done but it will not control the viral infection; therefore, recurrences are common.

Another type of warts in children is molluscum contagiosum, another viral infection of the skin and mucous membranes, which is by the molluscum contagiosum virus. It can be acquired by skin-to-skin contact, which may occur during play, in a swimming pool, or through sexual contact.

FOREIGN BODIES

Definition

Children sometimes introduce foreign bodies in the vagina.

Presentation

Vaginal discharge may sometimes be purulent. There may be dysuria or difficulty urinating.

Diagnosis

The physical examination confirms vaginal discharge and there may be introital redness. An ultrasound of the pelvis may confirm the diagnosis.

Treatment

Extraction under general anesthesia.

FUSION OF THE LABIA MINORA

Definition

The labia minora are normally separate from each other; so that, during examination, the urethral meatus and vaginal introitus are easily seen. The fusion or synechia of the labia are commonly seen in young prepubertal girls (Figure 10-10).

Presentation

Labial fusion is often asymptomatic, which is discovered during routine examinations. The fusion normally resolves at puberty in response to endogenous estrogens. The symptoms of urinary frequency, vulvovaginitis, urinary tract infections, or post-void dripping have been attributed to this condition. When treatment is deemed necessary, topical treatment

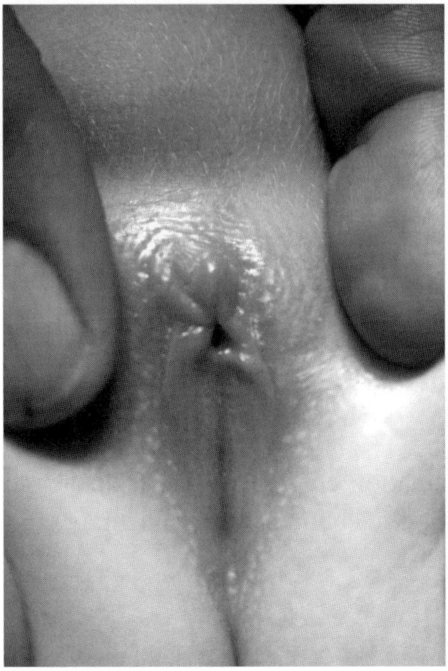

Figure 10-10. The fusion or synechia of the labia minora.

with estrogens or a steroid cream are usually effective. Surgical separation is rarely needed and it carries a high rate of recurrence.

FURTHER READING

Allouis M, *et al.* [Skène's duct cysts report of three cases in neonate (author's transation)]. *J Urol (Paris)* 1980; **86**(4):275–277.

Govindarajan M, *et al.* Magnetic resonance imaging diagnosis of Mayer-Rokitansky-Kuster-Hauser syndrome. *J Hum Reprod Sci* 2008; **1**(2):83–85.

Hillyer S, *et al.* Diagnosis and treatment of urethral prolapse in children: experience with 34 cases. *Urology* 2009; **73**(5):1008–1011.

Jones ME, *et al.* Recognizing rare disorders: aromatase deficiency. *Nat Clin Pract Endocrinol Metab* 2007; **3**(5):414–421.

Mayoglou L, *et al*. Success of treatment modalities for labial fusion: a retrospective evaluation of topical and surgical treatments. *J Pediatr Adolesc Gynecol* 2009; **22**(4):247–250.

Sarac A, Demir MK. Herlyn-Werner-Wunderlich syndrome: a rare cause of infertility. *Eur Radiol* 2009; **19**(5):1306–1308.

Chapter 11

Ambiguous Genitalia

Richard S. Hurwitz, Ricardo González,
and Barbara M. Ludwikowski

DEFINITION

The term "ambiguous genitalia" refers to external genital organs, which on examination cannot be determined to be clearly male or female. In most cases, the paediatric urologist is asked to see a newborn whose gender cannot be determined on the examination of the genitals.

This chapter describes the initial approach to the evaluation and management of children with ambiguous genitalia. Although in Western countries, most babies are seen at birth, in some parts of the world, the condition is hidden by the parents and children present later in life or adolescence posing special challenges. It must be kept in mind that there are life-threatening conditions that present with ambiguous genitalia. In these cases, prompt recognition after birth may be life-saving.

There are many other disorders of sex development (DSD), which do not present with ambiguous genitalia and will not be discussed in this chapter. For a complete discussion, the reader should consult specialised texts. In 2005, a new terminology has been proposed to designate the various types of DSD. For the purpose of clarity, whenever possible, we will give both the old and the new terminologies (Table 11-1).

Table 11-1. Proposed revised nomenclature.

Previous	Proposed
Intersex	DSD
Male pseudohermaphrodite	46, XY DSD
Female pseudohermaphrodite	46, XX DSD
True hermaphrodite	Ovotesticular DSD
XX male or XX sex reversal	46, XX testicular DSD
XY sex reversal	46, XY complete gonadal dysgenesis

CLASSIFICATION

The DSD categories associated with ambiguous genitalia include:

- 46, XX DSD, or female pseudohermaphrodite (virilisation of an XX individual),
- 46, XY DSD, or male pseudohermaphrodite (incomplete virilisation of an XY individual),
- gonadal dysgenesis,
- ovotesticular DSD or true hermaphrodite.

46, XX DSD, OR VIRILISATION OF AN XX INDIVIDUAL

The cause of virilisation of an otherwise normal female (XX karyotype) is prenatal exposure to androgenic agents. These agents can be endogenously produced by the foetus, the placenta, or the mother; alternatively, they may be exogenous in origin. Early (before the 12th gestational week) exposure to androgenic substances causes virilisation of the urethra and perineum, which leads to persistence of the urogenital sinus with fusion of the vagina and urethra, which open to the outside through a common channel (sinus). In addition, the clitoris hypertrophies whether by early or late gestation exposure to androgens. In severe cases, the urethra, may lie in the clitoris and the phallus resembles a hypospadiac or normal penis (see Chapter 10). Exposure to androgens after the 12th gestational week will lead to clitoral hypertrophy and scrotalisation of the labia majora, hyperpigmentation of the genital skin, and areolae.

The causes of virilisation of a female foetus include, in decreasing order of frequency:

- congenital adrenal hyperplasia (CAH) secondary to 21-hydroxylase deficiency,
- the intake of exogenous androgenic substances,
- the endogenous production of androgens by a maternal tumour,
- foetal-placental aromatase deficiency.

CAH Secondary to 21-Hydroxylase Deficiency

CAH represents the most common form of DSD, accounting for more than 60% of the cases. It is an autosomal recessive disorder in which the diminished activity or the lack of 21-hydroxylase (P450c21) results in the decreased production of cortisol with the accumulation of the precursors dihydro-epi-androsterone and androstenedione that have androgenic effect. The diminished production of cortisol leads to an increase in the production of ACTH by the pituitary, causing the enlargement of the adrenal glands and driving the production of precursors of cortisol with androgenic effect. In severe forms, the production of mineralocorticoids is also impaired and the condition can be life-threatening in the neonatal period. In 5% of the cases, other enzymes are involved but for the purpose of this section, we will consider only the 21-hydroxylase deficiency in females. In males, the external genitalia are normal but the metabolic effects are identical. The locus for the defective gene is 6p21.3.

The deficiency of other enzymes responsible to cortisol synthesis from cholesterol such as 11OH and 3β HSD are less frequently seen (see Figure 11-1).

Heredity

Persons affected by any form of the disease have two abnormal alleles, and both parents are usually heterozygous (or carriers). When both parents carry an abnormal allele, each child has 25% chance of having the disease, 50% chance of being a carrier like the parents, and 25% chance of having two normal genes.

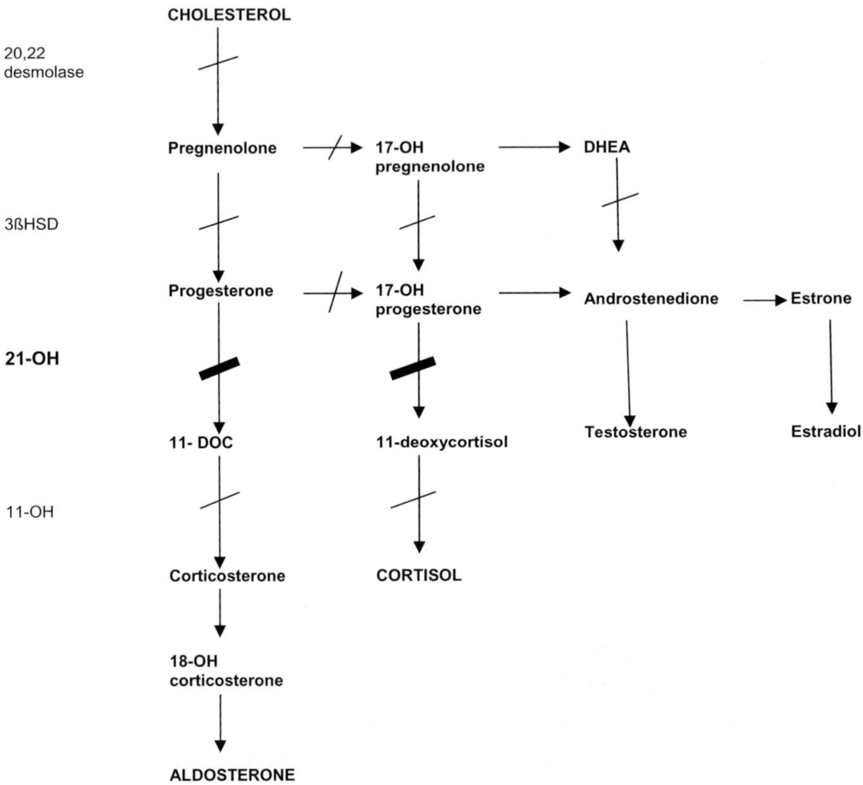

Figure 11-1. Chart depicting cortisol synthesis from cholesterol.

Presentation

The severity of the disease varies. In severe cases, salt wasting results from the lack of mineralocorticoids and in addition to having virilised external genitalia; girls in whom the condition was not suspected present with severe vomiting and dehydration in the first few weeks of life. The incidence of the salt wasting form of CAH is 1:15,000 births.

When mineralocorticoid production is sufficient to maintain normal sodium and potassium levels, the predominant clinical feature is the virilised genitalia. Five degrees of virilisation are generally recognised and classified according to Prader. In Stage 1, the clitoris is slightly enlarged and the vaginal introitus is narrow. In Stages 2 and 3, the clitoris is larger and there is a single vestibular opening (urogenital sinus). The length of the urogenital sinus (or how high the urethra and vagina join) is generally proportional to the degree of clitoral hypertrophy. In Stage 4, the genitalia resemble those of a boy with perineal or scrotal hypospadias and bilateral undescended testes. In Stage 5, the labial fusion is complete; the labial skin is rugated like the scrotum and the urethral meatus is at the glans or distal clitoral shaft resembling a penis (Figure 11-2). In all cases, there is hyperpigmentation of the genital skin. The urethra above the junction is invariably normal and the vagina may be of normal size or somewhat short. The internal genital organs are normal female.

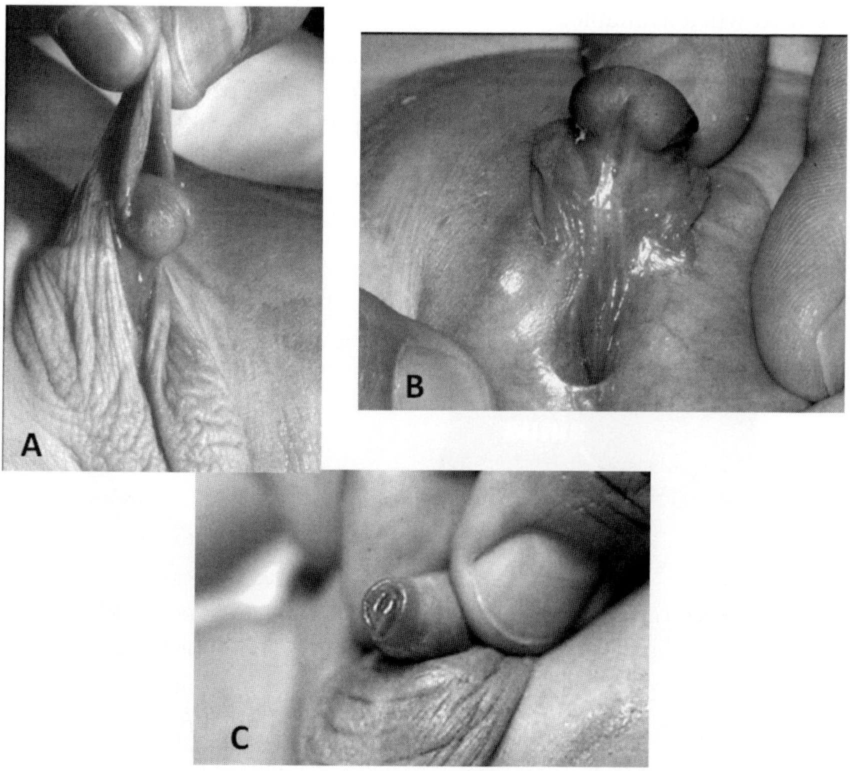

Figure 11-2. Genitals of patients with CAH. **(A)** and **(B)**: Prader IV, and **(C)**: Prader V.

The very mild forms may be overlooked at birth because of only slight virilisation and present in adolescence or adulthood with virilisation and infertility.

Diagnosis

The diagnosis of CAH should be suspected in all virilised babies without palpable gonads. Any newborn with virilised genitalia or a normal looking penis without palpable gonads should undergo an emergency evaluation including determination of 17 HO progesterone, a precursor of cortisol that reaches high levels in serum and urine when 21 OH is deficient (see Figure 11-1). A karyotype will confirm the chromosomal sex as female. The measurements of serum levels of cortisol and aldosterone should be obtained when available.

A genitogram, obtained by injecting contrast through the single opening of the urogenital sinus, will help define the anatomy. A pelvic ultrasound will reveal the presence of a uterus (Figure 11-3). The cervix uteri may be palpable on rectal examination.

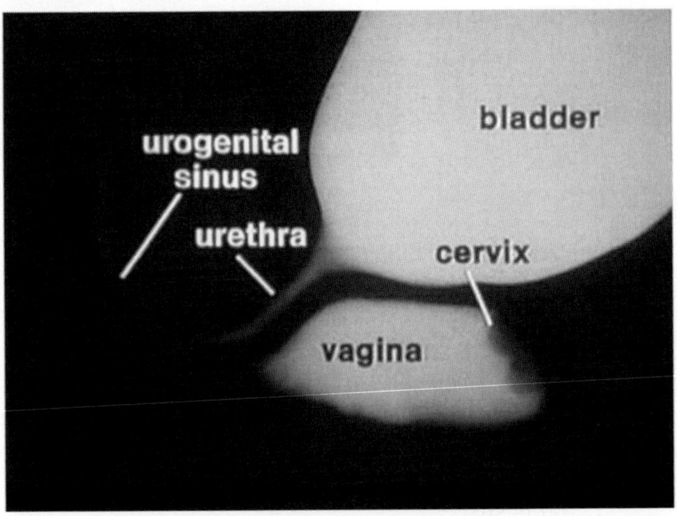

Figure 11-3. Retrograde genitogram in patient with CAH showing filling of the vagina with a cervical impression. The sinus is not demonstrated in this image.

Treatment

Gender assignment

Since females with CAH have normal sexual and fertility potentials, the gender assignment should always be female. Only the exceptional cases of extreme virilisation not recognised at birth that are raised as males who present late in childhood should be maintained in the assigned male gender.

Medical treatment

The medical management of CAH should be undertaken by the paediatric endocrinologist. Once steroid replacement therapy is established, surgical treatment should be considered.

Surgical treatment

The objectives of surgical correction are to create a feminine appearance of the external genitalia and to separate the openings of the urethra and the vagina. In cases of very large clitoris, careful clitoral reduction with the preservation of the clitoral innervation is necessary. There is some debate regarding the timing of the feminising genitoplasty. Some prefer to postpone it till puberty. On the other hand, in keeping with the guidelines used for hypospadias repair, which recommend it to be undertaken before 18 months of age, we prefer to perform the surgical correction as soon as the patient is stable from the endocrine viewpoint.

Girls who undergo vaginoplasty in infancy should be examined under anaesthesia at the onset of puberty to rule out vaginal stenosis that may cause retention of menstrual blood and difficulty with intercourse. If an introital stenosis is found, it is usually repaired with a minor operation.

Prenatal treatment

When the condition is suspected based on the family history and the diagnosis, the gender of the foetus is confirmed by molecular genetic analysis of foetal DNA. The administration of prednisone to the mother in early gestation will prevent or decrease virilisation of the foetus. Some concerns still exist regarding long-term effects on brain development.

The Intake of Exogenous Androgenic Substances

When CAH has been ruled out in a virilised female, a detailed history of the potential exposure of the mother to androgenic agents during gestation should be undertaken.

The Endogenous Production of Androgens by a Maternal Tumour

In these cases, the mother will have become virilised during gestation and the history will be available to the paediatric consultants.

Foetal-Placental Aromatase Deficiency

Aromatase (CYP19A1) is the enzyme responsible for the conversion of testosterone to oestradiol and androstenedione to oestron. The lack or diminished activity of aromatase in the placenta and a female foetus causes accumulation and high levels of the androgenic precursors of oestrogens resulting in virilisation of the foetus and the mother. The degree of masculinisation of both the foetus and the mother is variable. As opposed to the two previously described conditions, aromatase deficiency is associated with delayed puberty and infertility. Oestrogen replacement at the onset of puberty becomes necessary in most cases.

46, XY DSD OR MALE PSEUDOHERMAPHRODITE (INCOMPLETE VIRILISATION OF AN XY INDIVIDUAL)

The causes of undervirilisation of an XY individual include:

- defects in testosterone synthesis,
- defects in androgen action due to receptor deficiency,
- defects in androgen action due to 5α-reductase deficiency.

Presentation

A boy with one of the above-mentioned defects will present as an undervirilised male, with hypospadias, small size penis, and the testes although usually palpable may not be in the scrotum.

Defects in Testosterone Synthesis

The main causes include a deficit in one of the five enzymes required to convert cholesterol to testosterone, the lack of response to luteinising hormone (LH), or Leydig cell hypoplasia. The resulting low or absent levels of testosterone result in incomplete Wolffian duct development.

Although it is dihydrotestosterone (DHT) that is responsible for the virilisation of the external genitalia, the low levels of testosterone result in the lower production of DHT in the peripheral tissues with decreased or lack of virilisation.

Normal production of Müllerian inhibiting factor (MIF) results in the normal regression of the male Müllerian structures.

When testosterone is completely absent, the phenotype is female without upper vagina, uterus, tubes, or ovaries. In most cases, however, there is an incomplete virilisation of a male with hypospadias and undescended testes.

The diagnosis can be established by measuring testosterone levels in the first two months of life or by measuring testosterone levels following stimulation with human chorionic gonadotropin (HCG).

If these children are raised in the male gender, in addition to reconstructive surgery (see Chapter 19), testosterone replacement is needed to induce puberty and to maintain male sexual characteristics.

Defects in Androgen Action due to Receptor Deficiency

Abnormalities in the androgen receptor vary from *Complete androgen insensitivity* or *CAIS* (formerly known as testicular feminisation) to mild defects resulting in various degrees of undervirilisation.

In CAIS, the external genitalia are female and patients are raised as females. They usually present in childhood with inguinal hernias and an intra-abdominal testis is found during the surgical procedure or after puberty with amenorrhoea. The diagnosis may be made at birth in a phenotypic female with palpable gonads. The blood levels of testosterone and DHT are very high because the absence of receptors in the brain makes feedback inhibition impossible. The high levels of testosterone are converted partially to oestradiaol by the enzyme aromatase and breast development usually occurs at puberty.

The intra-abdominal testes are usually removed after the onset of puberty to prevent tumour development and at the same time allowing breast development. Vaginal enlargement may be needed after puberty.

Partial androgen insensitivity or *PAIS*: the phenotype ranges from a normal female with clitoromegaly, a male with hypospadias and cryptorchidism to a normal male phenotype with infertility. Former denominations for this syndrome included Reifenstein, Lubs, Gilbert-Dreyfus, and Rosewater syndromes.

The levels of testosterone and DHT are normal. In addition to undervirilisation of the external genitalia, the Wolffian structures may develop incompletely. The blood levels of testosterone, DHT, and oetradiol are elevated.

Depending on the phenotype at birth, the child may be raised as male or female. When raised as female, the testes should be removed before puberty because of the risk of malignant transformation (Table 11-2) and oestrogen replacement given. Vaginal reconstruction may become necessary after puberty.

Those individuals raised as males will need to undergo hypospadias repair, orchidopexy, and occasionally the surgical correction of gynaecomasty at puberty.

Defects in Androgen Action due to 5α-Reductase Deficiency

This disorder was formerly known as pseudovaginal perineoscrotal hypospadias. The enzyme 5α-reductase is responsible for the conversion of testosterone to DHT in the peripheral tissues. The virilisation of the foetal genitalia is dependent on the action of DHT on the androgen receptors. Testosterone itself plays no direct role; however, it only provides the

Table 11-2. Risk of germ cell malignancy according to diagnosis.

Risk group	Disorder	Malignancy risk %	Recommendation	No. patients
High	GD + Y intra-abdominal	15–30	Gonadectomy	>350
	PAIS non-scrotal	50	Gonadectomy	24
Intermediate	Turner + Y	12	Gonadectomy	43
	$17\beta-$HSD	28	Monitaor	7
	GD + T scrotal	Unknown	Biopsy and possible irradiation	0
	PAIS scrotal	Unknown	Biopsy and possible irradiation	0
Low	CAIS	2	Biopsy and possible irradiation	55
	Ovotest DSD	3	Testis tissue removal?	426
	Turner — Y	1	None	557
No	5α–Reductase	0	Unresolved	3
	Leydig cell hypoplasia	0	Unresolved	2

Abbreviations: GD: gondal dysgenesis; CAIS: complete androgen insensitivity; PAIS: partial androgen insensitivity.

substrate for the production of DHT. On the other hand, the pubertal changes of the male genitalia are effected directly by testosterone; conversion to DHT at this stage, it is not needed for further virilisation. To completely understand this disease, one must keep in mind that the virilisation of the internal genital ducts (Wolffian) depends on the ipsilateral action of testosterone and that regression of the female ductal structures (Müllerian) in the male are effected by MIF.

Depending on the degree of 5α-reductase deficiency, the phenotype ranges from normal female to various degrees of hypospadias, incompletely descended testes, and variable penile size (Figure 11-4). The

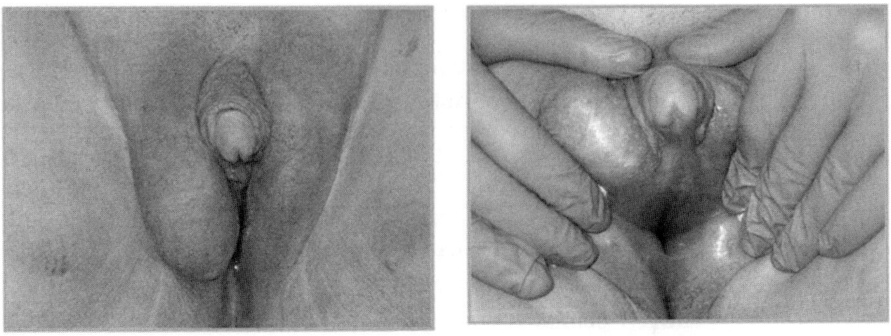

Figure 11-4. External genitalia in patient with partial androgen insensitivity.

condition is genetically transmitted and is common in the Dominican Republic where these children are often raised as girls. At puberty, under the influence of testosterone, the penis grows and patients develop male secondary sexual characteristics and usually revert to the male gender role.

The diagnosis is confirmed by an abnormally high ratio of testosterone to DHT. When raised as males, corrective surgery for the perineal hypospadias and cryptorchidism (see Chapters 18 and 19) is required.

GONADAL DYSGENESIS

These conditions include:

- mixed or asymmetrical gonadal dysgenesis,
- dysgenetic male pseudohermaphroditism,
- gonadal dysgenesis or Turner's syndrome,
- pure gonadal dysgenesis.

Mixed or Asymmetrical Gonadal Dysgenesis

This condition is characterised by the presence of ambiguous genitalia, a testis on one side and a streak gonad on the other. The karyotype is usually a 45XO/46XY mosaic, rarely can it be 46XY, other mosaic patterns are seen but a Y chromosome is always present. The streak gonad is composed of primitive gonadal tissue resembling ovarian stroma but follicles are absent.

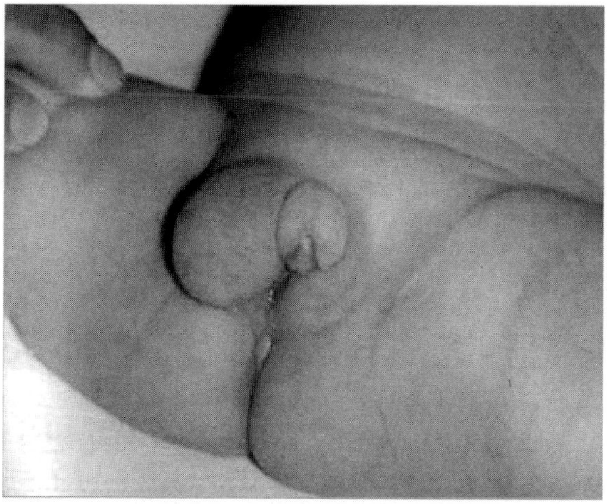

Figure 11-5. Patient with mixed gonadal dysgenesis. There is a very proximal hypospadias with a perineal open, a bifid scrotum, and a gonad in the scrotum.

The typical appearance of the genitalia is shown in Figure 11-5. There is a very proximal hypospadias with a perineal open, a bifid scrotum, and one gonad in the scrotum. About one-third of the patients have stigmata of Turner's syndrome. Adults with this condition have short stature and are invariable infertile.

Gonadal tumours develop in about 25% of cases (Table 11-2). The most common neoplasm is gonadoblastoma that can secrete sex steroids and cause hirsutism or gynaecomastia. Other tumours seen in this condition include seminomas and embryonal cell carcinoma. They occur more frequently in the testis than in the streak gonad but only when the gonad is intra-abdominal.

About 60% of the reported cases have been raised as females since the external genitalia are inadequately virilised, a uterus and a vagina are always present, fertility is not a consideration and most patients reach an adult stature of less than 150 cm.

If raised as female, early gonadectomy is recommended since tumours can develop in childhood and the testis will cause virilisation at puberty. Oestrogen replacement is necessary at puberty. The age for feminising genitoplasty is controversial.

For children with MGD raised as males, the genitalia should be surgically corrected (proximal hypospadias repair and consider the removal of Müllerian structures). All intra-abdominal gonads must be removed early with the exception of an intra-abdominal testis that is not associated with ipsilateral Müllerian structures and that can be brought down to the scrotum. Scrotal testes should be preserved.

Dysgenetic Male Pseudohermaphroditism

Patients with dysgenetic male pseudohermaphroditism share many features of MGD except that they have two dysgenetic testes instead of one testis and one streak gonad. These testes carry a high risk of tumour development and should be removed early. Both disorders share the same range of phenotypes and karyotypes. The management follow the guidelines outlined in MGD.

Gonadal Dysgenesis or Turner's Syndrome

Patients with Turner's syndrome have normal female external genitalia. It is discussed here briefly because the paediatric urologist may be consulted since horseshoe kidney is a frequent associated anomaly. The karyotypes are 45XO or 46XX/45XO. There are bilateral streak gonads with no risk of malignancy. The gonads should be removed only in cases of virilisation or if Y chromosome material is present. Other associated anomalies include short stature, webbed neck, and coarctation of the aorta. Patients not detected at birth (physical examination and webbed neck) present later in life with primary amenorrhoea.

Pure Gonadal Dysgenesis

In pure gonadal dysgenesis, the karyotype may be 46XX or 46XY. There is a normal female phenotype. In contrast with Turner's syndrome, the neck is not webbed and patients reach a normal stature. The gonads are bilateral and carry a high incidence of malignancy (Table 11-2) and should be removed. Although the Müllerian structures are present, the patients present with primary amenorrhoea.

OVOTESTICULAR DSD OR TRUE HERMAPHRODITE

The main feature of this condition is the presence of both ovarian and testicular tissues. In one-fifth of the cases, there are bilateral ovotestes; in two-fifth, a unilateral ovotestis and contralateral ovary or testis; and in another two-fifth, there is an ovary on one side and a testis on the other. The karyotypes found in ovotesticular DSD include: 46XY in 58%; 46XX/46XY in 13%; 46XY in 12%; and other mosaics in the rest.

The phenotype is variable including all gradations from male to female. The internal ductal system corresponds to the ipsilateral gonad. Most patients develop breast enlargement at puberty and 50% menstruate but fertility is rare. The incidence of gonadal tumours is 2.6% (see Table 11-2).

Neonatal gender assignment should be according to the appearance of the external genitalia but this remains controversial.

LATE PRESENTATION OF DSD

Although most cases of DSD are suspected and diagnosed shortly after the birth, the late presenting cases are occasionally encountered. Here, we list the main forms of late presentation DSD:

- previously unrecognised genital ambiguity,
- inguinal hernia in a female,
- delayed or incomplete puberty,
- virilisation in a female,
- primary amenorrhoea,
- breast development in a male,
- cyclic haematuria in a male,
- scrotal mass in a male with hypospadias.

INDICATIONS FOR LAPAROSCOPY AND GONADAL BIOPSY

Laparoscopy (or exploratory laparotomy) and gonadal biopsies are indicated in the following conditions:

- ovotesticular DSD,
- mixed gonadal dysgenesis,
- XY DSD with intraabdominal testes.

SUMMARY

We have discussed the main instances of DSD presenting with genital ambiguity. Patients with these conditions must be evaluated and treated using a multidisciplinary approach along with neonatologists, endocrinologists, geneticists, and ethicists. The potential liability and harm to the child that results from making a wrong decision will be minimised this way.

In the last few years, some patient advocacy groups have made recommendations that at times have been extreme in their opposition to surgical procedures to correct the ambiguity. These opinions, unsupported by data, have changed the way DSD is approached. Nevertheless, we should remember that the majority of cases of DSD are girls with CAH with a normal potential for successful female gender role, sexual function, and fertility. There seems to be no reason to vary from the classical treatment guidelines in this population.

FURTHER READING

Jednak R, Ludwikowski B, González R. Total urogenital mobilization. *J Urol* 2001; **165**(Part 2):2347–2349.

Mieszczak J, Houk CP, Lee PA. Assignment of the sex of rearing in the neonate with a disorder of sex development. *Curr Opin Pediatr* 2009; **21**:541–547.

Nimkarn S, Lin-Su K, New MI. Steroid 21 hydroxylase deficiency congenital adrenal hyperplasia. *Endocrinol Metab Clin North Am* 2009; **38**(4):699–718.

Vos AA, Bruinse HW. Congenital adrenal hyperplasia: do the benefits of prenatal treatment defeat the risks? *Obstet Gynecol Surv* 2010; **65**(3):196–205.

Chapter 12

Pediatric Genitourinary Trauma

Lisandro A. Piaggio

The increasing incidence of motor vehicle accidents (MVA) involving children in the last 50 years makes trauma, which is the leading cause of death in children older than one year, the leading cause of morbidity in all age groups in Western countries. Trauma to the urinary tract is second only to trauma of the nervous system in childhood injuries.

Lesions to the kidneys and urinary tract can present as isolated lesions, or more often, associated to multiple organ injuries. The initial management of the genitourinary trauma (GUT) is common to all traumatized patients and consists in patient resuscitation and stabilization. For initial attention of pediatric trauma, see specific bibliography. In this chapter, I will discuss specific features of the GUT. For practical purposes, I will divide in upper urinary tract (UUT): kidneys and ureters; lower urinary tract (LUT): bladder and urethra; and external genital lesions.

ETIOLOGY

Most GUT is secondary to MVA and falls. Small children are more commonly injured as pedestrians struck by a vehicle and older children and adolescents as passengers in an MVA. In the latter age group, participation in contact sports and assaults have gained importance in GUT.

In the initial attention of the patient, it is important to investigate the mechanisms of injury and the kinetic energy involved in it. Direct impact to the lumbar region or lower ribs, falls from height, deceleration injuries, and acute hyperextension to the lumbar vertebral column account for most of UUT lesions. Abrupt compression of the lower abdomen, especially with a full bladder in preschool age children, is responsible for most bladder ruptures. Penetrating injuries to the lower abdomen can injure the bladder. Urethral lesions are secondary to pelvic fractures after significant trauma or direct impact to the perineum. The external genitalia can be injured after direct impact (falls and sport participants) or in the context of multiple organ injury.

EVALUATION OF URINARY TRACT TRAUMA

The signs and symptoms that should make suspect urinary tract lesions after trauma are summarized in Table 12-1.

Laboratory analysis must include urinalysis to look for blood and hemoglobin. Initial blood counts would not accurately reflect blood loss, but can serve a baseline level for comparison.

Once the patient is stabilized, imaging studies should be obtained to evaluate intra-abdominal and retroperitoneal injuries. The gold standard for blunt abdominal and flank trauma today is computed tomography scanning (CT) (spiral or standard) with intravenous contrast and classification systems of these injuries are based on this technology. The main cause of death in pediatric trauma is the injuries to the central nervous

Table 12-1. Common signs and symptoms of GUT.

UUT	Skin lesions (contusions and abrasions) on lumbar region, flank, or hypogastrium
	Pain related to lower rib fractures or pelvic fractures
	Fractures of the vertebral pedicles
	Expansive flank mass and/or pain in the flank
	Tenderness on abdomen and renal fossa
	Macroscopic hematuria
LUT	Macroscopic hematuria
	Ecchymosis in the perineum in the shape of a butterfly (blood within the limits of Colles' fascia) suspect genital or pelvis bleeding
	Blood from the urinary meatus or vagina
	Inability to void
	Inability to pass a urethral catheter

system, which are usually evaluated with CT. According to the initial evaluation, the head, neck, thorax, abdomen, and pelvis can be scanned in the radiology suite and at the same time to look for visceral lesions, vascular lesions, and bone fractures and evaluate the vertebral column. CT is reliable to study UUT and associated injuries with few limitations. Solid organs such as the spleen, liver, and kidneys are best visualized, but for experienced radiologist hollow viscera lesions can be accurately diagnosed as well. Because of the relative infrequency of ureteral injuries, these lesions are often overlooked in the initial evaluation. The spiral CT is very fast and the ureters are not visualized in the first scan. A repeat scan in the excretory phase (10 minutes after the initial scan) is necessary to evaluate the ureters.

The retrograde urethrogram is the best study to image the urethra and a simple cystogram or a CT cystogram is adequate to evaluate bladder injuries. If there is any suspicious of urethral trauma (i.e. blood issuing from the urethral meatus), a retrograde urethrogram should be obtained. Once a urethral injury is ruled out, a catheter should be advanced through the urethra and the bladder is filled to distention with contrast. To make a good bladder evaluation, the amount of fluid instilled should be at least half of the estimated bladder capacity, which is in ml (age $+2$) $\times$ 30. Bladder infusion can stop once the total estimated bladder capacity is reached; voiding occurs or a total of 300 cc were instilled in a fully grown person. One should not rely on plugging an indwelling urethral catheter to get delayed CT images of the bladder with the excretion of the intravenous contrast. This may lead to misleading conclusions since, with this method, bladder distention is usually inadequate to evaluate for bladder leaks.

Ultrasonography (US) can be used to evaluate the kidneys and intra-abdominal solid organs. It is also useful to look for free intra-abdominal fluid or perinephric collections and also to evaluate the scrotal contents. Since the US machine can be taken to the bedside, is universally available, it avoids radiation, intravenous contrast, and sedation, it is ideal to get follow-up imaging studies and can be used in the shock room in the initial evaluation of the traumatized patient. In some countries, in which CT is not available on emergency basis, US continues to be the first-line imaging study for trauma evaluation. Although it is less sensitive than CT to identify UUT injuries, US can reliably show parenchyma renal fractures, renal hematomas, and urinomas, which misses only minor injuries. Doppler US can help in differentiating between vascularized (positive flow) or ischemic parenchyma or hematomas (negative flow), but it is not much reliable (low sensitivity) to determine renal pedicle injuries. Urinary collections are hypoechoic and can get echogenic sediment if they get infected (pus). Blood extravasations give mix images.

Intravenous pyelogram (IVP) can give useful information in the absence of CT scan. With lineal tomography, the kidney contour can be appreciated. Delayed or absent nephrogram on one side may be the result of renal pedicle injury. On excretory phase, calyceal or renal pelvis deformities can be appreciated as the results of tears or hematomas, and contrast material extravasations can help in the diagnosis of renal fracture and pelvic, ureteral, or bladder lesions. IVP has been mostly replaced by CT scan but still has a role in evaluating penetrating trauma to the kidney. If an unstable patient is taken immediately to the operating room before adequate imaging evaluation and nephrectomy is considered during the procedure, a one-shot IVP on the operating table is useful to document a contralateral functioning kidney.

Selective renal arteriography or venography is seldom used for the initial evaluation of trauma, but is useful to confirm renal pedicle injuries and is used in the anticipation of endovascular procedures.

BLUNT RENAL TRAUMA

The kidney is the most frequent site of GUT, which is resulting in half of all urinary system injuries. In around 10% of penetrating or blunt abdominal trauma, the kidney is injured. Kidney lesions are more common in boys than in girls (2:1). The most common type of injury to the kidney is blunt trauma (80–90%). In theory, the kidney in a child is more susceptible to blunt trauma than the kidney in an adult for several reasons (see Table 12-2). Recent studies have suggested adopting criteria similar to that of adult patients to determine what patient requires radiographic assessment.

The kidneys with congenital malformations (hydronephrosis), a baseline disease (tumors, cysts, stones), or abnormal location (pelvic kidney) are more vulnerable to blunt renal trauma than the normal kidneys. The

Table 12-2. Susceptibility of children to kidney injuries compared to adult.

Susceptibility to trauma	Larger kidney in proportion to body size Lower projection beyond the rib cage
Failed to provide a rigid protection	Ribs are more flexible
Less rigid support	Less development of abdominal and trunk muscles
Less buffer to injuries	Less retroperitoneal and peritoneal fats

incidence of congenital malformations in series of blunt renal injuries varies in different reports from 4 to 23%. Blunt renal injuries in children are seldom isolated (80% had other associated organ injuries). Surveys of renal trauma in children reveal associated liver or spleen injuries in 46%, closed head injuries in 35%, and orthopedic fractures in 21%.

Hematuria is a reliable sign of GUT lesion. Although there are situations (<3%) of significant UUT lesions that can initially present without hematuria such as complete ureteropelvic disruptions and renal pedicle injuries to the vessels, these situations — especially the last one — seldom present alone demanding imaging studies for complete patient assessment. Although hematuria will be present in the great majority of patients with renal lesions, the degree of hematuria does not correlate well with the severity of the injury. Only around one-third of the patients with gross hematuria after blunt renal trauma had a major renal injury and eventually a minor renal contusion may present with gross hematuria (see "rule of thirds" in Table 12-3). Clear urine alone cannot be used to decide which patients need evaluation for renal trauma. It is important to consider the history of injury, physical examination, consciousness of the child, and potential associated lesions. Radiographic imaging is recommended in all adult blunt trauma patients who present with either gross hematuria or hypotension. The child's superior ability to support blood pressure in the face of hypovolemia, compared to adults, makes hypotension an unreliable predictor of renal injury. Some authors recommend imaging studies in every child with significant blunt abdominal trauma and any degree of hematuria. Others suggest observation with bed rest for children with microhematuria and normal vital signs without CT scans.

Table 12-3. Rule of the thirds for hematuria after blunt renal trauma: only a third of patients with gross hematuria after blunt renal trauma will have a major renal injury; severe renal lesions will present with microhematuria in a third of patients and a third of patients with minor renal contusions will have gross hematuria.

General blunt trauma	Gross hematuria with major renal injuries	32%	1/3
Severe renal lesions	Gross hematuria	65%	2/3
	Microhematuria	32.7%	1/3
	No hematuria	2.3%	
Minor renal contusions	Gross hematuria	31%	1/3
	Microhematuria	66%	2/3
	No hematuria	3.4%	

Table 12-4. Current recommendations to get CT scan to detect UUT lesions.

- Gross hematuria,
- Microhematuria of more than 50 red blood cells per high power field associated with shock (systolic blood pressure < 90 mmHg),
- Blunt abdominal trauma with shock,
- Penetrating trauma and hematuria,
- Rapid deceleration injury or high velocity injury:
  - MVA at high speed,
  - pedestrian struck by bicycle or motor vehicle,
  - fall from height higher than 4.5 m,
  - direct impact on the abdomen or flank by a foreign body (baseball bat, helmet, etc.),
- Trauma that causes peritoneal signs; fractures of ribs, vertebral column, pelvis, or femur; or hematoma in the flank or perineum.

Eventually these patients can also be screened with US. The more conservative approach is justified with the fact that 80% of renal injuries are contusions and their detection may alter neither treatment nor outcome and a more severe damage is associated with significant trauma that will demand imaging studies. Current criteria to obtained imaging studies (CT) to detect lesions of UUT are summarized in Table 12-4.

The depth of the parenchymal tear into the kidney defines the stages of renal injury, as does the involvement and injury of the collecting system. The most severe forces cause the most severe injuries, such as shattered kidneys and renovascular injuries. The two more spread classifications of renal injury are the organ injury scale of the American Association for the Surgery of Trauma (Table 12-5) and the radiologic classification of renal injury (RCRI) (Figure 12-1). They are useful in differentiating the severity of the injury, but not in determining management.

Treatment of Blunt Renal Trauma

Contusions and minor lacerations are treated with bed rest until the gross hematuria or symptoms resolve. If there is pain and nausea, intravenous fluids are administered as necessary. Follow-up imaging studies are

Table 12-5. American Association for the Surgery of Trauma Classification System for Renal Injuries.

Grade 1 injuries:

- hematuria with normal imaging,
- contusions, and
- subcapsular and non-expanding hematoma without parenchymal laceration.

Grade 2 injuries:

- non-expanding perinephric hematomas confined to the retroperitoneum, and
- renal cortical lacerations less than 1 cm in depth without urinary extravasation.

Grade 3 injuries:

- renal cortical lacerations greater than 1 cm in depth without urinary extravasation.

Grade 4 injuries:

- parenchymal laceration extending through renal cortex/medulla and into collecting system,
- main renal artery or vein injury with contained hemorrhage, and
- segmental infarction without associated laceration.

Grade 5 injuries:

- shattered or devascularized kidney,
- complete avulsion or thrombosis of main renal artery or vein, and
- ureteropelvic junction avulsion.

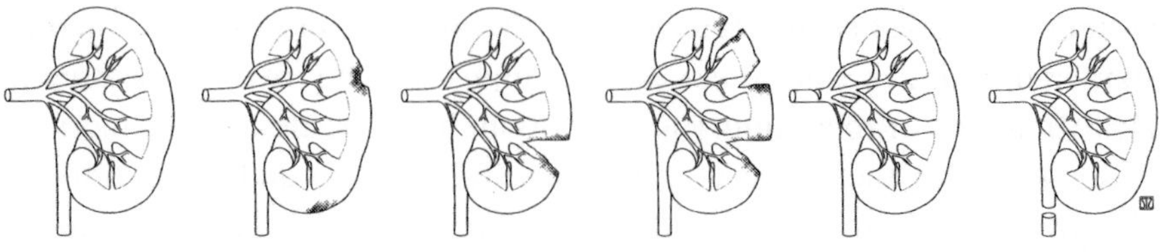

Figure 12-1. Classification of renal trauma. Renal injuries can be classified into four large categories based on imaging findings. **Category I**: renal injuries include minor cortical contusion, subcapsular hematoma, minor laceration with limited perinephric hematoma, and small cortical infarct. **Category II:** lesions include major renal lacerations extending to the medulla with or without the involvement of the collecting system and segmental renal infarct. **Category III:** lesions are catastrophic renal injuries and include multiple renal lacerations and vascular injury involving the renal pedicle. **Category IV:** injuries are ureteropelvic junction injuries.

usually unnecessary. With more severe lacerations (Grades II and III of RCRI), bleeding can be extensive and forming a large perinephric hematoma. If Gerota's fascia is intact, the bleeding may be tamponaded by the hematoma and the patient may stabilize. Repeated transfusions may be necessary if the bleeding persists, but shock is uncommon in children with isolated renal injuries. These patients need bed rest until pain and hematuria clear and imaging shows stabilization of the injury. Careful monitoring with blood counts and vital signs is mandatory.

With wide separation of the lacerated fragments (shattered kidney), there is massive bleeding and urine extravasation often filling the limits of Gerota fascia. The segments usually retain their blood supply and remain viable healing together in good alignment. Some authors advocate early repair and debridement of any devascularized segment, but this approach is controversial since it may end in an increase rate of nephrectomies. I recommend conservative approach unless the patient is hemodynamically unstable. Indications for surgery include persistent bleeding into an expanding or unconfined hematoma, massive urinary extravasation, and complete ureteropelvic disruptions. Non-massive urinary extravasations are better managed non-operatively, but if they do not begin to resolve by five days, some intervention is indicated (percutaneous drainage, ureteral stent, or both). In most series of children with blunt renal trauma, the majority of patients are successfully managed non-operatively, even with the most severe injuries. A small percentage (4%) initially originally treated non-operatively may require later surgery.

Renovascular Injuries

Renovascular injuries occur in 1 to 3% of all blunt renal traumas. They present with no hematuria since the parenchyma is usually not traumatized. The mechanism of injury is rapid deceleration of the kidney and stretching of the renal artery causing tearing of the intima, flaps raising, and secondary thrombosis (tunica media and adventitia are more elastic than the endothelium), which is ultimately leading to clotting of the artery and ischemia of the kidney. They are evidenced by CT by the lack of kidney perfusion (Figure 12-2). If possible, the patient should be taken immediately for surgical exploration and repair, but this is seldom the case since these patients present with multiple traumas and are frequently unstable. If the kidney has not been perfused for more than six hours, probably not

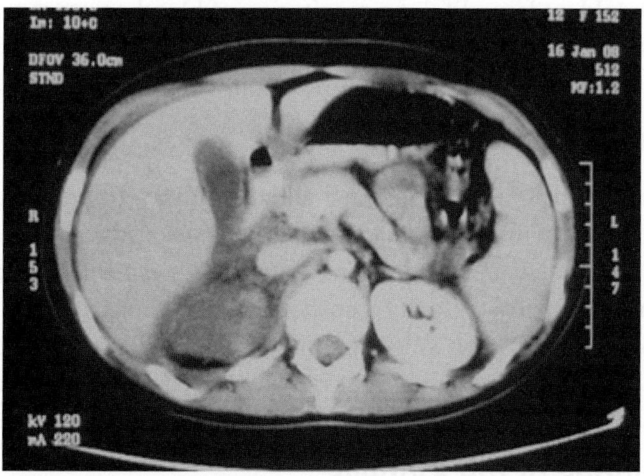

Figure 12-2. Contrast CT evidence — the lack of kidney perfusion of the right kidney after blunt abdominal trauma in a nine-year-old girl. Note the left renal artery extending from the aorta in this image (From: Dr. Julio Pratessi, Hospital es Dr. Andrés Isola, Puerto Madryn, Chubut, Argentina).

survive even with successful surgical repair. Full-thickness tears of the artery and vein are rare, require immediate surgery and have a very high mortality.

Complications of Blunt Renal Trauma

Complications are rare in the majority of blunt renal trauma, but in patients with severe renal lacerations and renal fractures can raise up to 30%, including hemorrhage, hypertension, urinoma, infection of hematoma or urinoma, and hydronephrosis. Increasing abdominal pain, fever, nausea, and hypotension or hypertension are the indications for follow-up imaging studies after blunt renal trauma regardless of the initial renal injury grade.

Delayed complications of blunt renal trauma in addition of the former are calculi, pseudoaneurysms, renal scars, and the loss of renal function. Devascularized renal segments or entire kidneys should only be removed if they cause problems, but this is seldom the case.

Functional loss in the damaged kidney may be progressive over time in the case of severely traumatized kidneys and probably is proportional to the grade of the original injury. Children who sustain significant injuries should undergo lifelong monitoring of blood pressure and routine urinalysis to look for proteinuria owing to renal deterioration.

Penetrating Renal Trauma

Penetrating renal injuries are almost all stab injuries or gunshot wounds. Although not as common as in adults, these types of lesions are seen with increased frequency in the pediatric patients — especially adolescents. Stab wounds and low-velocity gunshot wounds cause precise localized trauma to the kidney. High-velocity gunshot wounds cause damage at a considerable distance from the point of impact that can progress over time.

Stab Injuries of the Kidneys

In all stabbings that could potentially injure the kidney — in the lateral abdomen, flank, or lateral back — the kidney is damaged in only 15%.

The highest risk of injury to the kidney occurs when the patient is stabbed in the flank between the anterior and the posterior axillary lines, and reduces significantly with stabbings in the abdomen or back. Most renal stab wounds cause minor kidney injury. Associated organ trauma (liver, spleen, and colon) are found in 12–43% of patients. Hematuria is present in most patients with stab injuries to the kidneys, but as in blunt renal trauma, the degree of hematuria does not correlate well with the severity of the injury.

The imaging studies and management are similar than in blunt renal trauma. Since the separation of renal parenchyma is rare, CT imaging is not as helpful as in blunt renal trauma. IVP can demonstrate urinary extravasation. Angiography has been useful as a therapeutic tool to control bleeding with angiographic embolization. If available, it is the treatment of choice to stop bleeding in the stable patient with a high success rate. The complications of angiographic embolization are rare but include kidney loss.

In a stable patient with no active bleeding or persistent urinary extravasations, non-operative management is adequate, but around 40% of the patients with renal stab injuries will require surgical treatment. Indications for initial surgical intervention include the signs of associated intra-abdominal injuries such as peritonitis and hemodynamic instability. The common complications of penetrating trauma to the kidneys are secondary hemorrhage and vascular fistulas.

Gunshot Injuries of the Kidney

Gunshot wounds produce much more local kidney injury than stab wounds and are more likely to produce associated organ injuries (>90%). The signs of renal injury are the same as with stab injuries and include flank tenderness, flank mass, and hematuria. CT scan is necessary to evaluate all gunshot wounds that might involve the kidney, but 25% of patients may require emergency surgery before adequate imaging. In selected patients, renal gunshot wounds can be managed nonoperatively, but a larger proportion of patients will require surgical exploration compared with stab injuries and blunt trauma.

Sports Participation and Renal Injury

Although feared, team sports such as football and hockey, are rare causes of significant renal injuries and not associated with kidney loss. The most common sport causing blunt renal injury is bicycle riding. Other sports reported to have cause kidney loss are sledding, skiing, and rollerblading. The current recommendations of the American Academy of Pediatrics Committee on Sports Medicine and Fitness prohibiting children with a solitary kidney from participating in contact sports appear to be overly protective and need to be re-evaluated.

Retroperitoneal Hematomas

Emergency laparotomy in the case of severe trauma is indicated in the hemodynamically unstable patient. In these patients, the lack of preoperative imaging studies makes the finding of a retroperitoneal hematoma a decision challenge. In this scenario, a single-shot IVP may be useful (see above). If the IVP shows an intact functioning kidney and the hematoma is stable, it need not be opened. Severe injuries visible on IVP, expanding or pulsatile hematomas, the hematomas of retroperitoneal zone I (midline between renal pedicles), the findings of gross hematuria, or injury from a high-velocity gunshot wound should encourage the exploration of the hematoma. Any opening of a retroperitoneal hematoma is likely to be a bloody and potentially risky experience for the patient and the kidney.

Traumatic Ureteral Injuries

Any injury to the ureter is rare. Injury to the ureter occurs from trauma and the surgical injuries resulting from pelvic surgery. Most ureteral injuries in children are due to trauma, in contrast to adults, whose ureters are more likely to sustain surgical injury.

Penetrating Ureteral Trauma

The most common type of ureteral injury is due to gunshot wounds and are accompanied by associated intra-abdominal organ injury in 97% of cases. Stab wounds with knives are the second most common cause of ureteral injury. Delay in diagnosis is common. The most reliable method to diagnose ureteral trauma is direct visualization at the time of surgery and retrograde pyelogram. Hematuria is present in only 23 to 45% of patients with ureteral injuries.

Blunt Ureteral Trauma

Blunt injury to the ureter is very rare. Almost all are avulsion of the ureter from the renal pelvis at the ureteropelvic junction. They occurred in children because of the much more flexible trunk and spinal column when compared to adults. The mechanism of injury is extreme hyperextension followed by sudden deceleration and ureteral compression against a vertebral body in the scenario of severe trauma. More than half are diagnosed when complications occur (flank and abdominal pains, nausea, and fever secondary to urinoma). Hematuria is an unreliable sign. CT signs include medial extravasation of contrast material and transverse process fractures. Retrograde pyelogram is the most sensitive examination.

Treatment of Ureteral Injuries

The conservative management of ureteral trauma has become the rule. The percutaneous drainage of urinomas and nephrostomy tube drainage have been successful in the penetrating and blunt injuries of the ureter. The internal stenting of ureteral injuries without open surgery has also been successful.

Contusions discovered during surgical exploration do not need intervention, unless necrosis is possible. Partial lacerations of the ureter can be repaired primarily or they may be stented internally depending on their severity. Management of minor ureteral injuries is not affected by the location on the ureter.

The management of complete lacerations, avulsions, or crush injuries depends on the amount of ureter lost and the location along the ureter. If there is adequate healthy ureteral length, a primary ureteroureterostomy may be performed. If not, in a distal ureteral injury, a psoas bladder hitch, Boari flap, or nephropexy may be helpful to make a ureteroneocystostomy possible. Internal stenting and external draining are necessary in the repair of all significant ureteral injuries. If the injury is to the proximal ureter or midureter, transureteroureterostomy, autotransplantation, or ureteral replacement with bowel or appendix is the reasonable option. If the patient's general condition does not allow immediate repair, a temporary ureterostomy and delayed reconstruction is another option that provides good drainage without tubes.

Bladder Injuries

The bladder is seldom injured from suprapubic trauma, without a significant pelvic fracture, but lies in a less protected position in infants and children compared to adults. It is a more abdominal organ and lies exposed above the pubis, making it more susceptible to blunt trauma when the bladder is full. Only 10% of patients who sustain pelvic fractures have an associated bladder injury. Bladder injuries are more likely in patients who have multiple pelvic fractures, including a widened symphysis pubis and sacroiliac joint and fractures of the sacrum, iliac, and pubic rami.

The signs of bladder injury are suprapubic pain and tenderness, inability to urinate, and gross hematuria, which occur in 95% of cases. About half of the patients presenting with gross hematuria and pelvic fracture will have a bladder rupture. As with UUT trauma, LUT injuries seldom occur in isolation. The radiologic diagnosis of bladder injuries has been discussed in the evaluation of urinary tract trauma.

Bladder ruptures are described as intraperitoneal or extraperitoneal and differ in the site of injury, the mechanism of injury, and treatment. Intraperitoneal bladder rupture is more common in children because of the anatomical conditions explained above. When a child with a full bladder receives a direct impact in the lower abdomen, the acute increase in bladder pressure causes a rupture at the dome, where the bladder is not contained by the bony pelvis and is weaker. Since the bladder dome is covered by peritoneum, a tear in this area results in a communication with the peritoneal cavity. A third of bladder ruptures are caused by this mechanism of injury. They are commonly seen in MVAs when the child is wearing a lap seat belt. The urine is absorbed by the peritoneum causing nitrogen and creatinine, and sometimes potassium and sodium to increase in serum chemistry after a few hours of the injury. These findings are not seen with extraperitoneal bladder ruptures. It is widely accepted that if the urine is sterile, the signs of peritoneal irritation such as guarding and rebound are not as patent as in the case of rupture of a hollow viscera, but this has not always been my experience. The child usually presents in acute distress with abnormal abdominal findings on physical examination. Even after several hours of the injury, the child is not toxic and there are no signs of sepsis, but there is usually a moderate increase in body temperature and white blood counts. In addition, fever can occur.

The standard treatment of intraperitoneal bladder rupture consists of urgent surgical exploration, primary repair, and the irrigation of the peritoneal cavity. Drainage of the bladder with a suprapubic tube or a urethral catheter is mandatory. A peritoneal drain is left according to surgeon preference but can be avoided. Historically, the standard of the care of bladder surgery drainage has been suprapubic tube placement, but urethral catheters can be equally effective and safe. I believe that in a stable patient laparoscopic exploration to confirm diagnosis, looking for the associated injuries and bladder repair is the treatment of choice. More conservative treatments such as urethral catheter drainage and percutaneous peritoneal tube insertion under ultrasound guidance or bladder drainage alone have been reported to be successful with minimal morbidity. Delayed surgical repair may be necessary in some patients.

Extraperitoneal bladder rupture occurs almost exclusively with associated pelvic fractures. The cystogram reveals the extravasation of contrast material confined to the pelvis in a flame pattern. They are treated nonoperatively with urethral catheter drainage for 7 to 10 days. If there are bone fragments noted within the bladder, surgical exploration to removed them and debridement of non-viable tissue may be necessary. Complications such as bladder calculi, vesicocutaneous fistulas, persistent extravasation, and sepsis can occur.

Penetrating trauma secondary to gunshot wounds or stabbing is not common in children. Mortality secondary to extra-urinary injuries (rectosigmoid, small bowel, and iliac vessels) is high. Surgical exploration is necessary to treat associated injuries, the debridement of non-viable tissue, and bladder repair.

URETHRAL INJURIES

Urethral injuries are rare, since they need a high-energy trauma, such as when a pedestrian is struck by a motor vehicle. The bones of the pelvis and soft tissue of the perineum protect the posterior urethra, which is injured almost exclusively with pelvic fractures. Ten percent of pelvic fractures result in urethral injury. The types of pelvic fractures associated with urethral lesions are pubic arch (straddle) fractures combined with diastasis of the sacroiliac joint. The bulbous urethra injuries from straddle trauma such as falls onto a fixed object with one leg on either side, which occur with bicycles and fences. With this mechanism of injury, the urethra is crushed against the pubic rami. Since the urethra is not disrupted, usually, there is no extravasation of urine. Stenosis of bulbous urethra is found in horse riders and cycle riders because of repeated microtrauma to the posterior urethra. Penile urethral lesions are rare since its mobility protects it from injury; they are associated with other external genital injuries.

The most common clinical findings in patients with urethral injuries are gross hematuria or blood at the urethral meatus (Table 12-1). Occasionally, a patient may present with a full bladder and an inability to urinate. On physical examination, there can be perineal/scrotal swelling and ecchymosis resulting from extravasation of blood. The bleeding limited to the perineum within the limits of Colles' fascia in bulbous urethral injuries causes a classic butterfly pattern in the perineum. Digital rectal examination is also important and can reveal an absent or "high-riding" prostate with complete disruption of membranous urethra. If any of the above findings are noted on presentation, a retrograde urethrogram is indicated (Table 12-6). These classic findings may not be present initially and the possibility of a urethral injury is appreciated only after the trauma team is unable to place a urethral catheter.

Posterior Urethral Injuries

The membranous urethra connects the prostatic urethra above the pelvic floor with the bulbous urethra below it. It is fixed to the bony ring and is the portion of the urethra constantly injured with pelvic ring fractures. It

Table 12-6. Indications for retrograde urethrography after GUT.

- Blood at the urethral meatus,
- Inability to urinate,
- Perineal/scrotal ecchymosis,
- After blunt trauma to the penis gross hematuria or one of the above,
- Abnormal digital rectal examination,
- Penetrating trauma to the external genitalia, and
- Inability to place a urethral catheter after any kind of trauma.

can be lacerated or more commonly totally disrupted according to the severity of injury. Children can also have lacerations of the prostatic urethra and the disruption of the urethra at the bladder neck that does not occur in adults since these portions of the urethra are protected by the mature prostate. The hematoma and urinoma were formed after the injury forced the bladder away from the pelvic floor increasing the gap between the urethral edges. If the bladder neck is intact, the bladder may retain urine and become distended. If the bladder neck is injured, urine usually leaks out continuously and the bladder appears empty.

Evaluation of Urethral Injuries

Patients with pelvic fractures suspected to have urethral injuries have been involved in severe trauma and usually are unstable. Rectal examination to determine the position and fixation of the prostate should be performed after initial assessment in the emergency room. A retrograde urethrogram should be obtained before a urethral catheter is attempted if there is any suspicious of urethral injury (Table 12-6). Difficulty in passing a urethral catheter in a traumatized patient is an indication for radiologic evaluation of the urethra. If there is urinary retention and bladder emptying that are imperative before correct radiologic evaluation can be performed, a percutaneous suprapubic tube should be placed. The same scenario in the operating room can be managed with cystoscopic assistance for urethral catheter placement as well. If a catheter has been placed previously into the bladder, and urethral trauma is in question, the catheter should not be removed. A small feeding tube can be placed in the distal urethra along the bladder catheter and contrast material can be injected to outline the urethra for injury.

Management of Urethral Injuries

Bulbous urethral injuries are often uncomplicated by associated injuries and involve either observation or urethral catheter drainage. They may present later as a stricture in the injury site if it was not adverted at initial evaluation. Membranous urethral injuries are best managed with suprapubic catheter drainage and late urethral reconstruction since the patient is often unstable because of associated lesions. Immediate surgical repair of these injuries resulted in significant bleeding and high rates of incontinence and impotence, although it is recognized now that these sequelae are a result of the initial lesion and not secondary to the surgical repair. Injuries involving the bladder neck may be repaired to avoid secondary healing and fibrosis that can compromise the continence mechanism.

The better results of different reconstruction are obtained with urethral termino-terminal anastomosis. Excising the fibrotic scarred tissue to obtain vital ends of urethra in the area that is difficult to access is a challenge. It can be performed either through the perineum, transpubic approach, or combinations. The 10–30% of strictures that form postoperatively usually responds to dilation or endoscopic urethrotomy. Continence rate with this approach is above 90%, but unfortunately impotence is still very common.

Primary urethral realignment within a few hours of the injury is a viable option. It is performed by passing a catheter through the injured segment usually with the aid of an open cystostomy; with catheters, sounds, or the use of endoscopy. Even stricture develops in the majority of patients after catheter removal, proponents of this approach argued that the management of these strictures is easier than with initial diversion and delayed repair; with better or similar numbers in potency and continence rate. The patient suitable to this therapy is the one stable after trauma or that one going to the operating room for other treatment. If catheter cannot be passed, a suprapubic tube is left for delayed repair. Podesta (1997) recommends urethral realignment only in three situations: simultaneous bladder neck injury (with concomitant repair of bladder neck), associated rectal injury, and the incomplete rupture of posterior urethra.

The worst results occur in patients with prostatic urethra and bladder neck injuries, regardless of initial management. The 10–15% mortality rate in this group of patients underlines the multiple associated organ injury.

Injuries of the Female Urethra

Isolated injuries to the female urethra are rare. They are secondary to severe pelvic fractures and extensive soft tissue injuries to the vulva and vagina commonly after MVA. They are more common in girls than women. The vagina is usually injured at the same time. Common findings are vaginal bleeding, labial edema, and vulvar hematoma. Long-term urinary tract symptoms and sexual dysfunction are common.

Indications to investigate a urethral injury in a girl are similar than in boys (Tables 12-1 and 12-6). Concurrent bladder ruptures are common. A voiding study is necessary to rule out urethral injury since static cystograms may miss the lesion. If the bladder neck is intact, and a catheter can be placed through the urethra, initial management can be non-operative. If a catheter cannot be placed from the meatus, the same options are available as in boys.

SCROTAL TRAUMA

The scrotum and testicles can be subjected to both blunt and penetrating injuries. The physical examination can vary tremendously from a small area of ecchymosis to massive swelling and discoloration because of extensive hemorrhage. We recommend scrotal exploration in all cases where there is a large hematocele or the rupture of the tunica albuginea. Scrotal ultrasound can be used as an adjunct to the physical examination. This may reveal a heterogeneous appearance of the testicular parenchyma, suggestive of intratesticular hemorrhage, or the disruption of the tunica. If the ultrasound is inconclusive, one should still proceed with exploration if the physical examination is grossly abnormal.

PENILE INJURIES

The most common injury to the penis in the pediatric age is excessive skin loss secondary to circumcision. It, usually, can be managed conservatively with wound care and antibiotic ointments. Total penile denudation and glands or partial penile amputation should be treated immediately with surgery on a case bases. Total skin graft and primary penile or glands anastomosis with microsurgery have been described to be successful.

Accidental penile strangulation with human hair or a thread can occur in boys, especially while they are still on diapers. Since the baby usually is not in distress can be unadvertised until significant swelling develops. Careful examination is essential for a correct diagnosis since the edema can camouflage the constrictor agent that is usually at the penile base. The removal of the constrictor agent in the office is usually successful. If there is any doubt that the agent has been totally removed, immediate examination and treatment under anesthesia should be performed to prevent penile necrosis.

Domestic animal attacks are the severest form of penile lesions, since they usually course with tissue destruction and bacterial contamination. They should be treated with immediate surgical debridement and repair and broad spectrum antibiotics.

Straddle injuries with the seat toilette can occur in boys. They cause severe pain and rarely hematuria. If the patient is able to void after the trauma, it can be managed medically. If there is suspicion of urethral rupture, a retrograde urethrogram should be obtained. In the rare event that urine extravasations is demonstrated, a catheter placement under cystoscopic or radioscopic guidance should be placed.

GENITAL LESIONS IN GIRLS

Small tears or lacerations around the vaginal introitus, periurethral area, or the labia minora are common after straddle injuries. They may bleed profusely; but usually, they are superficial and commonly the bleeding has stopped before the arrival of a urologist for consultation. On the contrary, gentle pressure for a few minutes with wet sponges help in bleeding autolimitation. Patient cooperation and good light are essential to get a good perineal examination. Usually, the patient is very anxious and fears of feeling pain during examination or may be embarrassed and uncooperative. If a proper examination cannot be obtained, I have found sedation in the emergency room to be useful, especially if suturing a small wound with local anesthesia is anticipated. This is not necessary in the majority of cases. When examining the perineum, the clots should be removed with irrigation or gentle traction. If only superficial lesions are found, medical treatment with sit bath, ice packs, and non-steroidal anti-inflammatories are enough for healing. These lesions, usually, leave imperceptible scars. Bed rest is recommended for a few days until bleeding and secretions have completely stopped. Antibiotics are not necessary. If there is concern about an extensive lesion that may need surgical repair or impossibility to get an adequate examination, the patient should be taken to the operating room for examination under anesthesia. In cases of penetrating trauma, a voiding cystourethrography to rule out urethral and bladder injuries should be performed accordingly. On rectal examination, the indemnity of rectal walls and perineal muscles and anal sphincter tone should be checked. In cases of associated rectal injuries and in any other case of GUT and rectal injury, a protective colostomy to divert stool and broad-spectrum antibiotics are mandatory.

The possibility of sexual abuse must always be kept in mind when examining children with perineal trauma. When the details of the history do not match with physical findings or there is a history of repeated injury or associated genital or anal condylomata, an experienced sexual abuse team or social service should be consulted.

COMMENT FROM THE EDITORS

This comprehensive review of GUT leaves us with important messages. First, the management of trauma requires a team approach since many injuries involve many organ systems. Second, one should strive to be as conservative as possible with renal trauma while most bladder injuries require surgical repair. Regarding membranous urethral lesions associated with pelvic trauma, attempts at realignment should be left to the experts, who are seldom available in the acute situation. Placement of a suprapubic cystostomy leaving the urethral lesion intact and later seeking advice from experts seem the most prudent course of action in most cases.

FURTHER READING

Brown S, Elder J, Spirnak J. Are pediatric patients more susceptible to major renal injury from blunt trauma? A comparative study. *J Urol* 1998; **160**:138–140.

Brown S, Hoffman D, Jp S. Limitations of routine spiral computerized tomography in the evaluation of blunt renal trauma. *J Urol* 1998; **160**:1979–1981.

Casale A. Urinary tract trauma. In: *Pediatric Urology* (eds.) J Gearhart, R Rink, P Mouriquand. Philadelphia: Saunders, 2010, pp. 720–736.

Federle M. Evaluation of renal trauma. In: *Clinical Urography* (ed.) H Pollack Philadelphia: Saunders, 1989, pp. 1422–1494.

Husmann D. Diagnostic techniques in suspected bladder injury. In: *Traumatic and Reconstructive Urology* (ed.) J Mcaninch. Philadelphia: Saunders, 1996, pp. 262–273.

Husmann D. Pediatric genitourinary trauma. In: *Campbell-Walsh Urology* (eds.) A Wein, L Kavoussi, A Novick, A Partin, C Peters. Philadelphia: Saunders, 2007, pp. 3929–3945.

Jankowski J, Spirnak J. Current recommendations for imaging in the management of urologic traumas. *Urol Clin N Am* **33**:365–376, 2006.

Johnson B, Christensen C, Dirusso S, Choudhury M, *et al.* A need for reevaluation of sports participation recommendations for children with a solitary kidney. *J Urol* 2005; **174**(2):686–689.

Kawashima A, Sandler C, Corl F, West O, *et al.* Imaging of renal trauma: a comprehensive review. *RadioGraphics* 2001; **21**:557–574.

Livne PM, Gonzales ET. Genitourinary trauma in children. *Urol Clin North Am* 1985; **12**:53–65.

Mayor B, Gudinchet F, Wicky S, Reinberg O, *et al.* Imaging evaluation of blunt renal trauma: diagnostic accuracy of intravenous pyelography and ultrasonography. *Pedatr Radiol* 1995; **25**(3):213–218.

Mcaleer I, Kaplan G, Losasso B. Congenital urinary tract anomalies in pediatric renal trauma patients. *J Urol* 2002; **168**:1808–1810.

Mcaleer I, Kaplan G, Scherz H, Packer M, *et al.* Genitourinary trauma in the pediatric patient. *Urology* 1993; **42**(5):563–567.

Morey A, Bruce J, Mcaninch J. Efficacy of radiographic imaging in pediatric blunt renal trauma. *J Urol* 1996; **156**(6):2014–2018.

Ossandron Correa F, Lesiones de Riñón, uréteres y vejiga. In: *Trauma en Pediatría: Prevención, Diangóstico y Tratamiento* (ed.) A Iñón. Buenos Aires: Librería Akadia, 2009, pp. 1017–1030.

Osman Y, El-Tabey N, Mohsen T, El-Sherbiny M. Nonoperative treatment of isolated posttraumatic intraperitoneal bladder rupture in children — is it justified? *J Urol* 2005; **173**(3):955–957.

Perez-Brayfield M, Gatti J, Smith E, Broecker B, *et al.* Blunt traumatic hematuria in children. Is a simplified algorithm justified? *J Urol* 2002; **167**(6):2543–2546.

Podesta M, Medel R, Castrera R, Ruarte A. Immediate management of posterior urethral disruptions due to pelvic fracture: therapeutic alternatives. *J Urol* 1997; **157**(4):1444–1448.

Santucci R, Langenburg S, Zachareas M. Traumatic hematuria in children can be evaluated as in adults. *J Urol* 2004; **171**:822–825.

Slaton JW, Kropp KA. Conservative management of suspected bladder rupture after augmentation enterocystoplasty. *J Urol* 1994; **152**:713–715.

Smith E, Elder J, Spirnak J. Major blunt renal trauma in the pediatric population: is a nonoperative approach indicated? *J Urol* 1993; **149**:546–548.

Snyder C. Abdominal and genitourinary trauma. In: *Pediatric Surgery* (ed.) K Ashcraft. Philadelphia: Saunders, 2000, pp. 204–216.

Chapter 13

Hypertension in Childhood

José Alberto Ramírez

INTRODUCTION

Hypertension (HTN) is defined according to the guidelines recommended by the Fourth Report on the Diagnostic, Evaluation and Treatment of High Blood Pressure in Children and Adolescents in 2004. Implicit in these recommendations are the facts that blood pressure (BP) should be measured using a mercury sphygmomanometer and, in the asymptomatic patient, the BP should be above the 95th percentile for gender, age, and height on three occasions, each separated by at least a week. Therefore, HTN in children and adolescents, in contrast to adults, is not based upon outcomes, but is derived from databases of BP obtained in healthy children. This concept carries major clinical implications since there is the need for long-term studies in the prehypertensive patient, to assess natural course and evidence of target organ involvement.

Increasing evidence shows that the presence of HTN in childhood and adolescence is not benign. There appears to be a good correlation among body mass index (BMI), HTN, left ventricular hypertrophy (LVH), and early coronary artery disease in the adolescent. In fact, in children if the essential HTN is untreated, they may have vascular injury, LVH and increased intima-media thickness of the carotid and femoral arteries) at the time of diagnosis. Because nearly one of every six Americans has or develops HTN, pediatricians can play an important role in reducing the associated long-term cardiovascular (CVS) morbidity and mortality through the early identification, evaluation, and treatment of this disorder.

DIAGNOSIS OF HTN

Accurate measurement of the BP may be difficult in children because the readings vary significantly with cuff size, patient positioning, clinical setting, equipment used (mercury sphygmomanometer versus oscillometric methods), and the training of the observer. Children > 3 years old who are seen in a medical setting should have their BP measured. The dimensions for appropriate cuff size are presented in Table 13-1.

Normal BP is defined as when systolic BP (SBP) and diastolic BP (DBP) are < 90th percentile for the height, age, and sex of the child and adolescent. The classification of BP grades in children and adolescents is shown in Table 13-2.

The reliability of the measurements of DBP is an important issue in the evaluation of BP in children. Whether to use the K4 (muffling of the Korotkoff) or the K5 sound (disappearance of Korotkoff sounds) to define

Table 13-1. Recommended dimensions for BP cuff bladders.

Age range	Width (cm)	Length (cm)	Maximum arm circumference (cm)*
Newborn	4	8	10
Infant	6	12	15
Child	9	18	22
Small adult	10	24	26
Adult	13	30	34
Large adult	16	38	44
Thigh	20	42	52

*Calculated so that the largest arm would still allow the bladder to encircle arm by at least 80%.

Table 13-2. Classification of BP grades in children.

Normal	< 90th percentile
Prehypertensive	90th to 95th, or if BP exceeds 120/80 even if < 90th percentile up to < 95th percentile*
Stage 1 HTN	95th to 99th percentile + 5 mmHg
Stage 2 HTN	> 99th percentile + 5 mmHg

*This occurs typically at 12 years old for SBP and at 16 years old for DBP.

the auscultatory DBP is controversial. Nonetheless, the current standard for defining DBP is K5, and the BP tables provided in the Task Force Report, use K5 define the 90th and 95th percentiles for DBP. BP levels for the 90th and 95th percentiles of BP for boys and girls aged 3–17 years by the percentile of height are presented in Table 13-3.

EPIDEMIOLOGY

The current prevalence of pediatric HTN, although still uncertain, is likely to be far greater than the 1% quoted in the Task Force Reports.

School-based screening studies, in an urban US public school system, have demonstrated an estimated prevalence of HTN of 9.5% after three sets of screening, in conjunction with a prevalence of obesity of 23%.

Current data estimate that the prevalence of HTN in children and adolescents is 1.0 to 4.5%. In adults aged 20 to 34 years, HTN has been described to be present in 11.4% of men and 6.4% of women. If we trust

Table 13-3. BP levels for the 90th and 95th percentiles of BP for boys and girls aged 3–17 years by percentiles of height.

Boys					Girls				
		SBP/DBP (mm Hg) percentile of Ht					SBP/DBP (mm Hg) percentile of Ht		
Age (yrs)	BP	5th	50th	95th	Age (yrs)	BP	5th	50th	95th
3	90th	100/59	105/61	109/63	3	90th	100/61	103/63	106/65
	95th	104/63	109/65	113/67		95th	104/65	107/67	110/69
6	90th	105/68	110/70	113/72	6	90th	104/68	108/70	111/72
	95th	109/72	114/74	117/76		95th	108/72	111/74	115/76
9	90th	109/72	114/75	118/77	9	90th	110/72	113/73	116/75
	95th	109/72	114/75	121/81		95th	114/76	117/77	120/79
12	90th	115/74	120/76	123/79	12	90th	116/75	119/76	122/78
	95th	119/78	123/81	127/83		95th	119/79	123/80	126/82
15	90th	122/76	127/79	131/81	15	90th	120/78	123/79	127/81
	95th	126/81	131/83	135/85		95th	124/82	127/83	131/85
17	90th	127/80	132/82	136/84	17	90th	122/78	125/80	128/82
	95th	131/84	136/87	140/89		95th	125/82	129/84	132/86

that the prevalence of HTN in the late teen years is similar to that stated throughout childhood, it makes little sense that the incidence of HTN would suddenly increase three to five folds in early adulthood.

The incidence of HTN in children may vary based upon the patient's BMI, gender, ethnicity, and family history; all of which are risk factors that should be considered in any hypertensive child or adolescent.

The risk of systolic HTN was more than a two-fold increase in overweight children (BMI >85 percentile), compared to non-overweight children. In addition, the risk of dyslipemia increased with rising BP and BMI. Obesity also promotes the development of two other CVS risk factors: glucose intolerance and diabetes type 2. An increase in the weight for length in the first six months of life was associated with higher SBP at three years of life, particularly among the infants who were thin at birth. In the United States and Canada, the prevalence of HTN and pre-HTN is greater in boys than girls.

In children, as in adults, the incidence of HTN is affected by race and ethnicity. The prevalence of HTN in children and adolescents in US national surveys was 4.6, 4.2, and 3.3% in Mexican American, black, and white children, respectively, during the study period of 1999 to 2002.

A family history of HTN is present in as many as 70 to 80% of all patients with primary also referred to as essential HTN, and in 50% of hypertensive children. In patients with essential HTN, the elevated BP is thought to result from the interaction of multiple genes and the environmental factors. The best evidence for genetic factors influencing BP values comes from BP correlations within families:

- The BP correlation is stronger between parents and children, than between spouses.
- There is no significant BP correlation between parents and adopted children.
- Most studies in twins have shown that BP correlation is stronger between monozygotic twins than dizygotic twins or siblings.

Breastfeeding may be associated with lower BP in childhood. Those who were breastfed for six months had SBP that was 1.2 mmHg lower than in the infants who had been breastfed for less than six months, or not at all.

There are data suggesting a role for low birth weight in the development of essential HTN.

DIAGNOSTIC APPROACH

The complete differential diagnosis for persistent HTN in children can be extensive. However, the more common cause of HTN in children may be categorized into a few broad categories. As the potential cause of HTN in children is often age-dependant, the differential diagnosis can be further narrowed simply by focusing on diagnoses consistent with the age of the patient. The causes of pediatric HTN by age group are shown in Table 13-4.

As a general rule, the younger the patient is, the more severe the HTN is; the more likely it is that a secondary cause for the HTN is present. When the index of suspicion is very high for an underlying cause, an exhaustive evaluation may be necessary, and primary HTN would be diagnosed by exclusion. However, an extensive and invasive battery of

Table 13-4. Causes of pediatric HTN by age group.

Age group	Causes
Newborn/Infants	Renal infarct from umbilical artery catheter Prematurity with chronic lung disease Renal or vein thrombosis Coarctation of aorta
1 to 6 years	Renal scarring from UTI Coarctation of aorta Renal artery stenosis Glomerular diseases
6 to 12 years	Glomerular diseases Renal scarring from UTI Renal artery stenosis Primary HTN CKD
>12 years	Primary HTN Glomerular diseases CKD

diagnostic studies is not always indicated or appropriate for every patient whether or not a secondary cause is suspected.

The selected information for the evaluation of pediatric HTN are:

- medications that may cause HTN,
- obesity,
- neonatal history,
- symptoms and/or signs of HTN, general and/or specific to different organs,
- family history, and
- renal or endocrine symptoms and signs.

The neonatal history of selected findings can provide important information regarding possible complications during or in the early postnatal course, such as asphyxia, the use of an umbilical artery catheter, the occurrence of a renal vein thrombosis, maternal substance abuse, disparities between upper extremity and lower extremity pulses or BPs, abdominal bruits, abnormal urinalysis findings (hematuria and proteinuria), abdominal masses (hydronephrosis/obstructive uropathy), and bronchopulmonary dysplasia.

Although the essential HTN is becoming more prevalent in children, a secondary cause should be sought, especially in the preadolescent. The evaluation is guided by the history and the physical examination findings, to identify the symptoms or signs of HTN that may direct specific evaluation and to avoid unnecessary and invasive testings. The data gathered through the history and physical examination allow the clinician to select the most appropriate laboratory investigations in the next phase of evaluation.

Biochemical and imaging studies are used to address three primary organ systems: endocrine, renal, and CVS. Although high plasma renin activity or direct renin measurements suggest renal vascular disease, a low value may be even more significant because it implies the endocrine or genetic causes of HTN.

Low renin concentrations are present in the following disorders: (a) steroidogenic enzyme defects, and (b) non-steroidal defects (monogenic HTN), where an overactivity of the epithelial sodium channel (ENaC), either as a primary or secondary effect, leads to salt retention, volume expansion, and HTN.

Although these specific disorders are uncommon, the polymorphisms of the ENaC may be common and have been implicated in promoting essential HTN. In these entities, specific therapy with amiloride, gluco corticoids, or spironolactone may normalize the BP.

Because renal disorders are among the most common causes of secondary HTN in children, many studies are used to investigate the possibility of renal parenchymal or vascular disease. Acute and chronic renal diseases may be the cause of HTN.

There is no consensus on the best modality for renal vascular imaging, except that the gold standard is digital subtraction or conventional angiography with differential renal vein renin sampling. Other imaging modalities have limitations and may fail to detect intrarenal vascular lesions. Magnetic resonance angiography, computed tomographic angiography (CTA), isotope or renal nuclear medicine scanning, and renal ultrasonography with color Doppler may provide normal results in the face of significant segmental renal arterial disease. Despite the radiation and use of intravenous contrast, CTA may be considered in a non-emergent situation in lieu of other radiologic testing such as renal ultrasound and renal scans to exclude renal vascular disease.

CVS disorders, such as coarctation of the aorta and the mid-aortic syndrome, are important and often the overlooked causes of HTN in children. Investigations such as the measurement of serum lipids and echocardiography provide essential information about key CVS risk factors to guide therapeutic intervention. For example, LVH is a major indication for antihypertensive therapy, even for patients who have only borderline high BP readings.

In cases of suspected pheochromocytoma, 24-hour urinary measurement of catecholamines (fractionated metanephrine, epinephrine, and norepinephrine) or plasma catecholamines is appropriate. For functional localization of the neural crest tissue, nuclear imaging with I^{123} or I^{132} metaiodobenzylguanidine (MIBG scan) is performed.

In the Bogalusa Heart Study, a high plasma uric acid concentration was associated with high BP readings in childhood that may persist into adulthood. Interestingly, a serum uric acid value higher than 5.5 mg/dL was found in 89% of the children who had primary HTN, but only in about 30% of those who had secondary forms of HTN. None of the controls or patients who had white-coat HTN (WCH) had elevated values. The possible mechanisms for the relationship between hyperuricemia and HTN remain unclear.

Syndromes more frequently associated with HTN are: Cushing's syndrome, adrenal hyperplasia, Liddle's syndrome, Gordon's syndrome, neurofibromatosis, hyperthyroidism, pheochromocytoma, Cohn's syndrome, Williams' syndrome (elfin facies), and Turner syndrome.

ESSENTIAL HTN

Essential HTN is most common in older children and is a diagnosis of exclusion. It is more likely present in children who are postpuberal, have a family history of HTN, are overweight or obese, or have only mild HTN (BP at or just above the 95th percentile).

SECONDARY HTN

Almost all children (98%) younger than 15 years of age have a secondary cause, whereas 75% of adolescents have essential HTN. In a Polish review, 55% of children with sustained HTN had a known secondary cause. Sixty-eight percent were renal, while endocrine and renovascular diseases were 11 and 10%, respectively. In another observational series, 67% with HTN had a renal or renovascular disease, 23% had essential HTN, and 10% had non-renal causes. Glomerulonephritis and reflux nephropathy were the most common renal cause of HTN.

WHITE-COAT HTN

WCH or isolated office HTN is defined as office BP with more than 95th percentile, with normal values outside the clinical setting. Studies suggest a prevalence as high as 35% in children being evaluated for persistently elevated "casual" BP and approximately 44% in children with a positive family history of essential HTN. The prevalence of WCH is higher when the office values reveal borderline or mild stage 1 HTN, and much lower with moderate or severe stage 2 HTN. Recently, it has been shown that the left ventricular mass index in the patients with WCH, although less than in the patients with HTN, was increased in comparison to normotensive pediatric patients, a finding previously shown in multiple adult populations. About two-thirds of the children with WCH had either LVH detected by echocardiography or SBP greater than the 95th percentile for age, height, and gender during treadmill exercise.

The evaluation of BP pattern using the ambulatory BP monitor device (ABPM) allows the identification of patients with WCH.

A word of caution regarding the interpretation of the ABPM readings is necessary. The instrument uses, most of the time, the oscillometric method to measure BP. This, however, shows higher readings (5–10 mmHg) than the mercury sphygmomanometer. As a result, using daytime ABPM measurements, HTN will be overdiagnosed when applying task force criteria. Moreover, we do not have American normative data for ABPM. We are currently using, the Central Europe guidelines, which likely measure higher than those observed in the American children and adolescents.

Besides the diagnosis of the WCH, ABPM identifies patients with "masked HTN" (those whose BP may be within normal range in the office, but persistent HTN at home) and defines the presence of "dipping". In normal individuals, BP at night drops by 10–20%, when compared with the mean daytime readings. A large percentage of patients with essential HTN show "dipping", whereas all patients with secondary HTN do not.

SEVERITY OF HTN

The combination of the magnitude of the BP elevation and the presence of LVH are the proof of sustained HTN. The finding of LVH suggests risk for future CVS disease, which underscores the importance of recognizing and treating BP elevation in children and adolescents.

Hypertensive crisis, also known as hypertensive emergency, is defined by HTN accompanied by acute target-organ damage. Besides LVH, the other parameters that have been suggested to assess organ damage such as: cardiac diastolic dysfunction, carotid intima-media thickening, and microalbuminuria. Hypertensive urgency is defined by HTN without the presence of acute target-organ damage, although these patients may still manifest symptoms such as headache and nausea. Hypertensive crisis is fortunately uncommon in pediatrics, but does represent a potentially life-threatening medical emergency. Most children with hypertensive crisis have an underlying secondary cause for the HTN that is usually renal or renovascular in origin. It is uncommon to find essential HTN as the underlying cause for hypertensive crisis in children, although it can be seen in young African Americans.

TREATMENT OF HTN

Non-Pharmacologic Therapy

Lifestyle modifications or environmental changes must be implemented or at least attempted. Prevention of childhood obesity, reducing sodium intake (no added salt diet ~2 to 3 g/day or 88 to 132 mEq/day), and increasing physical activity are the three most important interventions.

Steps to reduce salt intake include limiting grocery purchases of salt-added foods, limiting meals from fast-food restaurants/take-outs, and not adding salt to cooking. A referral to a dietitian may improve compliance through education and follow-up re-evaluations. In general, BP responds to different types of activity in different ways.

During dynamic exercise (swimming, running, cycling, etc.), peripheral vascular resistance decreases, which results in an increase in SBP, a moderate raise in mean arterial pressure, and a fall in the diastolic value. In contrast to dynamic exercise, static or isometric exercise (weight or strength training) causes significant increases in SBP, mean BP, and DBP with no change in total peripheral resistance. The magnitude of the increase in BP during static exercise can exceed values for dynamic exercise significantly. Patients with WCH, pre-HTN, stage 1, and primary HTN should be advised to implement lifestyle changes and exercise.

Exercise restriction should be based on the possibility that an abrupt increase in BP may place the child or adolescent at a higher risk of a catastrophic event, exacerbate the BP effect on end-organ damage significantly, or contribute to sustained BP elevation.

Pharmacological Therapy

Pharmacological treatment should be started in patients with stage 2 HTN, patients with stage 1 and symptomatic when LVH is present, and in stage 1 HTN when BP is unresponsive to lifestyle changes.

There are two approaches to the use of antihypertensive medications in children. Some clinicians administer the drug until effect or side effects are observed. Others start a drug and, if there is no response at higher dose but in the absence of side effects, they add a second drug. Usually, as shown by several studies, the degree of HTN is closely related to the number of drugs used to control HTN.

Many antihypertensive drugs are available for children, although clinical trials are limited, and most recommendations are based on extrapolation from adult dosage recommendations or clinical experience. In our opinion, the preferable adverse effect and compliance profiles support the use of ACEs, ARBs, and calcium channel blockers (CCBs) as first-line therapy. Although beta blockers (propranolol and atenolol), an alpha and beta blocker (labetalol), direct vasodilators (hydralazine and minoxidil), and central alpha agonists (clonidine) have been used in pediatrics, they should not be considered first-line medications except under specific circumstances (i.e. clonidine in central HTN).

Hypertensive patients fall into two categories: those with volume HTN, due predominantly to sodium retention and increased intravascular volume, and those patients who present mainly peripheral vasoconstriction, most of the time mediated by angiotensin II.

The drugs that are efficacious in patients with volume-dependent HTN are diuretics and CCBs. The drugs that improve vasoconstriction are ACEs, ARBs, CCBs, and beta blockers.

After defining the underlying pathophysiologic mechanism of the HTN, we proceed with a step approach. For those with volume-dependent HTN, diuretics and CCBs are indicated as starting therapy. The other medications such as beta blockers are introduced if there is no control of BP. For those with high renin HTN either ACEs or ARBs is the initial therapy of choice. The addition of diuretics or the combination of ACEs and ARBs comprises the next step in case of failure to respond to the initial therapy. The approach does not apply to those patients with pheochromocytoma (phentolamine) or central HTN (clonidine).

Drugs currently in use for the treatment of hypertensive emergency are: sodium nitroprusside at a starting dose of 0.25–0.3 μg/kg/min to a maximum dose of 10 μg/kg/min, nicardipine 0.5–1 μg/kg/min to a maximum 5 μg/kg/min, Enalapril at 5–10 μg/kg/dose to a maximum of 20 mg/day,

Table 13-5. Recommended antihypertensive agents for the treatment of HTN in children and adolescents.

Class	Drug	Dose	Interval	Maximum dose
Diuretics	Amiloride	0.4–0.6 mg/kg/day	q.d.	20 mg/day
	Hydrochlorothiazide	0.5–1.0 mg/kg/day	q.d.–b.i.d.	3 mg/kg/day
	Furosemide	0.5–2.0 mg/kg/dose	q.d.–b.i.d.	6 mg/kg/dose
	Spironolactone	1.0 mg/kg/day	q.d.–b.i.d.	3.3 mg/kg/day
ACE Inhibitors	Captopril	0.3–0.5 mg/kg/dose	b.i.d.–t.i.d.	6 mg/kg/day
	Enalapril	0.1–0.6 mg/kg/day	q.d.	0.6 mg/kg/day
	Ramipril	2.5–6.0 mg/day	q.d.	10 mg per day
	Lisinopril	0.08–0.6 mg/kg/day	q.d.	0.6 mg/kg/day
ARS Blockers	Losartan	0.75–1.44 mg/kg/day	q.d.	1.4 mg/kg/day
	Valsartan	2.0 mg/kg/day	q.d.	2.7 mg/kg/day
CCBs	Amlodipine	0.06–0.3 mg/kg/day	q.d.	10 mg/day
	Nifedipine	0.25–0.5 mg/kg/day	q.d.–b.i.d.	3 mg/kg/day
B blockers	Atenolol	0.5–1.0 mg/kg/day	q.d.–b.i.d.	2 mg/kg/day
	Propranolol	1.0 mg/kg/day	b.i.d.–t.i.d.	8 mg/kg/day
Vasodilators	Hydralazine	0.25 mg/kg/dose	b.i.d.–t.i.d.	7.5 mg/kg/day
	Minoxidil	0.1–0.2 mg/kg/day	b.i.d.–t.i.d.	1 mg/kg/day

q.d., once a day; b.i.d., twice a day; t.i.d., thrice a day.

and Phentolamine 0.05–0.1 mg/kg/dose to a maximum of 5 mg/dose. Antihypertensive drugs for the outpatient management of HTN in children of 1 to 17 years of age are listed in Tables 13-4 and 13-5.

CONCLUSIONS

The prevalence and the severity of HTN is increasing in both children and adolescents. These observations suggest that the trend of decreasing CVD observed over the past 50 years may be reversed, as the current population of hypertensive children and adolescents become adults. Although progress has been made with regard to children with HTN in terms of definition and in developing guidelines for the pharmacological treatment, much remains to be done. If physicians who care for hypertensive children seek to promote health that extends beyond the traditional pediatric age range, early recognition for HTN clearly must begin in childhood.

COMMENT FROM THE EDITORS

The treatment of arterial HTN in children falls mainly in the realm of the pediatric nephrologist and occasionally the cardiologist. Nevertheless, the pediatric urologist will come across many hypertensive children in her/his practice and knowledge of the topic is important. Correct BP measurement in children should be available in all pediatric urology clinics.

FURTHER READING

Flynn JT, Tullus K. Severe hypertension in children and adolescents: pathophysiology and treatment. *Pediatr Nephrol* 2009; **24**:1101–1112.

National High Blood Pressure Education Program Working Group on High Blood Pressure in Children and Adolescents. The fourth report on the diagnosis, evaluation, and treatment of high blood pressure in children and adolescents. *Pediatrics* 2004; **114**(2 Suppl 4th report):555–576.

Nehal US, Ingelfinger JR. Pediatric hypertension: recent literature. *Curr Opin Pediatr* 2002; **14**:189–196.

Part Two

Common or Unique Conditions

Chapter 14

Ureteral Obstruction

Miguel A. Castellán

Congenital obstruction of the ureter most commonly occurs at the proximal (ureteropelvic junction (UPJ)) and the distal end of the ureter. Congenital midureteral obstructions are considerably less frequent.

URETEROPELVIC JUNCTION OBSTRUCTION

Definition

UPJ obstruction is defined as an obstruction of the flow of urine from the renal pelvis to the proximal ureter. This obstruction leads to elevated intrarenal backpressure, the dilatation of the collecting system and hydronephrosis. UPJ obstruction is the commonest cause of prenatal hydronephrosis in the foetal kidney, with an annual incidence of 5 per 100,000. The challenge for the paediatric urologist is the postnatal management since not all hydronephrotic kidneys are obstructive; a patient may have an enlarged renal collecting system without obstruction. One of the critical decisions in managing patients with prenatally detected hydronephrosis is identifying the beginning of renal decompensation before the onset of permanent kidney damage.

Aetiology

UPJ obstruction may be caused by an intrinsic narrowing at the junction between the ureter and the renal pelvis or extrinsic compression by a lower pole renal vessel. The precise mechanism that causes primary UPJ obstruction remains unknown.

Intrinsic obstruction secondary to a narrow segment with muscular discontinuity is the commonest cause. It has been attributed to an interruption in the development of the circular musculature of the UPJ or an alteration of the collagen and composition between and around the muscle cells at the level of the UPJ. The asymmetry of ureteral wall musculature may produce a functional discontinuity of the muscular contractions at this level that inhibit the natural peristaltic emptying of the renal pelvis into the ureter. When examined at the time of surgical repair, these segments are often narrower in caliber than the normal distal ureter. Although the lumen is physically patent, it is non-elastic and poorly distensible.

The other causes of intrinsic UPJ obstruction include ureteral valves, mucosal folds, or ureteral polyps. Another anatomical cause of obstruction is an abnormal insertion of the ureter into the renal pelvis, impairing the drainage from the renal pelvis; however, in many cases, it is difficult to distinguish if this is the cause or a consequence of the hydronephrosis.

Extrinsic compression of the UPJ by an abnormal crossing of lower pole vessel is most common in adult patients. Reported incidence in different series has varied between 15 and 50% of cases. It is unclear if the aberrant vessel causes obstruction or if it is associated to a hydronephrotic kidney. Renal dilatation and hydronephrosis may distort renal vasculature architecture and predispose the entrapment of the ureter by a lower pole vessel.

Presentation

UPJ obstruction occurs in all paediatric age groups. In developed countries, the majority of paediatric cases are identified *in utero*. Hydronephrosis is present in approximately 1 per 1500 live births (see Chapter 1). UPJ obstruction represents 45 to 65% of cases of foetal hydronephrosis (Figure 14-1). In this age group, most of the infants are asymptomatic. When not suspected prenatally, infants may present with palpable mass, which is failure to thrive or a urinary tract infection (UTI). About 50% of the abdominal masses detected in infancy were renal in origin and 40% of these are secondary to UPJ obstruction.

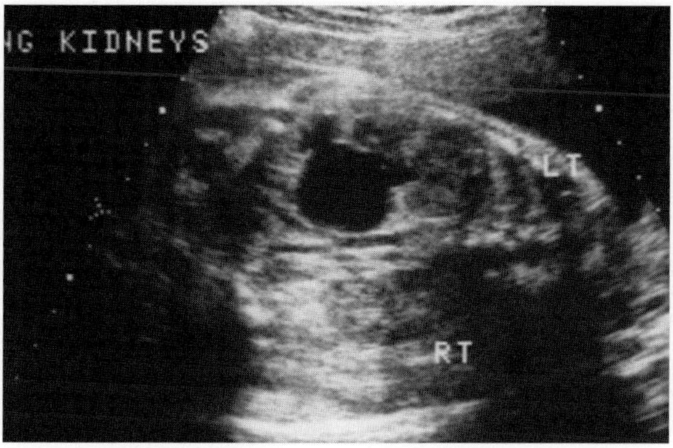

Figure 14-1. Prenatal US showing unilateral grade 2 hydronephrosis.

The male to female ratio is 3–4:1 and the lesion is unilateral in 90% of cases. Left kidney is generally more affected than the right (approximately 67%). In older children, most anomalies are discovered because of symptoms. In older children, symptoms include episodic flank pain, haematuria, abdominal mass, or UTI. Sometimes, upper abdominal pain is associated with nausea or vomiting related to intermittent UPJ obstruction. Usually, this is the result of intermittent obstruction brought on by a high fluid load (Dietl's crisis). Haematuria may be associated with a history of minor trauma.

When UPJ obstruction is found in kidneys with double collecting system, the lower pole moiety is almost always the segment affected. UPJ obstruction can also be associated to other congenital anomalies, including imperforate anus, contralateral multicystic dysplastic kidney, congenital heart disease, VATER syndrome, or esophageal atresia.

Diagnosis

Renal ultrasonography (RUS), because of its wide availability and noninvasive nature, has become the primary initial tool for the identification and evaluation of pre- and postnatal hydronephrosis.

All children with prenatal hydronephrosis should have a postnatal RUS (Figure 14-2). Children with bilateral severe prenatal hydronephrosis

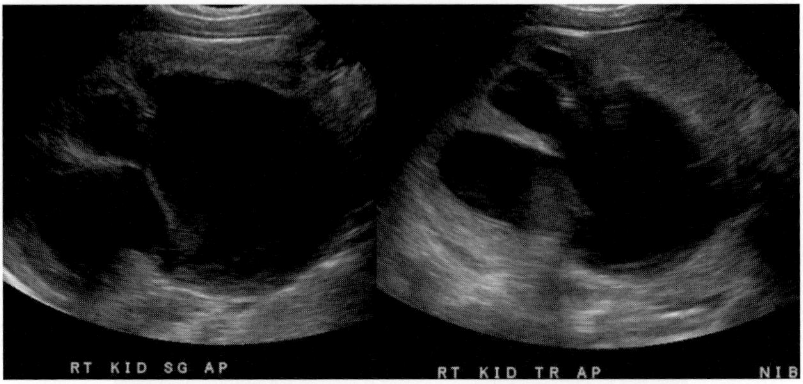

Figure 14-2. Postnatal US (A: longitudinal view, B: transverse view) showing grades 3–4 hydronephrosis in a patient with UPJ obstruction.

and children with prenatal diagnosis of hydronephrosis of any degree in a solitary kidney should have a postnatal RUS prior to discharge from hospital. However, ideally, the first postnatal RUS should not be performed within the first 48–72 hours, as relatively low urine output during this period may underestimate the degree of hydronephrosis. Therefore, in this situation, if the RUS is normal and the serum creatinine is dropping appropriately, a repeated RUS should be performed between two and four weeks. The remainder of children with antenatally detected hydronephrosis should have an RUS performed between 7 and 30 days.

According to the findings on the postnatal ultrasound, hydronephrosis can be graded as follows (Society for Fetal Urology Grading).

- 0 — Intact central complex,
- 1 — Slight separation,
- 2 — Further separation; one or few calyces may be visualised,
- 3 — Pelviectasis and fluid-filled calyces seen throughout kidney, normal parenchyma, and
- 4 — Grade 3 with large dilated calyces and thinned parenchyma.

A prominent extrarenal pelvis without calyectasis is usually a benign physiologic variant. Only grades 3 and 4 are felt to be clinically significant with respect to obstruction. Serial RUS evaluations can provide another useful parameter in helping to follow-up hydronephrosis by monitoring its grade, longitudinal growth of the affected kidney, and changes in the growth rate of the normal kidney.

In cases presenting with intermittent abdominal or flank pain, it is important to perform the RUS during an attack of pain.

Another important diagnostic tool is the isotopic diuretic renography, which is a functional study that can help define whether obstruction exists. Agents commonly used for renal evaluation include Tc 99m DTPA and Tc 99m MAG 3 (Figure 14-3). DTPA is only filtered by the glomeruli an provides an indirect means of measuring the GFR. MAG 3 is filtered by the glomeruli and also secreted by the proximal tubules with a higher extraction fraction than DTPA. MAG 3 remains essentially in the intravascular space and gives superior anatomic

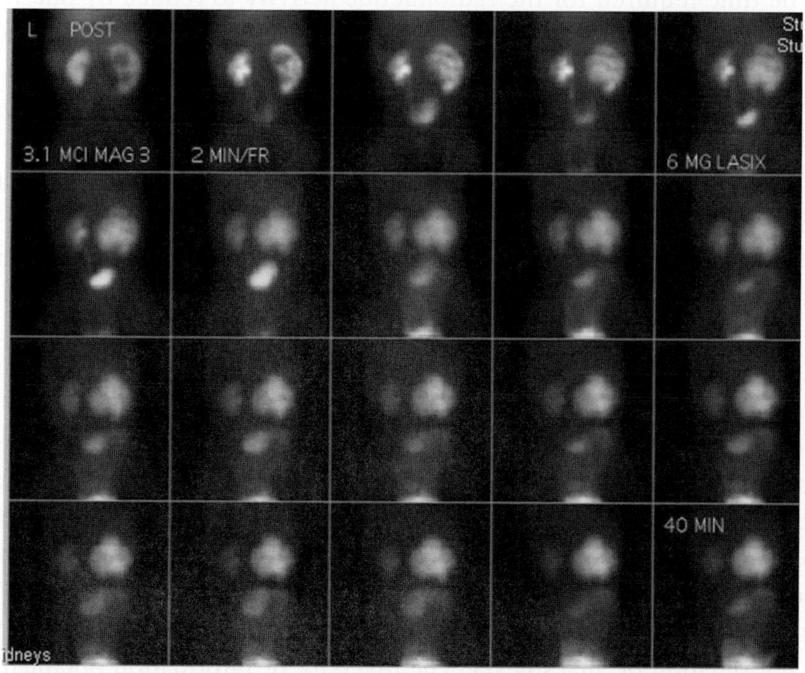

Figure 14-3. Diuretic MAG 3 renal scan demonstrating retention of radiotracer in right kidney in a patient with RT UPJ obstruction (see 40 minutes image).

details on the scan images. Both can distinguish total and individual renal function and both can determine the drainage time of the radioisotope from the renal pelvis. Some institutions prefer the diuretic to be given prior the tracer, some with the tracer, and the others give the diuretics when the renal pelvis is full of tracer (15–20 minutes after tracer). A postmicturition image at the end of the dynamic diuretic renogram should be taken or a bladder catheter should be inserted for the test. A differential renal function of >10% between kidneys is thought to represent significant renal impairment on the affected side. The measurement of differential renal function with DTPA or MAG 3 must be done promptly (1–3 minutes) after the injection of the radionuclide. Occasionally, it is desirable to obtain a more accurate measure of cortical activity and a DMSA scan is recommended. The washout curve is another tool that helps in the diagnosis and extension of obstruction. The washout half-time (T1/2) is the time required for the radionuclide activity to reduce by one-half (calculated from the diuretic renogram). In the hydronephrotic kidney, if the washout is rapid after diuretic is given, the patients are said to have a dilated non-obstructive kidney. If the washout is delayed (>20 minutes), it is interpreted as obstructive. If the washout is between 15 and 20 minutes, then the study is indeterminate (Figure 14-4).

The main role of the VCUG in infants is to rule out vesicoureteral reflux and in boys to evaluate the posterior urethra. Patients with prenatal diagnosis of hydronephrosis have an increased risk of associated VUR (8.5–15%).

Ultrafast MRI urography is another diagnostic method used in paediatric patients in some centres. It offers unique advantages for evaluating renal blood flow, anatomy, and urinary excretion. Contrast material used is gadopentetate dimeglumine and is usually injected 15 minutes after furosemide. MRI does not involve ionising radiation and can be used for follow-up of patients with suspected obstruction. The main disadvantages of the study are the elevated cost and the need for heavy sedation or anaesthesia. The diversity of information obtained in a single study makes MR urography an attractive method for the assessment of UPJ obstruction.

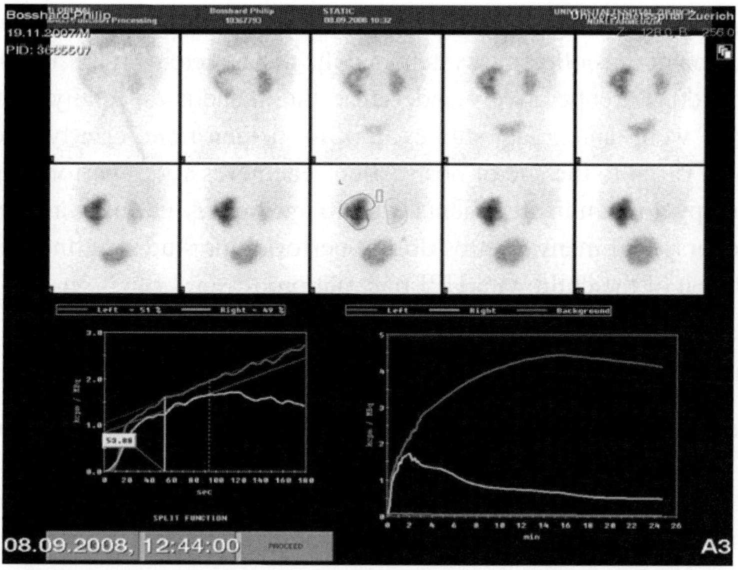

(A)

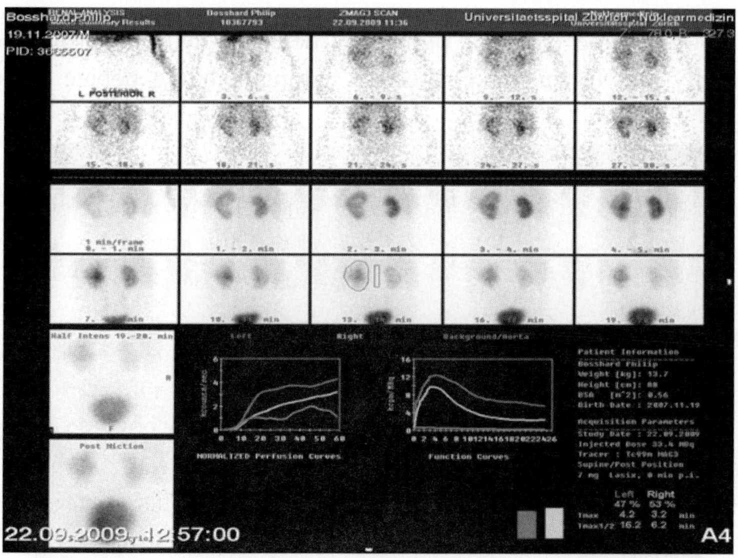

(B)

Figure 14-4. Curves on a diuretic renogram. **(A)** A normal curve on the right side and no drainage on the left suggestive of obstruction. **(B)** Improvement of the drainage curve after pyeloplasty.

Antegrade or retrograde pyelography gives an excellent anatomic evaluation of the collecting system and the distal ureter (Figure 14-5). The study is done preoperatively under anaesthesia and is especially useful in patients were antegrade studies fail to demonstrate clearly ureteral anatomy distal to the site of obstruction. The necessity of performing retrograde pyelogram in all patients prior to pyeloplasty has been a source of controversy and many centres do not perform this study routinely in the evaluation of the child with UPJ obstruction.

Management

In cases of symptomatic children or those with decreasing or decreased renal function, the surgical correction of the obstruction is clearly indicated. However, in many infants with prenatally detected dilatation, the optimal management may be controversial.

Observation

About 50% of the cases of prenatally detected hydronephrosis persist postnatally and in this case, there is a long-standing debate as to the

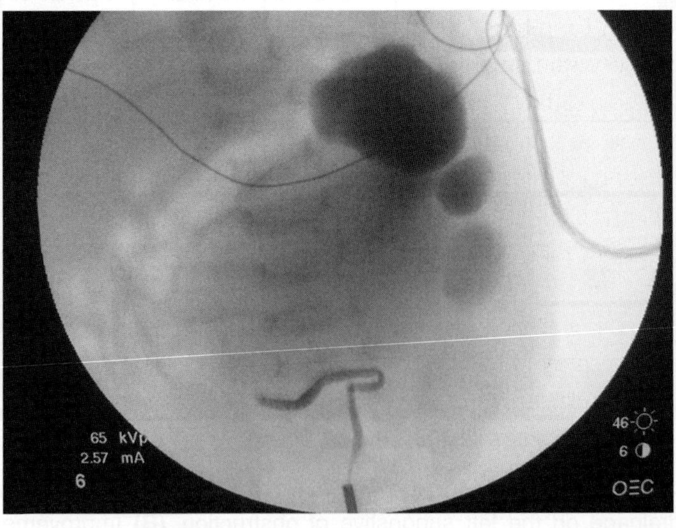

Figure 14-5. Retrograde pyelogram demonstrating UPJ obstruction.

optimal management. Not all congenital hydronephrotic kidneys develop progressive loss of function if left untreated. Many kidneys remain functionally stable and hydronephrosis tend to resolve over time. Most of the times, an observational approach can be adopted in patients with unilateral hydronephrosis, with a function greater than 40% in the affected side, even if the washout is delayed. This group of patients need to be closely monitored for the criteria such as surgical intervention that include functional deterioration, evidence for worsening the degree of dilatation, or the development of symptoms. Approximately, 23% of congenital hydronephrotic kidneys monitored by an observational approach ultimately require surgical intervention.

Observational protocol should consist of serial RUS, at three-month intervals in the first year of life and then yearly RUS and diuretic renogram until certain the hydronephrotic kidney's function is stabilised. Longer term follow-up and follow-up in adulthood are lacking in patients managed by an observational approach.

Surgery

In the last several years, different surgical techniques have been published for the correction of UPJ obstruction. In infants and young children, open pyeloplasty still remains the standard procedure, but in some centres, the use of laparoscopic pyeloplasty has been extended to infants. In older children and adults, laparoscopic or robotic-assisted laparoscopic pyeloplasty is now the treatment of choice.

Dismembered pyeloplasty (Anderson-Haynes) remained the procedure of choice for the surgical correction of UPJ obstruction whether done openly or laparoscopically (Figure 14-6A and 14-6B). The procedure involves the excision of the obstructing segment and the anastomosis of the normal upper ureter to a dependent portion of the renal pelvis. The open operation may be performed through a flank, dorsal lumbotomy, or anterior extraperitoneal technique. When done laparoscopically, in infants, the transperitoneal approach is preferred. In older children and adult patients, laparoscopic pyeloplasty or robotic-assisted laparoscopic pyeloplasty is emerging as a new standard in the treatment of UPJ obstruction. A perirenal drain is usually placed adjacent to the repair site.

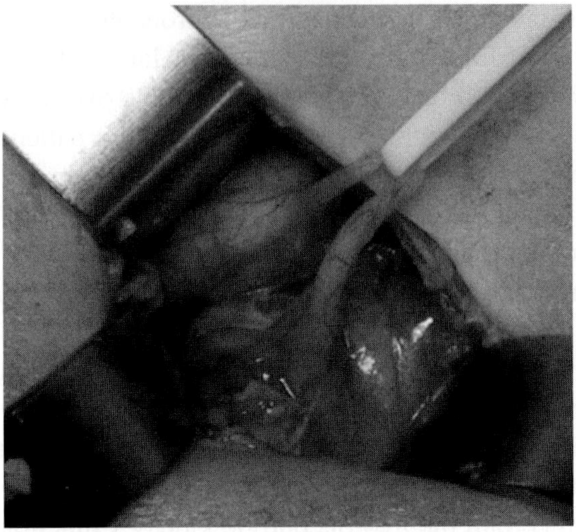

(A)

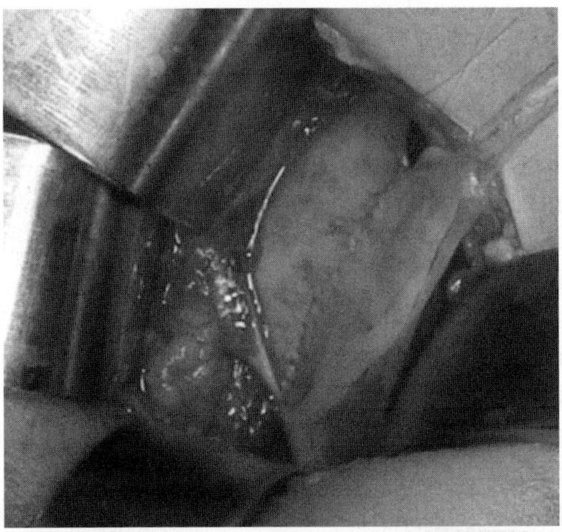

(B)

Figure 14-6. **(A)** Operative picture showing UPJ obstruction. **(B)** Operative picture showing open dismembered pyeloplasty. The UPJ was excised, the proximal ureter is spatulate, and one side of the anastomosis is completed.

The decision of whether to leave a transient ureteral stent in the postoperative period is based on the personal preference of the surgeon. A bladder catheter can also be used in the immediate postoperative period to help further reduce the risk of urine leak.

Prognosis and Long-Term Complications

Renal US is usually obtained 4–6 weeks after the procedure. Success is defined by US as improvement in hydronephrosis, with an overall decrease in the degree of pelvicaliectasis. Serial RUSs are recommended for the first year after surgery and should be continued less frequently thereafter if results show a tendency to normalise (Figure 14-7). A diuretic renogram may be obtained six months after the pyeloplasty or earlier if the degree of dilatation on the RUS does not improve. Stabilisation or improvement in renal function and a decrease in washout time are also good signs that define success. This renogram established a new baseline, which is helpful for long-term outcome. The success rate of dismembered pyeloplasty exceeds 94%. The commonest long-term complications include recurrent UPJ obstruction, UTI, and urinary stone formation.

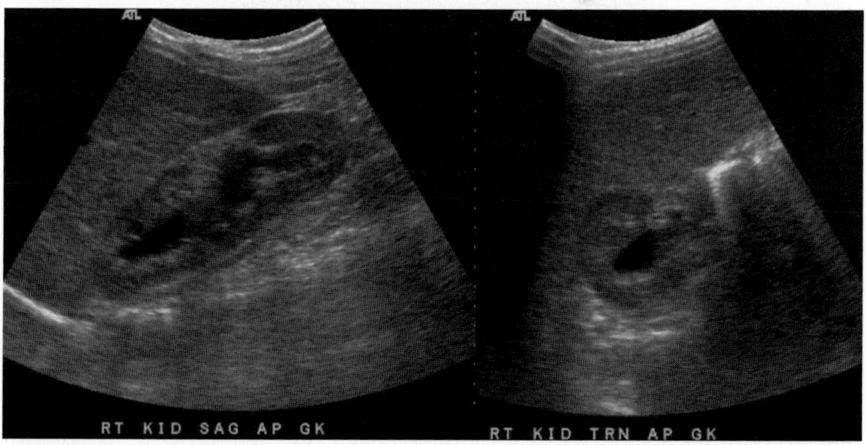

Figure 14-7. Postoperative US after dismembered pyeloplasty (left: longitudinal view, right: transverse view), in same patient as in Figure 14-2, showing improvement in hydronephrosis grade.

Current Controversies

Identification of the beginning of renal decompensation before the onset of permanent kidney damage is still one of the current controversies. Newer imaging modalities or biochemical markers should help us in the future to better distinguish those patients with hydronephrosis that will progress to renal injury from those with hydronephrosis and no significant ureteral obstruction.

PRIMARY OBSTRUCTIVE MEGAURETER (POM)

Definition

A dilated ureter measuring more than 7 mm is called a megaureter. Megaureters may be caused by obstruction, reflux, a combination thereof, or may have no discernable cause. Therefore, they are classified as obstructed, refluxing, both refluxing and obstructed, or non-obstructive and non-refluxing. POM is defined by the presence of an enlarged ureter (>7 mm diameter) caused by a congenital obstruction of the distal ureter. Similarly, to the management of UPJ obstruction, the challenge arises in differentiating non-obstructive megaureter with obstructive megaureter. Many dilated ureters may not represent a threat to their renal moieties and can be followed-up expectantly. POMs may result from altered peristalsis that prevents the normal flow of urine (functional obstruction) or a narrow segment resulting in mechanical obstruction.

Aetiology

The exact cause of distal congenital ureteral obstruction is unknown. Primary obstructed megaureters enter the bladder in a normal location on the trigone, with the ureteral orifice appearing unaffected. The commonest finding is a distal adynamic ureteral segment that affects the free efflux of urine resulting in a functional obstruction. Several investigators agree that there is an alteration in the organisation and relationship of smooth muscle and extracellular matrix at the affected distal ureter. Histologic and ultrastructural abnormalities include the predominance of circular smooth muscle with an increased collagen deposition between the muscle bundles. In POM, there is a predominance of collagen type 1 deposition at the affected segment. All these structural abnormalities lead to a disruption in myoelectrical propagation and peristalsis causing functional obstruction. Partial obstruction in the abnormal distal segment of the ureter leads to progressive dilatation and hydronephrosis. Other less common causes of POM include congenital ureteral strictures and ureteral valves.

Presentation

The incidence of obstructed megaureter is 1 per 10,000 population. At present, most POMs are incidentally diagnosed prenatally. Prenatal RUS suggests UVJ obstruction in upto 23% of patients with prenatal diagnosis of hydronephrosis. The other forms of presentation include vague abdominal pain, haematuria, UTI, or abdominal mass. The male-to-female ratio is 1.2–4.8:1 and has a slight predilection for the left side (1.7–4.5:1). Obstruction is bilateral in 10–20% of obstructed megaureter cases. In up to 10–15% of children, the contralateral kidney may be absent or dysplastic.

Diagnosis

A renal and bladder ultrasound is the best initial study for a child with a suspected urinary tract abnormality (Figure 14-8). In neonates with prenatal diagnosis of hydronephrosis, postnatal imaging is usually done after the first 48 hours of life. Hydronephrosis can be graded according to the Society of Fetal Urology. The presence of a dilated distal ureter differentiates UVJ from UPJ. It can also help in defining the extent of the hydroureter and the presence of collecting system duplication. Longitudinal and transverse sonographic images at the bladder level can detect distal ureteral dilatation, the presence or absence of ureterocele, and bladder configuration, size, and thickening. Other useful clinically relevant data include the presence or absence of calculi, echogenic debris suggesting infection, and the location and condition of other renal units. The evaluation of ureteral jets by colour Doppler has been suggested as an indirect evidence of the degree of obstruction.

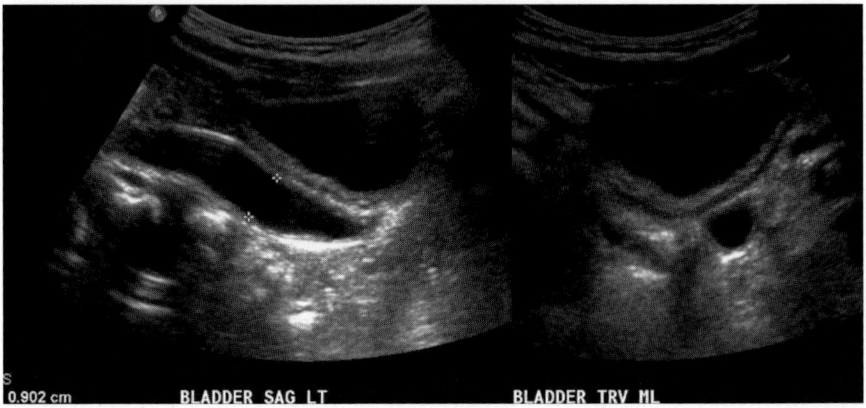

Figure 14-8. US of the pelvis (A: longitudinal view, B: transverse view) showing left megaureter in a patient with POM.

A voiding cystourethrogram (VCUG) is an essential element in the evaluation of a megaureter as part of the workup for ureterohydronephrosis, to rule out reflux. High-grade reflux alone can result in a megaureter. The VCUG is also necessary to assess the anatomy of the bladder and urethra, which can help in the diagnosis of the other causes of ureteral dilatation, such as bladder outlet obstruction or neurogenic bladder.

A diuretic renogram allows the assessment of individual renal function and provides the objective parameters of drainage and obstruction. Technetium Tc 99m diethylenetriamine pentaacetic acid (DTPA) or technetium Tc 99m mercaptotriglycylglycine (MAG 3) is the most widely used radioisotopes (Figure 14-9). Renal scanning is used to assess renal blood flow, relative function, and drainage. It is also helpful in predicting the capacity for functional recovery prior to surgery. The scanning area should ideally include the lower ureters in all patients with megaureters. Some studies are not easy to interpret, and possibly the most useful information is provided when there is no obstruction and the renal function is good. A half-time clearance of greater than 20 minutes is highly suspicious for obstruction. Exact definitions of obstruction do not exist and serial examinations are often required to establish an accurate treatment approach. A relative decrease in renal function (<35%) and a delayed half-time clearance of the radioisotope (T1/2·20 minutes) are strong indicators for surgical correction.

Antegrade or retrograde pyelography as well as MRI can be used to define precisely the anatomy of the ureter (Figure 14-10).

Management

The natural history of primary non-refluxing megaureter is a tendency of gradual reduction of dilatation over several years. Initial management therapy should include antibiotic prophylaxis. This is particularly true for infants who are susceptible to renal damage with concomitant infection.

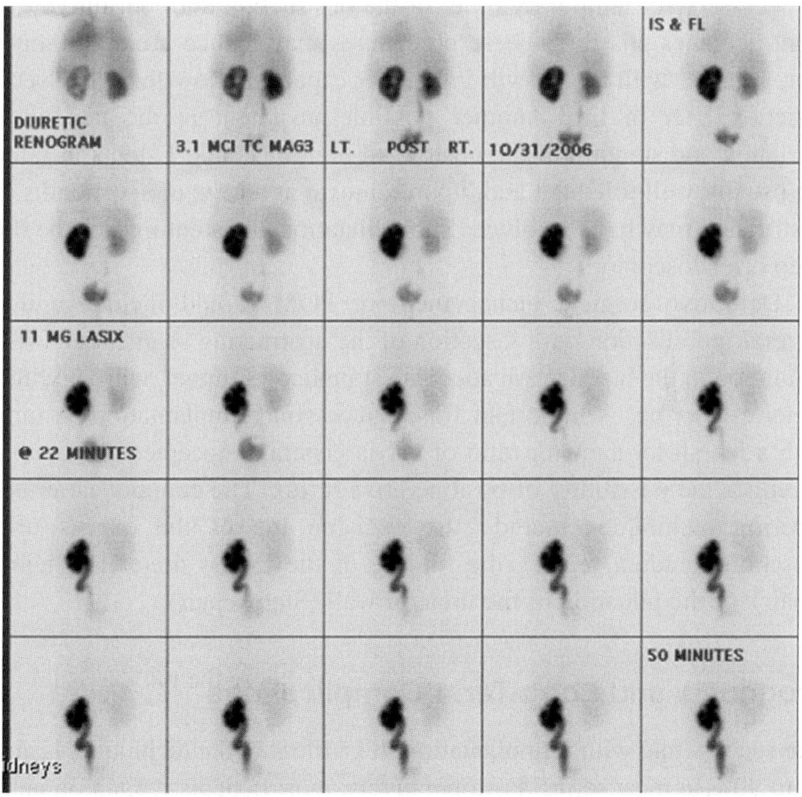

Figure 14-9. Diuretic MAG 3 renal scan demonstrating the retention of radiotracer in left kidney and ureter in a patient with LT POM (see 50 minutes image).

As long as the renal function of the involved kidney is normal and there are no UTIs, expectant management is preferred. Periodic imaging is used to monitor the degree of dilatation and differential or individual renal function. Antibiotic prophylaxis is recommended in the first year of life.

Significant predictors of future need for surgical correction include grades three to four hydronephrosis, diameter of retrovesical ureter > 1 cm and decreased individual renal function (<40%). Neonates and infants may present clinically with UTI that does not respond to antibiotics alone or with bilateral MOP or a MOP in a solitary functioning kidney with elevated creatinine. In those cases, temporary diversion, such as a distal cutaneous ureterostomy, or construction of a direct anastomosis between the dilated ureter and the bladder (refluxing ureteroneocystostomy) may be necessary for temporary relief of the obstruction until definitive treatment becomes possible. These procedures may reduce ureteral diameter that, together with the growth in bladder capacity, allow for a safe reconstruction later in life. Another possible treatment in the newborn is dilatation and stenting of the obstructed ureter. Double J stents in infants are usually well tolerated and, upon removal at an age of six months, the obstruction may have resolved. Such dilatation and stenting may be done open or endoscopic.

Definitive surgical management of POM should include a distal ureteral mobilisation with resection of the obstructing segment and reimplantation in the bladder. An adequate submucosal tunnel, with or without ureteral tapering, is important for a successful reimplantation. A tunnel with a length-to-diameter ratio of 5:1 is generally accepted as necessary to reduce the possibility of postoperative reflux. The commonest ureteral tapering techniques include the excision the of the excess ureter (Bischoff/Hendren repair), the folding of the excess ureter (Kalicinsky repair), or the plication of the ureteral wall (Starr repair).

Prognosis and Long-Term Complications

The success rate with reimplantation, regardless of the technique, is about 80 to 90% in most series. Postoperatively, most patients remain on antibiotic prophylaxis until repeat studies have confirmed the resolution of the obstruction. The commonest complications include ischaemic ureteral

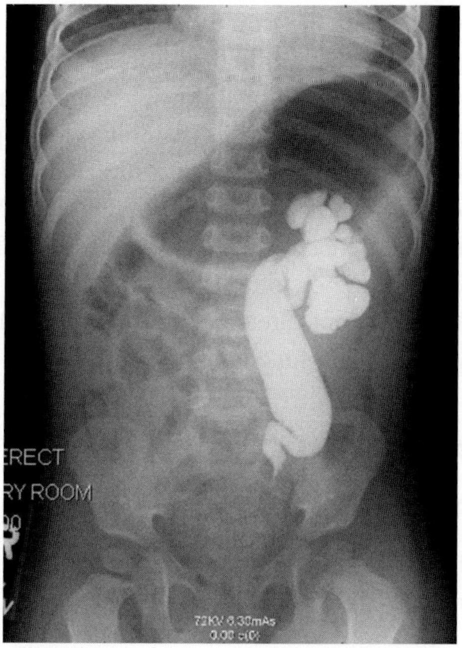

Figure 14-10. Retrograde pyelogram demonstrating retention of contrast material in left kidney and ureter in a patient with LT POM.

stricture or fistula, urinary extravasation, vesicoureteral reflux, ureteral kinking, or obstruction.

Future and Current Controversies

As in UPJ obstruction, exact definitions of obstruction do not exist and serial examinations are often required to establish an accurate treatment approach. Minimally invasive surgery and the application of improved laparoscopic and robotic techniques to reconstructive paediatric urology are promising and can give new treatment strategies for MOP.

SINGLE SYSTEM URETEROCELES

A ureterocele is a cystic dilatation of the terminal ureter. Single system ureteroceles is almost always intravesical and are also called orthotopic or simple.

Although usually found in the adult population, they are occasionally encountered in children. Most commonly simple intravesical ureteroceles in children are found incidentally or following a UTI. The degree of obstruction tends to be less severe than in children with duplicated systems. Ultrasonography confirms the presence of a ureterocele inside the bladder with varying degrees of hydronephrosis (Figure 14-11). A MAG 3 renal scan can confirm the presence of and the degree of obstruction. Treatment options include endoscopic puncture or transvesical incision and reimplantation of the ureter. Single system ectopic ureteroceles are more common in males and tend to be associated with non-functioning renal units.

MIDURETERAL OBSTRUCTION

Retrocaval and Retroiliac Ureter

Persistence of the right posterior cardinal vein results in the typical retrocaval ureter. The right side is affected except in cases of situs

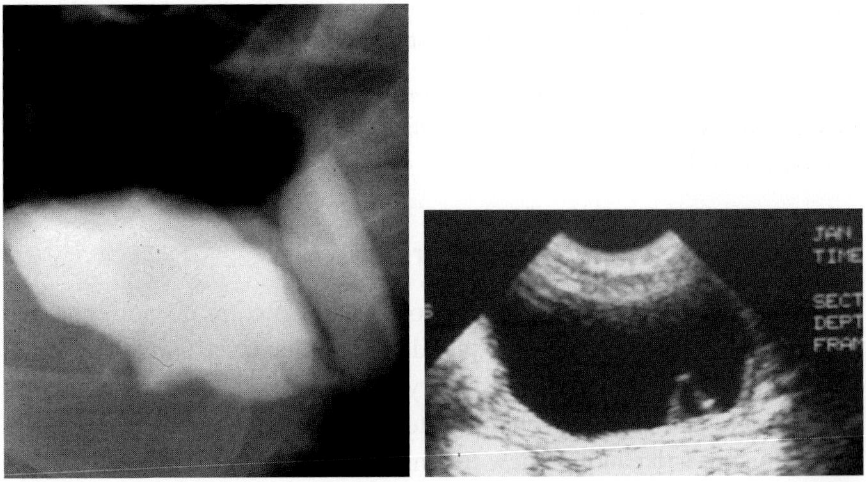

(A) (B)

Figure 14-11. Single system intravesical ureterocele causing hydronephrosis in a newborn. **(A)** VCUG shows a filling defect in the bladder. **(B)** VCUG shows a dilated distal ureter and a typical thin-walled, round, and fluid-filled structure within the bladder.

inversus. The ureter typically deviates medially behind the inferior vena cava at the level of L3. Symptoms tend to present later in life, typically in the fourth decade and include UTI, pain, calculus, or haematuria. US, CT scan, or MRI have been useful in defining these vascular anomalies. A retroiliac ureter is rare and may occur on either or both sides, typically at the L5 level. Surgical correction is performed only when these anomalies are obstructive and usually consists of a dismembered ureteroureterostomy.

Ureteral Valves

Diaphragmatic annular valves are a rare cause of ureteral obstruction. They consist of transverse folds of redundant mucosa that contain smooth muscle. They should be differentiated with the transverse folds observed in newborns, which are non-obstructive lesions that tend to disappear with time as the ureter grows. The valves are distributed throughout the length of the ureter. Renal US and MAG 3 renal scan and/or excretory urography should be obtained to evaluate the degree of obstruction. Surgical treatment includes resection of the obstructive segment and primary anastomosis. To prove the diagnosis, the longitudinal sections of the obstructed ureteral segment should be studied histologically.

COMMENT FROM THE EDITORS

This excellent review highlights the accepted knowledge regarding ureteral obstruction. The challenge for the paediatric urologist facing an asymptomatic child with prenatally detected dilatation of the upper urinary tract is to determine when this represents a risk to the kidney or to the child's well being. This field is evolving. For those children requiring correction of a UPJ obstruction, we prefer the laparoscopic approach although at present the only demonstrable advantages of this approach for children under three years of age are cosmetic. An intriguing development for the treatment of POMs is endoscopic dilatation as advocated by some Spanish surgeons. Validation of this approach from other centres is needed before this treatment can be universally applied.

FURTHER READING

Acharya SK, Jindal B, Yadav DK, Singha S, Bagga D. Retrocaval ureter: a rare cause of hydronephrosis in children. *J Pediatr Surg* 2009; **44**(4):846–848.

Cerwinka WH, Damien Grattan-Smith J, Kirsch AJJ. Magnetic resonance urography in pediatric urology. *J Pediatr Urol* 2008; **4**(1):74–82.

Chacko J, Piaggio LA, Neheman A, González R. Pediatric laparoscopic pyeloplasty: lessons learned from the first 50 cases. *Endourol* 2009; **23**(8):1307–1311.

Conway JJ, Maizels M. The "well tempered" diuretic renogram: a standard method to examine the asymptomatic neonate with hydronephrosis or hydroureteronephrosis. A report from combined meetings of The Society for Fetal Urology and members of The Pediatric Nuclear Medicine C. *J Nucl Med* 1992; **33**(11):2047–2051.

Duel BP, Vates TS, Heiser D, Barthold JS, González R. The utility of antegrade pyelography prior to pyeloplasty via dorsal lumbotomy. *J Urol* 1999; **162**:174–176.

Eskild-Jensen A, Gordon I, Piepsz A, *et al.* Interpretation of the renogram: problems and pitfalls in hydronephrosis in children. *BJU Int* 2004; **94**:887–892.

Fernbach SK, Maizels M, Conway JJ. Ultrasound grading of hydronephrosis: introduction to the system used by the Society for Fetal Urology. *Pediatr Radiol* 1993; **23**(6):478–480.

Koff SA. Pathophysiology of ureteropelvic junction obstructions. *Urol Clin North Am* 1990; **17**:263–272.

Lee RS, Retik AB, Borer JG, Peters CA. Pediatric robot assisted laparoscopic dismembered pyeloplasty: comparison with a cohort of open surgery. *J Urol* 2006; **175**(2):683–687.

Liu HY, Dhillon HK, Yeung CK, *et al.* Clinical outcome and management of prenatally diagnosed primary megaureters. *J Urol* 1994; **152**:614–617.

Ransley PG, Dhillon HK, Gordon I, *et al.* The postnatal management of hydronephrosis diagnosed by prenatal ultrasound. *J Urol* 1990; **144**:584–587.

Rossi E, Salas JR, Aucatoma FC, Muñoz MO, Fochs LM. Congenital ureteral valves: two new cases and a review of the literature. *J Pediatr Urol* 2007; **3**(5):344–349.

Salem YH, Majd M, Rushton HG, Belman AB. Outcome analysis of pediatric pyeloplasty as a function of patient age, presentation and differential renal function. *J Urol* 2006; **175**(2):683–687.

Shukla AR, Cooper J, Patel RP, Carr MC, Canning DA, Zderic SA, *et al.* Prenatally detected primary megaureter: a role for extended follow-up. *J Urol* 2005; **173**(4):1353–1356.

Stehr M, Metzger R, Schuster T, Porn U, Dietz HG. Management of the primary obstructed megaureter (POM) and indication for operative treatment. *Eur J Pediatr Surg* 2002; **12**(1):32–37.

Chapter 15

Duplication Anomalies and Ureterocele

Barbara M. Ludwikowski and Ricardo González

Duplications of the renal collecting system may be complete or partial. They are complete when two ureters remain separate to their distal ends and partial when they join before entering the bladder (bifid ureter or ureter fissus). Complete duplication of the ureter occurs in 0.2% of live births and it has a strong hereditary tendency. Partial duplications are even more common. In about 20–50% of cases, the anomaly is bilateral. Duplications *per se* are not pathological but certain conditions are frequently associated with duplicated collecting systems. Duplications are found in 8% of children presenting with a urinary tract infection (UTI). In duplications, the upper moiety ureter enters the bladder in a more caudal position than the lower moiety ureter or ends up in an ectopic position outside the bladder (Weigert–Meyer rule). The upper moiety ureter may exhibit obstruction from a ureterocele or ectopia. The lower moiety ureter is in a more cephalad position in the bladder and tends to reflux. Some of the pathologic conditions associated with duplicated systems include (Figure 15-1):

- vesicoureteral reflux (VUR),
- ureteropelvic junction obstruction (UPJO),
- ureteroceles, and
- ectopic ureter.

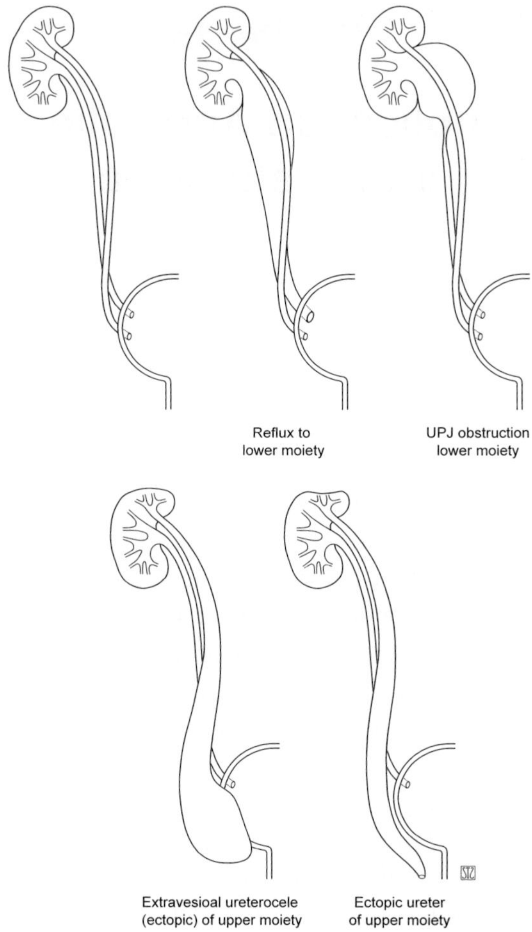

Figure 15-1. Some of the pathologic conditions associated with duplicated systems include vesicoureteral reflux to the lower moiety, ureteropelvic junction obstruction to the lower moiety, the obstruction of the upper moiety from a ureterocele, and the obstruction of the upper moiety from an ectopic ureter.

Although all of these conditions occur in non-duplicated systems as well, when present in duplicated systems, they present unique diagnostic and therapeutic challenges and opportunities and therefore deserve to be discussed separately. Some, such as ectopic ureters and ureterocele, are more prevalent in duplicated systems. The same conditions not associated with duplication are discussed in Chapters 14 and 16.

VESICOURETERAL REFLUX

About 10% of cases of VUR are found to occur in duplicated collecting systems and that spontaneous resolution occurs slower or happens less frequently than in single ureters.

VUR is discussed in detail in Chapter 16 and the basic concepts of presentation, diagnostic evaluation, and management will not be repeated here.

When reflux exists in a duplicated system, it is usually to the lower moiety or to both but almost never to the upper alone, except in cases of urethral ectopia of the upper ureter, in which case reflux to this segment may be seen during voiding.

Diagnosis

The typical radiographic appearance of reflux into the lower moiety ureter is the so-called "drooping lily", which is seen when the contrast medium fills the lower system and not the upper. The most cephalad calyx seen is not the true upper calyx, which is not opacified, giving the impression that the axis of the kidney is tilted outwards (Figure 15-2).

Treatment

In general, treatment options for reflux into duplicated systems are the same as for single ureters with the following exceptions. The expectant treatment period may be shortened given the lower expectation of spontaneous resolution. If the lower moiety has no function, as determined on the DMSA scan, a lower pole nephrectomy should be considered. Depending on experience and facilities available, this can be done openly or, preferably, laparoscopically. For higher-grade reflux to the lower moiety alone, a laparoscopic or open anastomosis of the refluxing lower pole ureter to the upper pole ureter can be considered.

URETEROPELVIC JUNCTION OBSTRUCTION

The evaluation and treatment of UPJO are discussed in detail in Chapter 14. In this section, we discuss some unique features of UPJO in the presence

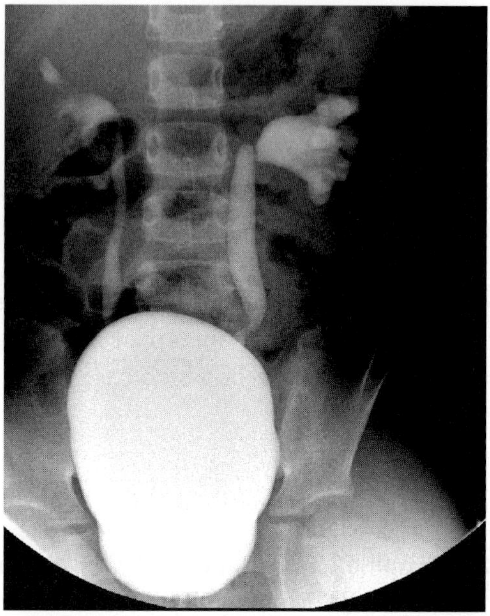

Figure 15-2. The typical radiographic appearance of reflux into the lower moiety ureter is the so-called "drooping lily", which is seen when the contrast medium fills the lower system and not the upper during cystourethrography. The most cephalad calyx seen is not the true upper calyx, which is not opacified, giving the impression that the axis of the kidney is tilted outwards.

of duplication. Most cases of UPJO have been reported on the lower moiety but it can also occur in the upper moiety alone. When surgical treatment is indicated (see Chapter 14), one can choose a laparoscopic or open pyeloplasty, but an anastomosis of the obstructed to the non-obstructed moiety can be considered (pyelo-pyelostomy or pyelo-ureterostomy).

URETEROCELE

Definition

A ureterocele is a cystic dilatation of the distal ureter, which protrudes into the bladder and usually causes ureteral obstruction. Ureteroceles can be associated with or without duplications. The cystic dilatation can be

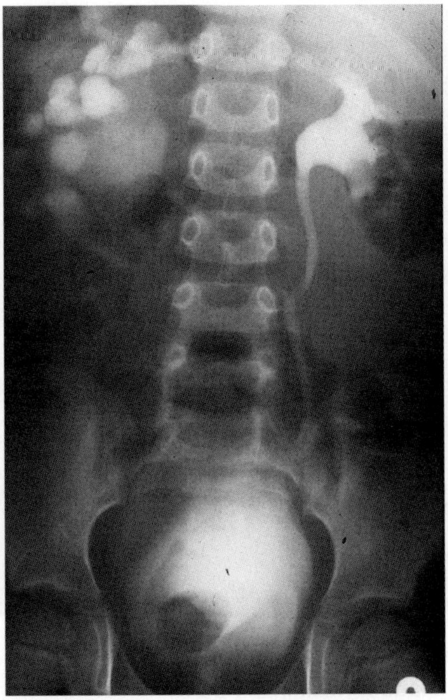

Figure 15-3. Intravesical ureterocele on the right side seen as a defect of filling in the bladder in an excretory urogram (rarely used today).

confined to the bladder (Figure 15-3) or extend distally beyond the bladder neck (Figure 15-4). Single system ureteroceles are discussed in Chapter 14.

In the cases of duplication, the ureterocele invariably involves the ureter of the upper moiety. There may be reflux to the lower moiety ureter and occasionally to the contralateral ureter. The ureterocele may obstruct the bladder neck and the contralateral ureter. Rarely, ureteroceles can occur on both sides. The moiety obstructed by the ureterocele may have normal, decreased, or no function.

Presentation

The commonest form of presentation is a UTI, although in many places where prenatal ultrasonography is done routinely, prenatal suspicion is

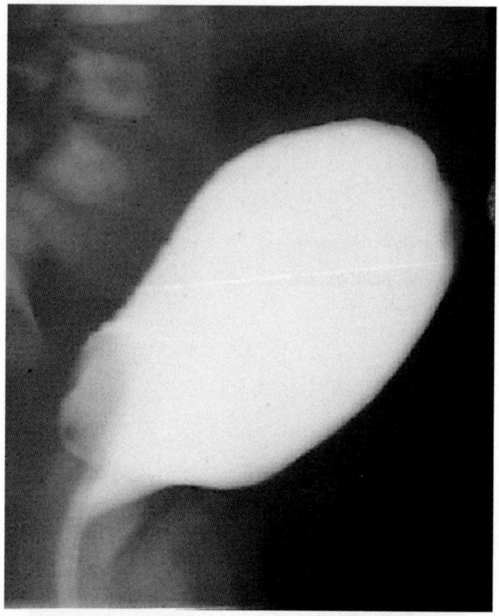

Figure 15-4. Extravesical ureterocele seen as a posterior defect of filling that extends distal to the bladder neck in a VCUG.

more common. Newborn girls may present with a mass prolapsing from the urethral meatus (see Chapter 10) and older children with urinary retention.

Diagnosis

The diagnosis of a ureterocele and duplication is established on ultrasonography (Figure 15-5). It is important to examine the bladder full and empty in every child evaluated for a UTI or in whom a duplication of the upper collecting system is found. A voiding cystourethrogram is essential to detect the presence of reflux and to determine the caudal extension of the ureterocele. Dilute contrast medium should be used to avoid obscuring the defect of filling characteristic of these lesions. A renal scan using DMSA, MAG 3, or DTPA are needed to evaluate the function of the renal moieties involved. When the interpretation of imaging studies is unclear, the distal extension of the ureterocele can be determined by

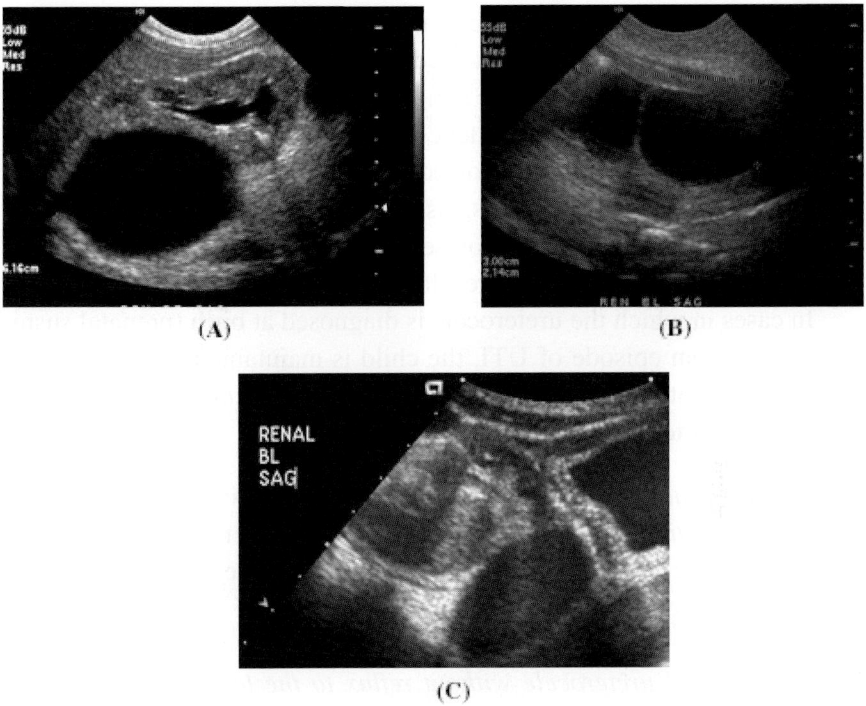

Figure 15-5. **(A)** A markedly dilated upper pole collecting system (left side in the picture) with normal lower pole moiety. **(B)** The cystic lesion and the bladder characteristic of a ureterocele. **(C)** A much dilated ureters with echogenic material (purulent urine) cephalad to the bladder (seen on the right side of the picture).

cystourethroscopy. Magnetic resonance urography (MRU) can also be used to clarify the anatomy in difficult cases.

Management

The goals of treatment are to prevent infections and to protect the renal moieties that are not involved by the ureterocele. A secondary goal is to preserve the function of the involved moiety in the unusual case in which the function is worth preserving. The treatment must be tailored to the individual patient. Universal endoscopic puncture of all ureteroceles as practiced in some centers is ill-advised and only adds to the final number of procedures needed to solve the problem. There are reports in the literature suggesting that prenatally detected ureteroceles without reflux need no treatment other than prophylactic antibiotics for several years; however, in most centers, the surgical treatment of ureteroceles is the norm. In one series of selected patients followed without surgery, about one-third required surgery because of UTIs. As opposed to what is proposed below, some authors do not hesitate to preserve a poorly functioning upper pole moiety; however, the long-term results of doing so are not known.

In cases in which the ureterocele is diagnosed at birth (prenatal suspicion) or after an episode of UTI, the child is maintained on antibacterial prophylaxis until definitive treatment is undertaken. The following scenarios need to be considered.

1a. *Intravesical ureterocele without reflux to the lower moiety and with good function of the upper moiety.* In the upper moiety functions, endoscopic puncture may provide the definitive treatment. Reflux may develop in about 20% of the cases and if the child develops UTIs, ureteral reimplantation may be necessary.
1b. *Intravesical ureterocele without reflux to the lower moiety and no function of the upper moiety*. If the upper moiety has no function, upper pole nephrectomy, open or laparoscopic, is the definitive treatment. The leftover collapsed intravesical ureterocele does not cause problems.
2a. *Intravesical ureterocele with reflux to the lower moiety and with good function of the upper moiety.* In these cases, when the upper pole has acceptable function, the most efficient therapeutic measure is to do an intravesical procedure consisting of ureteral reimplantation of both ureters and excision of the ureterocele.
2b. *Intravesical ureterocele with reflux to the lower moiety and no function of the upper moiety.* Alternatively, if the upper pole has no function, an upper pole nephroureterectomy and reimplantation of the lower moiety ureter has to be considered.
3a. *Extravesical ureterocele* (*ectopic ureterocele*) *with no reflux to the lower pole moiety and with good function of the upper moiety*. A simple ureteroureterostomy done openly or laparoscopically anastomosing the obstructed upper ureter to the normal lower moiety ureter

is curative. The anastomosis can be done high or at the level of the iliac vessels. Advocates of high anastomosis (near the renal pelves) do so to avoid the so-called yo-yo reflux. In our experience, with low anastomosis, this has not been a problem.

3b. *Extravesical ureterocele (ectopic ureterocele) with no reflux to the lower pole moiety and no function of the upper moiety.* In these cases, upper pole nephrectomy, open or laparoscopic, is the definitive treatment. Endoscopic puncture in these cases leads to reflux to the upper moiety ureter and the possible need of a subsequent intravesical operation that is avoided in most cases if a partial nephrectomy is done.

4a. *Extravesical ureterocele (ectopic ureterocele) with reflux to the lower pole moiety and with good function of the upper moiety.* In this rare situation, the child should be maintained on prophylactic antibacterial until a bladder level operation consisting of the excision of the ureterocele and the reimplantation of both ureters is done. If the upper pole ureter is much dilated, a better option is to perform an end-to-side ureteroureterostomy of the upper moiety ureter to the less dilated lower moiety ureter just above the bladder and reimplantation of the lower ureter.

4b. *Extravesical ureterocele (ectopic ureterocele) with reflux to the lower pole moiety and with no function of the upper moiety.* As in scenario 3b, an upper pole nephrectomy is recommended but in this case, it should be followed by the excision of the ureterocele and the reimplantation of the lower ureter in the same or subsequent operation.

These options are summarized in Table 15-1.

Specific Indications for Endoscopic Puncture of the Ureterocele

In addition to the treatment of intravesical ureteroceles, single or with duplication in cases without reflux, the endoscopic puncture or the incision of the ureterocele is useful in the cases of sepsis that is not responding well to antibiotic therapy. In this situation, depending on the

Table 15-1. Treatment options for ureteroceles in duplicated collecting systems.

Upper moiety function	Intravesical ureterocele without reflux to the lower moiety	Intravesical ureterocele with reflux to the lower moiety	Extravesical ureterocele without reflux to the upper pole moiety	Extravesical ureterocele with reflux to the upper pole moiety
Good	Endoscopic puncture	The ureteral reimplantation of both ureters and the excision of the ureterocele	Ureteroureterostomy done openly or laparoscopically anastomosing the obstructed upper ureter to the normal lower moiety ureter	The excision of the ureterocele and the reimplantation of both ureters is done
Poor or none	Upper pole nephrectomy, open or laparoscopic	Upper pole nephroureterectomy and the reimplantation of the lower moiety ureter	Upper pole nephrectomy, open or laparoscopic	Upper pole nephrectomy and the excision of the ureterocele and the reimplantation of the lower ureter

anatomy, the incision may be a temporary measure until the child is well enough for a definitive operation. Endoscopic puncture is also useful in the cases of prolapsing ureterocele in newborns and when a ureterocele obstructs the bladder neck and causes the dilatation of the other moieties.

ECTOPIC URETER WITH DUPLICATION

Definition

When the distal opening of the ureter is not in the normal location at the corner of the trigone. Lateral ectopias are responsible for VUR since the more cephalad and lateral position of the ostium tend to shorten the tunnel. That is why in duplications, the lower moiety ureter tends to enter the bladder in more cephalad and lateral position refluxes more often (see Section "Vesicoureteral reflux"). However, in this section, we shall deal with clinically significant caudal ectopia. In caudal ectopia, the ureter may enter the bladder neck, urethra, and, in female, the vestibule, vagina, and, rarely, the uterus. Rectal ectopias are exceptional in both sexes. In males, the ureter may enter the prostatic urethra, the vas, or the seminal vesicle. Ectopic ureters opening outside the bladder or urethra tend to be obstructed and often associated with non-functioning renal moieties.

Presentation

As in all situations, in which there is ureteral obstruction, presentation with sepsis in infancy or childhood is possible. In males, UTIs are the only complications of ureteral ectopia. In females, paradoxical incontinence, which is dribbling of urine in between normal voidings, is characteristic of an ectopic ureter that enters in the distal urethra, vestibule, or vagina; thus, bypassing the sphincter mechanisms (see Chapter 5). If the urine produced by the moiety subtended by the ectopic ureter is minimal in volume, mild vaginal discharge or vulvar pruritus may be the presenting symptom. In males, the ectopic ureter never enters the urethra caudal to the sphincter mechanism; therefore, incontinence is never a symptom. Prenatal detection of duplication with upper pole dilatation is becoming the commonest form of presentation in the developed world (see Chapter 1).

Diagnosis

Once the presence of an ectopic ureter is suspected, it can be confirmed by a renal and bladder ultrasound. Typically, one finds a duplicated system with upper pole dilatation and a dilated ureter extending behind the bladder and beyond the bladder neck (Figure 15-6). Examination with a full bladder is important to detect the dilated distal ureter. Often, the dilatation is more pronounced distally and, in fact, the upper pole moiety may be barely discernible on ultrasonography. In cases of strong suspicion based on clinical presentation that cannot be confirmed with ultrasonography, an

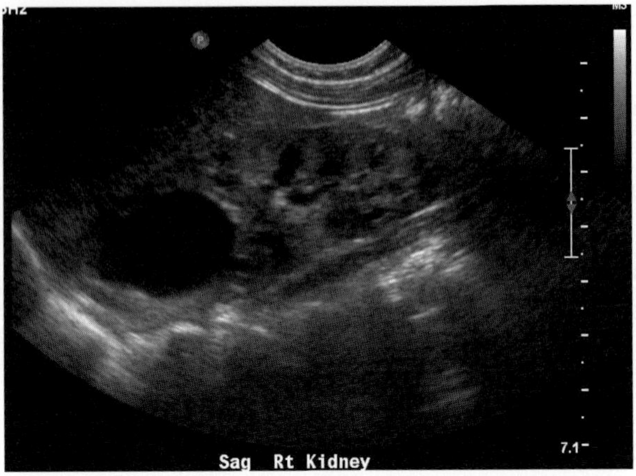

(A)

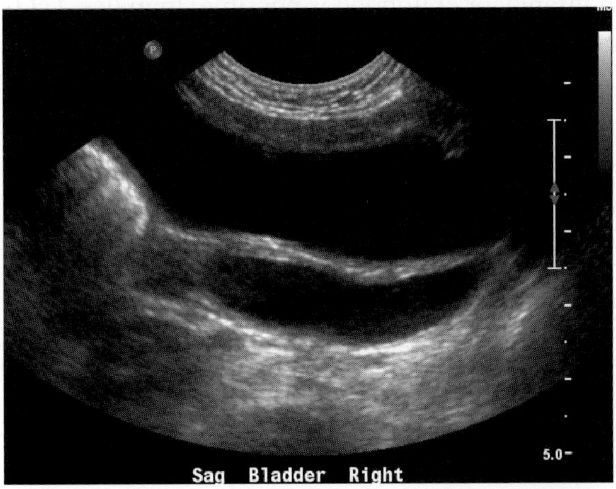

(B)

Figure 15-6. **(A)** A markedly dilated upper pole collecting system (left side in the picture) with normal lower pole moiety. **(B)** The dilated ureters coursing behind the bladder to enter in an ectopic position.

MR urogram is very helpful. Rarely, in difficult cases or when MRI is not available, a CT scan can also help. In most cases, in which the upper pole is visible sonographically, a nuclear renal scan is done to determine the function of the upper pole. A micturition cystourethrogram can show reflux during voiding to an upper pole moiety with a proximal urethral ectopia.

Management

The goal of treatment is to prevent infections and to correct incontinence if present. If the upper moiety is non-functioning, an upper pole nephrectomy is curative. There is no need to remove the entire ureter. Less than 5% of children will later require further excision of the distal stump of the ureter because of infection. The rationale for not removing all ureters completely is that the removal of the distal ureteral segment, as it goes through the pelvic floor, is difficult and carries the risk of injuring the urinary sphincter mechanism. If the upper moiety has function, the upper pole ureter can be anastomosed to the lower moiety ureter in the pelvis in an end-to-side fashion. Both procedures can be done openly or laparoscopically (see Section "Ureterocele").

FURTHER READING

Estrada Jr. CR, *et al.* Nomograms for predicting annual resolution rate of primary vesicoureteral reflux: results from 2462 children. *J Urol* 2009; **182**:1535–1541.

Glassberg KI, *et al.* Suggested terminology for duplex systems, ectopic ureters and ureteroceles. *J Urol* 1984; **132**(6):1153–1154.

González R, Piaggio LA. Initial experience with laparoscopic ipsilateral uretero-ureterostomy in infants and children for duplication anomalies of the urinary tract. *J Urol* 2007; **177**:2315–2318.

Horst M, Smith GH. Pelvi-ureteric junction obstruction in duplex kidneys. *BJU Int* 2008; **101**:1580–1584.

Jednak R, *et al.* A simplified technique for upper pole heminephrectomy in duplex kidneys. *J Urol* 2000; **164**:1326–1328.

Piaggio L, *et al.* Comparison of laparoscopic and open partial nephrectomy for duplication anomalies in children. *J Urol* 2006; **175**:2269–2273.

Siomou E, *et al.* Duplex collecting system diagnosed during the first six years of life after a first urinary tract infection: a study of 63 children. *J Urol* 2006; **175**(2):678–681.

Shekarriz B, *et al.* Long term outcomes based on the initial surgical approach for ureteroceles. *J Urol* 1999; **162**:1072–1076.

Chapter 16

Vesicoureteral Reflux

Maria J. Martínez Urrutia, Pedro López Pereira, and Enrique Jaureguizar Monereo

DEFINITION

Vesicoureteral Reflux (VUR) is defined as the abnormal retrograde flow of urine from bladder to ureter and into the collecting system of the kidneys. VUR may be associated with Urinary Tract Infection (UTI), hydronephrosis, abnormal kidney development, and renal parenchymal scars.

EPIDEMIOLOGY

Reflux may occur as an isolated entity or with other associated anomalies of the genitourinary tract.

VUR is a common childhood problem with high prevalence. It can be detected in 0.4–1.8% of healthy children. It is 10 times as common in white children as in the black children and children with red hair have an increased risk. The incidence in population with UTI ranges from 30 to 50%. VUR is more prevalent in male newborns; after one year of age, it is commoner in females than in males. The incidence of VUR decreases as patient age increases.

Although it has a definite genetic component, the exact mode of inheritance remains unknown. Researchers hypothesize that VUR is an autosomal dominant defect with a variable penetrance. About 34% of the patients who have this condition have also affected siblings.

PATHOPHYSIOLOGY AND ANATOMY

The normal mechanism of the ureterovesical junction includes oblique insertion of the intramural ureter, an adequate length of the intramural portion of the ureter, and strong detrusor support. This structure prevents the reflux. The intramural tunnel length-to-ureteral diameter ratio is 5:1 for a healthy non-refluxing ureter.

The ureter is composed of three muscular layers: an inner longitudinal layer, a middle circular layer, and an outer longitudinal layer. The inner longitudinal layer of smooth muscle passes through the ureteral hiatus, continues distally beyond the ureteral orifice into the trigone, and intertwines with the smooth muscle fibers of the contralateral ureter, forming the Bell muscle of the trigone and posterior urethra. The middle circular muscle fibers, outer longitudinal muscle fibers, and periureteral adventitia merge with the bladder wall in the upper part of the ureteral hiatus to form the Waldeyer sheath. This sheath attaches the extravesical portion of the ureter to the ureteral hiatus.

When the bladder fills, it is distending and thinning its wall and the intramural portion of the ureter also stretches and becomes compressed against the detrusor backing. This process allows a continual urine antegrade flow off, preventing retrograde flow from the bladder to the kidney (flap-valve mechanism) and this mechanism prevents reflux. The competence of this passive flap-valve mechanism is probably reinforced at the time of voiding by active elongation of the intravesical ureter within Waldeyer sheath.

The embryonic position of the ureteric bud is the key to the occurrence of this defect. When the ureteric bud is closer to the bladder than the mesonephric duct is, the resulting submucosal ureteral tunnel will be shorter than normal, which is resulting in a malfunctioning flap-valve mechanism that is more likely to produce VUR (Figure 16-1).

The human kidney contains two types of renal papillae: simple or convex and compound or concave. The latter is predominate at the polar region of the kidney. These papillae possess gaping orifices that are perpendicular to the papillary surface that remain open when intrarenal pressure increases. These gaping orifices allow free intrarenal reflux (Figure 16-2). However, simple papillae possess an oblique ductal orifice that closes when intrarenal pressure increases and does not allow

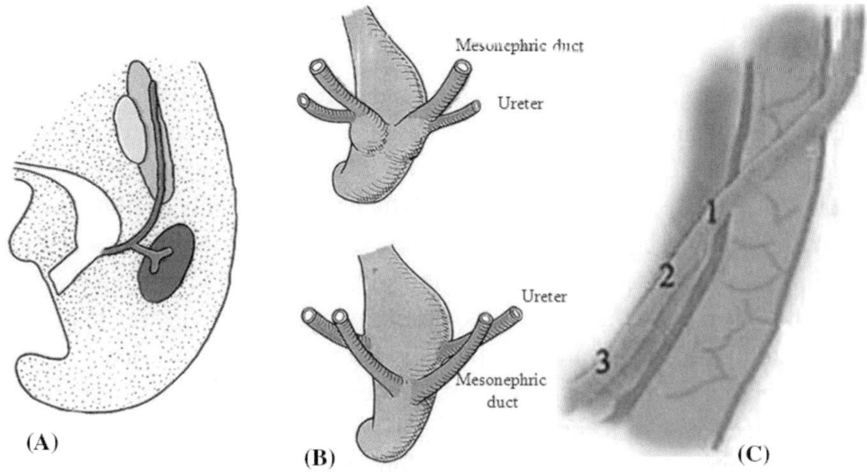

Figure 16-1. **(A)** Metanephric system in a five-week-old embryo. **(B)** Dorsal view of urogenital sinus. **(C)** Ureterovesical junction: (1) reflux; (2) possible reflux; (3) no reflux.

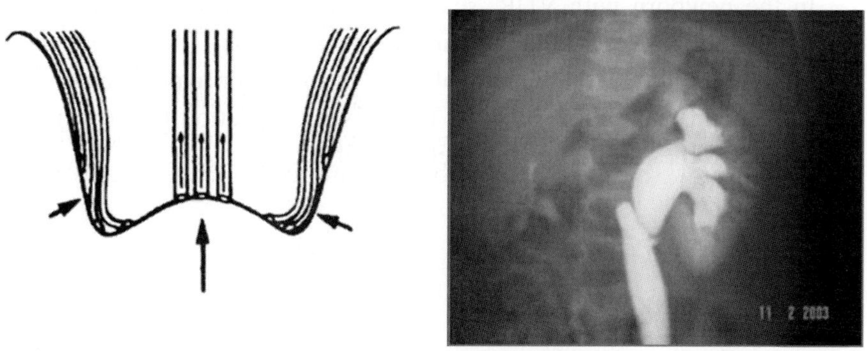

Figure 16-2. Intrarenal reflux. Anatomy of concave papilla (Ransley PG, *Urol. Res.* 1977; **5**:61–69).

intrarenal reflux. This intrarenal reflux is a result of intrarenal papillary anatomy.

In 1975, Ransley and Ridson (1981) confirmed the Tanagho studies, showing that reflux could be experimentally created in animals by modifying the ureteral junction. In later studies, they were able to show the correlation among reflux, renal papilla anatomy, pyelonephritis, and renal injury.

Intrarenal reflux of infected urine appears to be the main cause of renal damage associated with VUR. The presence of bacterial endotoxins activates the host's immune response and the release of oxygen-free radicals. The release of free radicals and proteolytic enzymes results in fibrosis and scarring of the affected renal parenchyma during healing. Initial scar formation at the infected polar region distorts the local anatomy of neighboring papillae and converts simple papillae into concave papillae, perpetuating further intrarenal reflux and additional renal scarring.

Intrarenal reflux of sterile urine (under normal intrapelvic pressure) has not been shown to produce clinically significant renal scars. Nevertheless, it may also lead to the formation of a renal damage lesion when there is high intravesical pressure.

Children with overactive bladder and voiding dysfunction (VD) generate high intravesical pressure, which can exacerbate pre-existing VUR or cause secondary VUR.

In the newborn with VUR, scars associated with high grade reflux have been detected before the occurrence of infection. These congenital scars are thought to be the regions of focal dysplasia or hypoplasia resulting from abnormal nephrogenesis. There is a correlation between renal dysplasia and the position of the ureteral orifice.

TYPES

Primary Reflux

Primary reflux is caused by a congenital abnormality of the intravesical ureter. This part of ureter may not be long enough to enable to close sufficiently to prevent urine reflux or the ureter may be inserted abnormally into the bladder. Primary reflux often resolves as the child grows and the ureter lengthens.

Secondary Reflux

Secondary reflux is the consequence of some other bladder pathology that leads to a decompensation of a normally formed ureterovesical junction.

Neurogenic bladder, posterior urethral valves, and non-neurogenic bladder dysfunction are the conditions that are typically associated with secondary reflux. The treatment of these patients depends on the management of the underlying causes with the expectation that as the problem is resolved, the reflux may remit.

PRESENTATION

The commonest symptom of VUR is UTI, and pyelonephritis is the initial presentation in most cases. VUR is detected in 30% of children with recurrent urinary infection. Other symptoms might include failure to thrive, nocturnal and diurnal enureses, and high blood pressure and proteinuria (pyelonephritis may result in kidney damage and renal failure). Reflux nephropathy is defined as the clinical triad: renal scar, hypertension, and VUR.

Hydronephrosis observed on a prenatal ultrasonography may be the first indication of VUR and a large number of neonates are evaluated for prenatal hydronephrosis. Reflux is the cause of the hydronephrosis in about 10% of these children.

DIAGNOSTIC METHODS

VUR is commonly diagnosed after UTI. A urine culture with more than 100,000 bacterial colonies should be considered as UTI.

Once the acute illness is resolved, the diagnosis of reflux can be considered. VUR is a radiographic diagnosis and the gold standard study is the voiding cystourethrogram (VCUG). Other recommended tests for VUR evaluation include: renal-bladder ultrasonography, nuclear renal scan, and urodynamic study.

Voiding Cystourethrogram

A standard VCUG allows accurate diagnosis and grading of the degree of reflux. Furthermore, it provides clear anatomic detail. VUR is graded based on the appearance of contrast in the ureter and upper collecting system beside the severity of calyceal changes, ureteral dilatation, and redundancy. The voiding phase of the cystography is considered the most important part of the test for assessing reflux (Figure 16-3). The VCUG also helps to evaluate the lower spine and whether the child has excessive feces in the colon. This finding could indicate the existence of a functional problem. The International Reflux Grading System was adopted in the early 1980s (Figure 16-4).

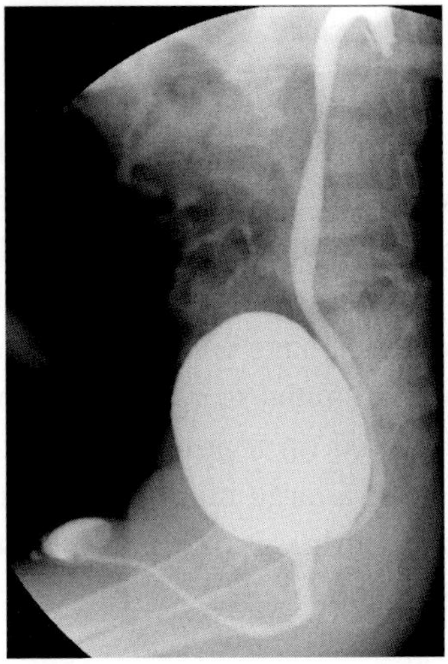

Figure 16-3. VCUG of a patient with Grade III VUR. Note that phimosis was observed in this boy.

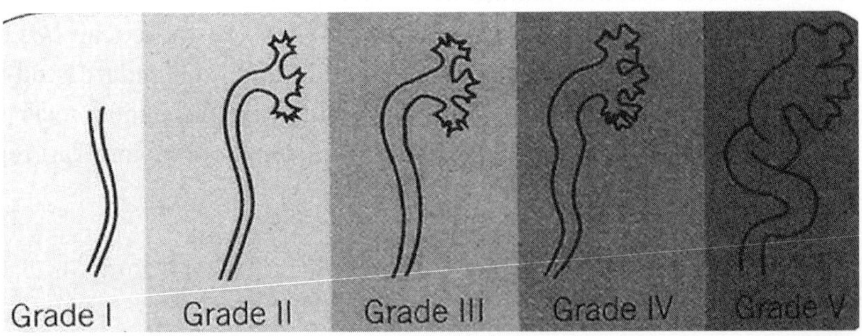

Figure 16-4. International reflux classification. Grade I: appearance of contrast in the ureter only. Grade II: contrast in the ureter and renal pelvis without dilatation of calyces. Grade III: mild calyceal dilatation without ureteral tortuosity. Grade IV: moderate calyceal dilatation and blunting. Grade V: severe calyceal dilatation with ureteral tortuosity.

Nuclear Cystography

It is also possible to show the presence of VUR by radioisotope cystogram, but this technique is insufficient to show the grade of reflux and urethral anatomy. However, it implies a lower radiation exposure and offers increased sensitivity. This study could be indicated during follow-up in a patient with known reflux, after surgery or even for the diagnosis of sibling reflux.

Cystosonography

Echocystography (US cystography) with galactose-based contrast medium is a useful tool for the diagnosis of VUR. Its ability to detect reflux is similar to that of conventional VCUG in cases of high-grade reflux and it may be a complementary technique to VCUG (follow-up studies, first examination in girls and screening of high-risk patients).

Ultrasonographic Scan

Renal ultrasonography is necessary to examine upper urinary tract morphology, dilatation, parenchymal thickness, and echogenicity. The evaluation of the bladder (prevoid, postvoid, and bladder wall thickness) provides additional information about the lower urinary tract and bladder function.

Nuclear Renal Scan

Technetium-99-m-dimercaptosuccinic acid (DMSA) is considered the best nuclear agent for visualizing the cortical tissue, evaluating renal function, and revealing the presence of renal scars. Acute pyelonephritis or chronic renal scars can be detected with this technique. Pyelonephritis impairs renal tubular uptake of radionuclide isotope, causing cortical photon defects on the DMSA scan. Persistent photopenic defects on the DMSA scan represent renal scarring and irreversible renal damage (Figure 16-5). One-third of patients with VUR have renal scars.

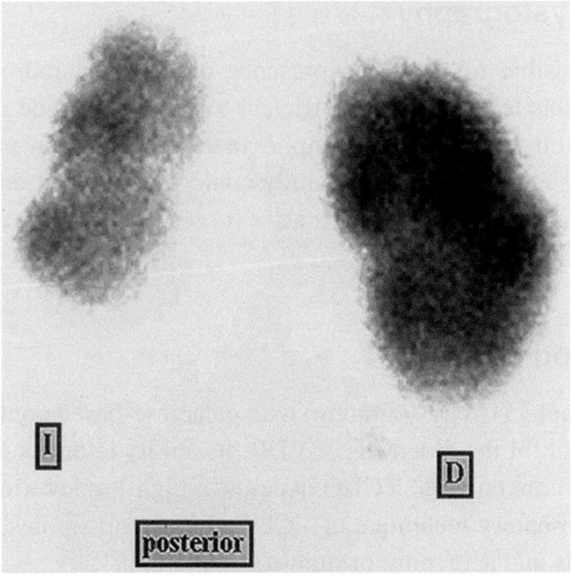

Figure 16-5. DMSA scan shows photopenic areas and scar in the lateral aspect of left kidney.

Urodynamic Study

A urodynamic evaluation should be done in children with a history of incontinence, frequency, urgency, and recurrent UTI. VD is a common finding in children evaluated for UTI and may be associated with VUR. The observation that high intravesical pressures occur during dysfunctional voiding has led the speculation that VUR could develop in these circumstances. This is similar to the occurrence of reflux in high-pressure neurogenic bladders.

Dysfunctional voiding is the result of voluntary contractions of the external sphincter by the child in an attempt to stop leakage of urine by involuntary detrusor contractions. It causes higher intravesical pressures during storage and voiding (Figure 16-6). High intravesical pressure may cause the reflux of urine, especially during voiding. If VD does cause reflux, it probably occurs by the compromise of a borderline ureterotrigonal structure. As the dysfunction becomes more severe, a functional outlet obstruction involves causing distortion of the urine outflow and resulting in increased residual postvoiding urine. UTI may be the result of this

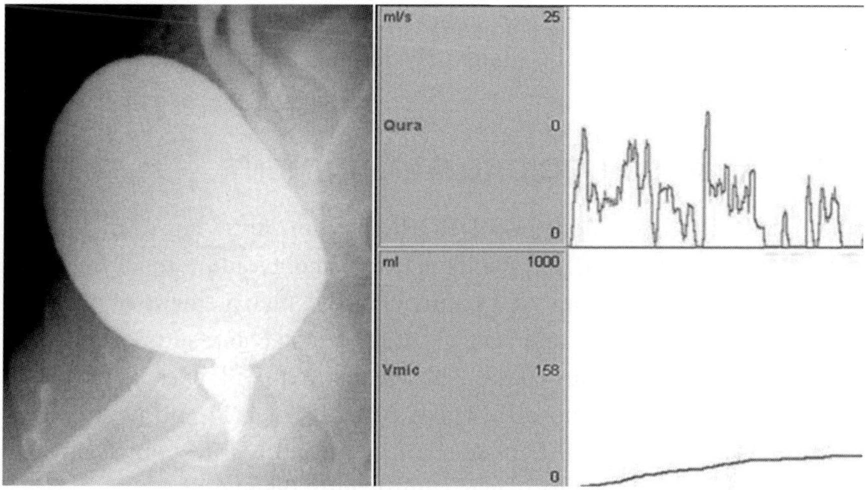

Figure 16-6. Dysfunctional voiding in a girl with reflux. "Spinning top" deformity of the bladder neck. Flow curve characteristic of voluntary sphincter contraction during voiding.

pathologic mechanism. There are two dysfunctional voiding patterns: bladder overactivity and high-pressure bladder with ineffective emptying.

Urodynamic evaluation with the monitoring of intravesical pressure can be done at the same time as the VCUG.

Other Diagnostic Tests

Cystoscopy

Cystoscopy plays a very limited role in VUR diagnosis. It is specially indicated when the anatomy of the urethra, bladder, or upper tract is incompletely defined by a prior radiographic evaluation.

Laboratory Studies

The following studies are recommended in all neonates who are born with antenatal or postnatal hydronephrosis:

- Urinalysis and urine culture to rule out UTI.

- Serum creatinine level and serum electrolytes at least after 24 hours after birth, because the child may have a dysplastic kidney on the affected side.

MEDICAL AND SURGICAL MANAGEMENT

The goals of management in VUR patients are: allowing normal renal growth, preventing UTI, and pyelonephritis, and avoiding renal failure.

There are two options of treatment in the management of children with VUR; conservative and surgical treatments. The results of randomized prospective studies have shown the equivalence of the two treatments. There were no differences in terms of UTI and new or progressive scar formation between either group. However, following surgical repair, pyelonephritis was significantly decreased.

Conservative Treatment

The aim of conservative treatment is to keep the urine sterile and wait for the spontaneous resolution of reflux during growth. While we are waiting for this to happen, the children are protected from UTI using low doses of daily antibiotic prophylaxis (one-third of the normal therapeutic dose). Amoxicillin, cephalosporin, trimethoprim-sulfamethoxazole, and nitrofurantoin have proven the most useful with minimal side effects.

The advice to give antibiotic prophylaxis to all children with VUR is based on the fact that prophylaxis reduces the incidence of renal scars after pyelonephritis.

During the course of conservative treatment, any fever, unexplained illness, or urinary tract symptom must be evaluated with urine culture. A breakthrough urinary infection, in spite of continuous antibiotic prophylaxis, is a dangerous situation.

A recent study from Columbia University shows that compliance with continuous antibiotic prophylaxis therapy is very poor. The overall rate of compliance was 41% with only 17% of patients having antibiotic coverage over at least 80% of the year following diagnosis of VUR and less than 10% having antibiotic coverage throughout the entire year.

The age until which the conservative treatment should be maintained remains a controversial issue. With the increasing age the probability of

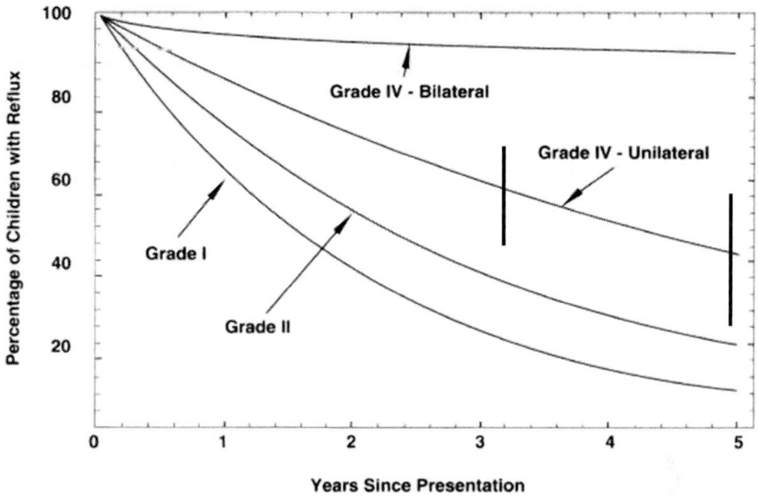

Figure 16-7. The chance of spontaneous resolution of reflux in children younger than five years (Elder *et al.*, 1997).

spontaneous resolution decreases. There is no point on insisting on a conservative treatment for patients after the age of five (Figure 16-7).

Surgical Treatment

The aim of surgery is to stop the reflux. The surgical options include an open surgical approach, endoscopic injection of a bulking agent, and laparoscopic correction.

Open Surgery

Ureteral reimplantation or ureteroneocystostomy is the definitive method of correcting primary reflux, especially in the setting of anatomic abnormalities. Multiple different antireflux techniques have been performed. The aim is to mobilize the distal segment of the ureter and to place it under a tunnel of bladder submucosa in order to restore the flap-valve mechanism that is designed to prevent VUR. Mostly the techniques fall into one of two main categories: intravesical reimplantation, in which the bladder is opened and the ureters are dissected intravesically, and extravesical

Table 16-1. Open surgical antireflux procedures.

Extravesical	Intravesical	Extra- and intravesical
Lich-Grégoir, 1961	Hucht-1, 1952	Paquin, 1959
Detrusorrhaphy, 1971	Glenn-Anderson, 1967	Mathisen, 1964
	Cohen, 1975	Politano-Leadbetter, 1985
	Gil-Vernet, 1984	
	Kelalis, 1985	

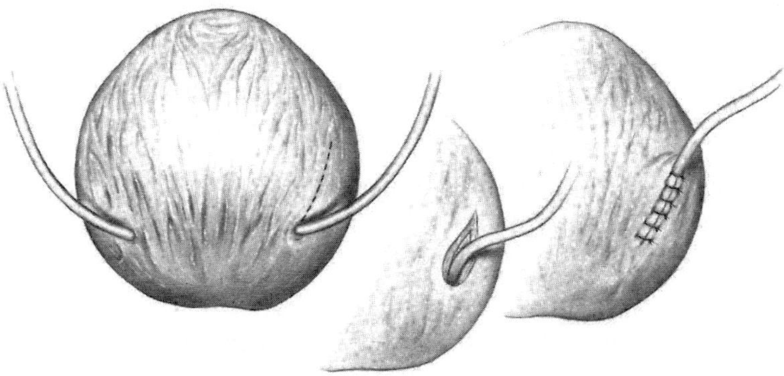

Figure 16-8. Lich-Grégoir technique.

reimplantation, in which the ureters are dissected away from the bladder wall without opening the bladder and left attached to the bladder mucosa to be reimplanted under mucosa flaps (Table 16-1).

Extravesical reimplantation: Lich-Grégoir technique

The incision of the bladder muscle is performed cephalad and lateral to the ureteral hiatus and along the natural course of the ureter. The extension of the incision depends on the diameter of the ureter. The ureter is placed into the mucosal bed and overlying muscle is closed (Figure 16-8). This procedure has particular advantages and applicability in renal transplantation. Although this technique has been applied successfully in many patients, including those with ureteral duplication, the presence of a suprahiatal diverticulum (Hutch's diverticulum) could be a contraindication. Detrusorrhaphy is a modification of the Lich-Grégoir procedure that incorporates ureteral advancement into the repair.

Intravesical reimplantation: *Cohen technique*

This is the most widely open procedure used today. The ureters are mobilized transvesically and separate submucosal tunnels are created for each ureter, so that each ureter opens on the side that is opposite to its hiatus (Figure 16-9). Glassberg *et al.* (1985) recommended a modification of the

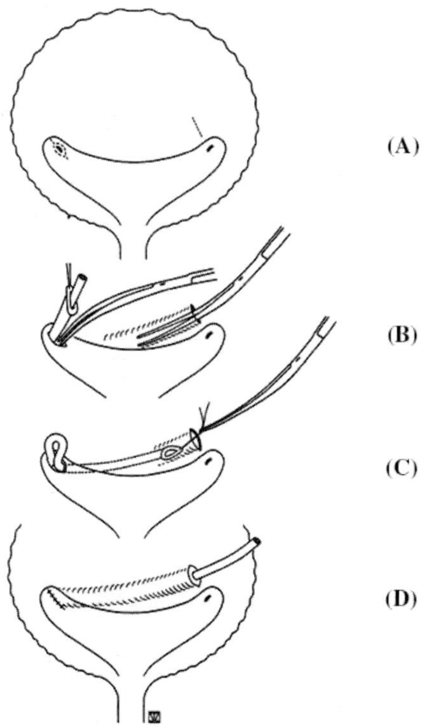

Figure 16-9. Cohen technique. **(A)** Circumferential incision around the ureter orifice. Ureter is freed by sharp dissection. **(B)** The site of the new orifice is chosen superior and lateral to the contralateral orifice. **(C)** Submucosal tunnel is fashioned cephalad to the trigone. **(D)** The ureter is advanced through the tunnel. Modified from Cohen (1977).

original technique for patients with dilated ureters and small bladder. This modified technique involves incising the bladder at the superolateral margin of the hiatus and mobilizing the peritoneum cranially. This incision allows the ureter to enter the bladder in a more superior and lateral position, thus creating a longer tunnel.

Intravesical and extravesical reimplantation: Politano-Leadbetter technique

The ureter is mobilized intravesically and pulled extravesically to be brought inside the bladder through a new hiatus that lies superior and lateral to the original ureter hiatus. The lateral umbilical ligament should be transected to prevent kinking of the ureter. After the ureter has been brought through its new superior and lateral hiatus, a submucosal tunnel is developed from the side of the new hiatus to the site of the original ureteral hiatus.

There is no clear documentation of any of the many techniques being superior to the others in terms of VUR resolution. The success rate of ureteral reimplantation is higher than 95%, and close to 100% for the lower grades of reflux.

Potential complications due to the ureteral reimplantation of the ureters include bleeding in the retroperitoneal space, hematuria, infection, ureteral obstruction, injury to adjacent organs, and persistent reflux. These occur in less than 1% of cases.

Persistent reflux

The persistent reflux of the reimplanted ureter and the development of a novo reflux on the contralateral side are usually temporary and resolve spontaneously. Transient postoperative reflux is usually caused by the detrusor instability of the healing bladder. The persistent reflux of the ipsilateral ureter in the absence of secondary causes is usually caused by a technical error. Some technical problems are inadequate ureteral mobilization, short intramural tunnel, inadequate anchoring of the ureter, and inappropriate placement of the ureteral orifice. Reoperation or endoscopic treatment must be considered.

Ureteral obstruction

Most postoperative ureteral obstructions resolve spontaneously. However, a temporary ureteral stent left postsurgically could avoid this problem. Ureteroscopic dilatation and stent placement may correct mild obstruction or stenosis. Nephrostomy is rarely required.

Hematuria

Gross hematuria after reimplantation is common, but is often self-limited and requires no intervention.

Endoscopic Treatment

In 1981, Matouschek described the technique of subureteral implantation of a bulking agent to correct reflux, and the technique was subsequently popularized by O'Donnell and Puri. The principle of the procedure is to inject, under cystoscopic guidance, a biocompatible bulking agent underneath the intravesical portion of the ureter in a submucosal location (Figure 16-10).

The bulking agent elevates the ureteral orifice and distal ureter in such a way that the lumen is narrowed, which is preventing regurgitation of urine up the ureter but still allowing its antegrade flow. Several bulking agents have been evaluated. These include polytetrafluorethylene (PTFE or teflon), collagen, autologous fat, polydimethylsiloxane, silicone, chondrocytes, and

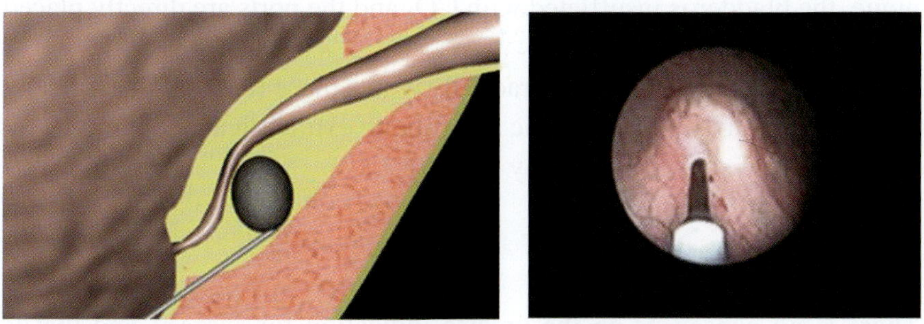

Figure 16-10. Endoscopic treatment of reflux.

a solution of dextranomer/hyaluronic acid (deflux). Following Food and Drug Administration (FDA) approval of the use of dextranomer hyaluronhic acid copolymer for the treatment of primary VUR, a growing number of physicians have begun to consider endoscopic treatment as an alternative to the undefined duration of prophylactic antibiotics. Endoscopic treatment provides a high success rate in children with reflux that decreases with an increasing grade (Grade II, 78%; Grade III, 72%; Grade IV, 63%; and Grade V, 51%). If the first endoscopic treatment is unsuccessful, a therapeutic option is to perform a second endoscopic treatment. Shifting or disappearance of the implant is the most frequent causes of failure.

Two injections (retreatment) can be performed, bringing the aggregate rate of resolution to 85%.

Complications are rare with the procedure and transient ureteral obstruction and UTIs are the most commonly reported.

Laparoscopic Antireflux

In the last decade, there has been a shift to performing ureteric reimplantation using a laparoscopic approach in order to provide all the advantages of a minimally invasive technique with long-term results similar to traditional open ureteric reimplantation. Robot-assisted laparoscopy has complemented and overcome some of the limitations of conventional laparoscopic techniques. The Lich-Grégoir method is the most popular laparoscopic extravesical approach.

Laparoscopic transvesical ureteric reimplantation (Cohen procedure) using a pneumo-vesicoscopic approach is gaining popularity. In this technique, the bladder is insufflated with CO_2 and the ports are directly placed within the bladder.

Laparoscopic surgery has gradually won a place for itself in surgically dealing with VUR. Laparoscopic and robotic extravesical and intravesical surgeries have shown good early results.

Indications for Surgery

There is no consensus on the precise indication for surgery, and that is why it is difficult to select the ideal treatment for each patient. The current policy is to prescribe prophylactic antibiotic treatment for prolonged periods (24–36 months) in the expectation of spontaneous maturation by the ureterovesical junction and the resolution of the VUR. If the patient suffers from recurrent breakthrough infections, or if there are signs of continued deterioration of the renal mass, endoscopic correction or surgical reimplantation should be offered. The aim of the treatment is to stop the reflux. This does not necessarily mean that the progression of renal damage is halted or that further UTI are prevented.

In cases where the reflux has caused severe damage to the kidney (relative function less than 10%), nephroureterectomy may be done.

Prognosis and Long-Term Complication

All patients with a history of reflux should be monitored for life even if the reflux resolves. In the operated and non-operated patient group, the risk of further recurrent UTI may persist. Susceptibility to UTI continues for a number of years in many girls and women. However, postoperative UTIs are primarily afebrile. Long-term follow-up studies of up to 20 years confirm the ongoing risk of UTI, including febrile UTIs (46–52%), as well as the development of hypertension (6%).

By the time surgical correction has been performed, some children have already have significant kidney damage. When kidney deterioration has been demonstrated, the pediatric nephrologist must provide careful surveillance with appropriate medication and dietary restriction.

The role of bladder function in the outcome of reflux is significant starting from the first year of life. In the youngest infants, abnormal bladder function can be present at birth, whereas in older children, it may be acquired and learned during the toilet-training years. Appropriate management of the VD often results in the resolution of the reflux. The studies of Sillén (1999) have shown that resolution of reflux in the infant correlated with the normalizing of bladder functions with aging.

Current Controversies

Significant advances in our understanding of the pathogenesis of reflux have taken place and, although the surgical management of reflux has largely been perfected, many questions remain unresolved.

- Do we need to correct all refluxing renal units?
- Can prophylactic antibiotics safely be discontinued in children with VUR?
- Should older girls with persisting reflux be allowed to come off prophylaxis?

At the beginning, it was held that because reflux does not naturally occur in human beings, when it was diagnosed, especially when it was associated with UTI and pyelonephritis, it seemed logical to advocate the surgical correction of all reflux.

Later, it was recognized that most cases of reflux may resolve spontaneously with time and growth. Surgery was reserved, thereafter, for the cases that did not or could not resolve with time (antibiotics and observation in many and surgery in some cases).

To date, the current debate concerns whether we can further refine this paradigm, so that only patients vulnerable to pyelonephritis and renal scarring are considered candidates for surgery or some other invasive therapy.

The most of our beliefs and practice regarding VUR are still based on "low-evidence" sources and evidence-based medicine (EBM) does not yet have sufficient arguments to establish a recommendation for diagnosis and treatment of VUR.

There is no consensus in the case of persistent asymptomatic VUR, regarding the indication and duration of antibiotic prophylaxis or the best treatment.

There is consensus to the effect on the fact that any symptomatic UTI should be immediately treated by adequate antibiotics without delay. If the appropriate treatment is postponed, renal damage may occur.

COMMENT FROM THE EDITORS

Five decades after the recognition of the relationship among reflux, UTIs, and scarring, we are still debating how best to evaluate and treat these children. The authors have reviewed the state of the art knowledge on the topic and the current accepted practice for management. We must rely on the ongoing prospective trials to better define the optimal therapy of VUR in the future.

FURTHER READING

Beetz R, Maunhardt W, Fisch M, *et al.* Long-term follow-up of 150 young adults surgically treated for vesicoureteral reflux in childhood: the ongoing risk of urinary tract infections. *J Urol* 2002; **168**:704–707.

Cohen SJ. The Cohen reimplantation technique. *Birth Defects Orig Artic Ser* 1977; **13**(5):391–395.

Cohen SJ. Ureterozystoneostomie, eine neue antirefluxu-technik. *Aktvel Urol* 1975; **6**:1–7.

Danies SL, Hodgson NB. Management of reflux in total duplication anomalies. *J Urol* 1971; **105**:720–724.

Decter RM. Update on vesicoureteral reflux: pathogenesis, nephropathy and management. *Rev Urol* 2001; **3**(4):172–178.

Elder J, Diaz M, Caldamone A, *et al.* Endoscopic therapy for vesicoureteral reflux: a meta-analysis. I. Reflux resolution and urinary tract infection. *J Urol* 2006; **175**:716–722.

Elder JS, Peters CA, Arant Jr BS, *et al.* Pediatric Vesicoureteral Reflux Guidelines Panel summary report on the management of primary vesicoureteral reflux in children. *J Urol* 1997; **157**(5):1846–1851.

Gil-Vernet JM. A new technique for surgical correction of vesicoureteral reflux. *J Urol* 1984; **131**:456–458.

Glassberg KI, Laungani G, Wasnick RJ, Waterhouse K. Transverse ureteral advancement techniques of ureteroneocystostomy (Cohen reimplant) and a modification for difficult cases (experience with 121 ureters). *J Urol* 1985; **134**(2):304–307.

Glenn JF, Anderson EE. Distal tunnel uretal reimplantation. *J Urol* 1967; **97**: 623–626.

Greenfield SP, Wan J. The relationship between dysfunctional voiding and congenital vesicoureteral reflux. *Curr Opin Urol* 2000; **10**(6):607–610.

Hensle T, Grogg A, Eaddy M. Pediatric vesicoureteral reflux: treatment patterns and outcomes. *Nat Clin Pract Urol* 2007; **4**(9):462–463.

Hoebeke P, Van Laecke E, Van Camp C, *et al.* One thousand videourodynamic studies in children with non-neurogenic bladder sphincter dysfunction. *BJU Int* 2001; **87**(6):575–580.

Hutch JA. Vesicoureteral reflux in the paraplegic cause and correction. *J Urol* 1952; **97**:623–626.

Kelalis PP. Surgical correction of vesicoureteral reflux. In: *Clinical Pediatric Urology*, 2nd Edn. (eds.) PP Kelalis, LR King, AB Belman. Philadelphia: WB Saunders Co., 1985, pp. 381–419.

Kramer S. Vesicoureteral reflux. In: *Clinical Pediatric Urology*, 4th Edn. (eds.) A Belman, L King, S Kramer. London: Martin Dunitz, 2002, pp. 749–810.

Lich R, Howerton LW, Davis LA. Recurrent urosepsis in children. *J Urol* 1961; **86**:554–558.

Mackie GC, Awang H, Stephens FD. Duplex kidney: a correlation of renal dysplasia with position of the ureteral orifice. *J Urol* 1975; **114**:274–280.

Mathews R, Carpenter M, Chesney R, *et al.* Controversies in the management of vesicoureteral reflux: the rationale for the RIVUR study. *J Pediatr Urol* 2009; **5**:336–341.

Mathisen W. Vesterovesical reflux and its surgical correction. *Surg Gynecol Obstet* 1964; **118**:965–971.

Matouschek E. Die behandlung des vesikorenalen reflues durch transurethrale einspritzung von teflonpaste. *Urologe* 1981; **20**:263–264.

Mouriquand P. Surgical treatment of vesicoureteric reflux. In: *Operative Pediatric Surgery*, 6th Edn. (eds.) L Spitz, AG Goran. New York: Edward Arnold, 2006, pp. 783–792.

O'Donnell B, Puri P. Treatment of vesicoureteric reflux by endoscopic injection of Teflon. *Br Med J* 1984; **289**:7–9.

Paquin AJ Jr. Ureterovesical anastomosis: the description and evaluation of a technique. *J Urol* 1959; **82**:573–583.

Politano VA, Leadbetter WF. An opertive technique for correction of vesicoureteral reflux. *J Urol* 1958; **79**:932–941.

Puri P. Vesicoureteral reflux: endoscopic correction. In: *Operative Pediatric Surgery*, 6th Edn. (eds.) L Spitz, AG Goran. New York: Edward Arnold, 2006, pp. 779–782.

Ransley PG. Intrarenal reflux anatomical, dynamic and radiological studies — Part I. *Urol Res* 1977; **5**:61–69.

Ransley PG, Risdon RA. Reflux nephropathy: effect of antimicrobial therapy on the evolution of the early pyelonephritis scar. *Kidney Int* 1981; **20**:733–742.

Report of a meeting of physicians at the Hospital for Sick Children of London. Vesicoureteric reflux: all in the gene? *Lancet* 1996; **348**:725–728.

Sillén U. Bladder dysfunction in children with vesicoureteric reflux. *Acta Paediatr Suppl* 1999; **88**(431):40–47.

Smellie JM, Normand IC. Reflux nephropathy in childhood. In: *Reflux Nephropathy* (eds.) J Hodson, P Kincaid-Smith. New York: Masson Publishing, USA, 1979, pp. 14–20.

Smellie JM, Barratt TM, Chantler C, *et al.* Medical versus surgical treatment in children with severe bilateral vesicoureteric reflux and bilateral nephropathy: a randomised trial. *Lancet* 2001; **357**:1329–1332.

Thakre AA, Sreedhar B, Yeung CK. Laparoscopy in the management of pediatric vesicoureteral reflux. *Indian J Urol* 2007; **23**(4):414–419.

Wheeler D, Vimalachandra D, Hodson E, *et al.* Antibiotics and surgery for vesicoureteric reflux: a meta-analysis of randomised controlled trials. *Arch Dis Child* 2003; **88**:688–694.

Wingberg J, Bollgren I, Kallenins G, *et al.* Clinical pyelonephritis and focal renal scarring: a selected review of pathogenesis, prevention and prognosis. *Pediatr Clin North Am* 1983; **29**:801–814.

Yeung CK, Godley M, Dhillon HK, *et al.* The characteristic of primary vesicoureteric reflux in male and female infants with prenatal hydronephrosis. *Br J Urol* 1997; **80**(2):319–327.

Chapter 17

Urethral Obstruction

Miguel L. Podesta

POSTERIOR URETHRAL VALVES

Definition of the Disease

Posterior urethral valves (PUVs) is the most common cause of congenital lower urinary tract obstruction in the male pediatric population, ranging from 1/4000 to 1/7500 births. This congenital anomaly varies in severity and is associated with structural and functional changes of the entire urinary tract, including renal dysplasia, urinary back pressure damage, and the alterations of renal and bladder functions. In more severe cases, lower urinary tract obstruction can result in the deterioration of fetal renal function and progressive oligohydramnios, which may lead to pulmonary hypoplasia with a high risk of perinatal morbidity and mortality.

Etiology

Young and co-workers (1919) reported three types of congenital urethral valves. Type I: two obliquely oriented mucosal folds that extend downward and laterally from the lower border of the verumontanum around the membranous urethra to meet at the 12 o'clock position. Type II consists of folds or ridges of mucosa that branch off from the verumontanum toward the bladder neck. Type III presents a transverse diaphragmatic membrane on the same level as, or even below, the verumontanum. Interestingly, the latter valve type does not originate from the crista urethralis. Type I valves occur more frequently than Type III and may result from the defects of the integration of the Wolffian ducts into the urethra during fetal development, whereas the latter valve type may represent the failure of canalization of the urogenital membrane. Most pediatric urologists believe that Type II valves are not obstructive. More recently, Dewan *et al.* (1997) proposed that Types I and III are the variations of a single entity and described them as a membrane within the lumen of the urethra below the verumontanum with a pinhole opening.

Anatomical Consequences of Urethral Obstruction by PUV

Since the degree of obstruction caused by urethral valves varies from one patient to another, a wide range of secondary changes are observed in the urinary tract above the level of the urethral lesion. The posterior urethra is significantly elongated and dilated (Figure 17-1). The bladder neck is

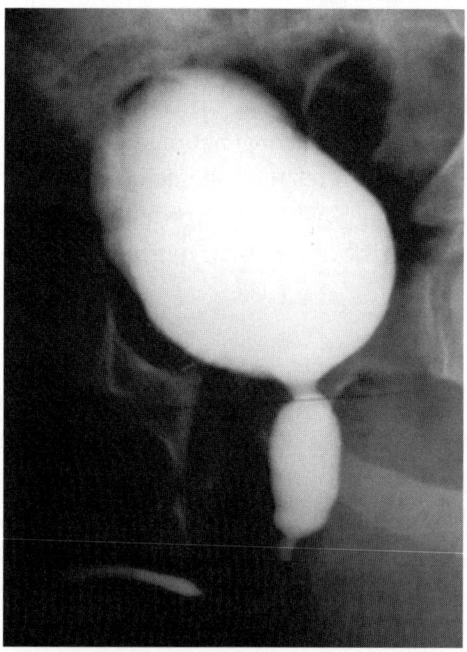

Figure 17-1. VCU in a young infant showing dilated posterior urethra with a narrow bladder neck secondary to PUVs. Note the diminished anterior urethral lumen below the valves.

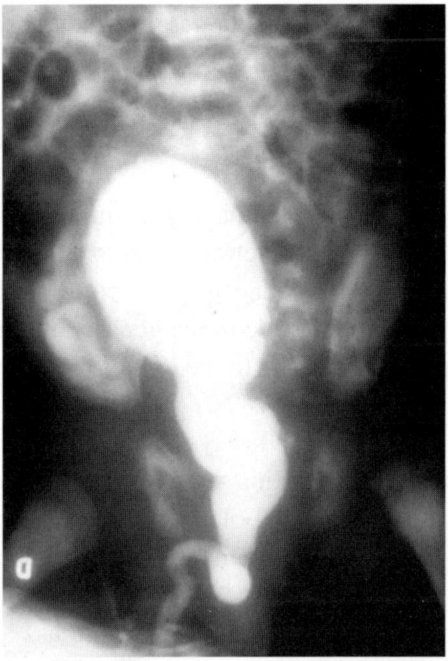

Figure 17-2. Oblique view of VCU showing grossly dilated posterior urethra and bladder neck due to urethral valves. Note the thickened bladder wall and right vesicoureteral reflux.

hypertrophic, sometimes grossly open but often narrow and prominent (Figure 17-2). Detrusor thickening is frequently associated with sacculation of the bladder wall and the ureters are usually dilated and tortuous. Unilateral or bilateral vesicoureteral reflux is present in approximately half of the patients. Finally, varying degrees of hydronephrosis and unilateral or bilateral dysmorphic kidneys are a common finding.

Experimental studies in fetal animals that underwent *in utero* surgically induced severe urethral obstruction have shown that the obstruction early in gestation can result in renal cystic dysplasia whereas the obstruction in the later stages of pregnancy may induce bladder enlargement and hydronephrosis. Thus, we may interpret that renal dysplasia results from early and severe urethral obstruction during gestation.

An alternative explanation by Henneberry and Stephens (1980) postulates a correlation of renal morphology with the ureteral orifice position, which also applies to non-duplicated ureters in fetuses with partial urethral obstruction, with or without vesicoureteral reflux. These authors believe that the ureteral meatus location may be a determining factor in the development of renal dysplasia in PUV patients. Thus, it seems that kidney damage in the patients with PUV may be caused by different pathogenic mechanisms.

It is important to recognize voiding dysfunction disorders in PUV patients even after the successful relief of the obstruction. Mitchell (1982) and Parkhouse *et al.* (1988) advanced the hypothesis that severe bladder dysfunction plays a significant role in the genesis of the progressive deterioration of the upper tract leading to the loss of renal function and urinary incontinence.

The mechanism behind bladder dysfunction in the patients with congenital valve obstruction remains incompletely understood. There is evidence indicating that abnormal bladder function is related to the poor development of bladder wall components as a response to the severity of outlet obstruction during gestation. Ultrastructural studies have shown that obstructed bladders have increased muscle mass and connective tissue. Moreover, there seems to be more of the stiff collagen tissue (type I) than malleable collagen (type III). A second factor that may contribute to bladder function inadequacy is prolonged bladder defunctionalization in patients with upper tract diversion. A final contribution to bladder malfunction may be attributed to the increased number of ureteral reimplantation procedures needed for undiversion reconstruction.

Presentation

Prenatal

The widespread use of obstetric ultrasound examinations has enabled the identification of urological anomalies such as PUVs before birth. Two thirds of the newborns with bladder outlet obstruction are now detected in this way. PUV is suspected in male fetuses with bilateral hydroureteronephrosis associated with a persistent enlarged bladder and dilatation of the posterior urethra with or without amniotic fluid volume modifications. The detection of progressive oligohydramnios before 24 weeks of intrauterine life is associated with a high incidence of pulmonary hypoplasia and poor renal function outcome. The detection of cortical cystic changes or the absence of corticomedullary renal parenchyma differentiation by prenatal ultrasonography suggests renal dysplasia; however, it should be noted that the absence of renal cysts does not exclude dysplastic renal changes (see Chapter 1).

Clinical

A spectrum of symptoms and signs results from the degree of urinary obstruction, the presence of infected urine, and the renal function impairment in different combinations. Neonates with severe urethral obstruction accompanied by oligohydramnios may develop respiratory distress in the first days of life or have a urinoma or urinary ascites secondary to spontaneous bladder or calyceal fornix rupture (Figure 17-3). Other

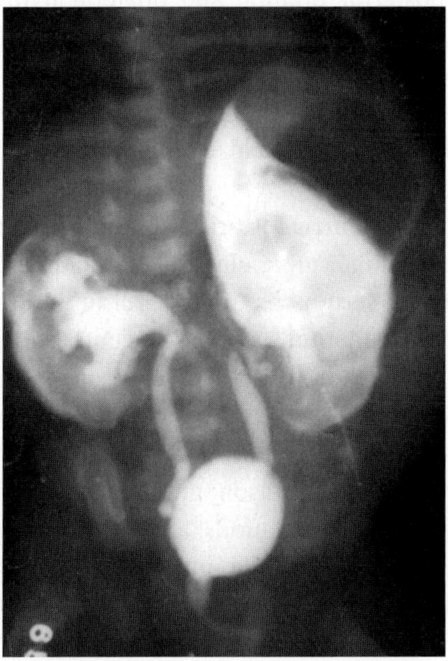

Figure 17-3. VCU in a neonate shows dilated posterior urethra above PUV with bilateral dilating vesicoureteric reflux. Observe severe left renal urinoma and right perirenal urinary extravasation due to fornix leak of urine.

neonates may have bladder distention, urinary dribbling associated with dehydration, and metabolic acidosis.

Associated urine infection is responsible for high peaks of temperature, palpable abdominal or flank mass, decreased urinary stream, or even failure to thrive. In such cases, intestinal manifestations (vomiting and diarrhea) often accompanied by jaundice and irritability due to compromise of the central nervous system may accompany the clinical picture.

In older children, obstructive voiding symptoms, hematuria, recurrent urinary tract infection, and renal function deterioration are common findings.

Diagnostic Methods

As previously mentioned, the antenatal diagnosis of PUV can be suspected in male fetus when high-resolution transabdominal or transvaginal sonography studies detect bladder distension, hypertrophy of the bladder wall, dilated posterior urethra, and bilateral hydronephrosis. These newborns should be investigated in the first day of life by repeat ultrasonography and voiding cystourethrogram (VCU).

It must be emphasized that initial postnatal assessment begins with a complete medical history, physical examination, biochemical analysis, and imaging studies.

Biochemical analysis includes urine culture, determinations of serum creatinine, urine creatinine, urea, electrolytes, and acid–base evaluation. As would be expected, serum creatinine level in the first 24 hours of life reflects maternal renal function since the placenta is responsible for clearance of creatinine and urea nitrogen. However, an estimate of the patient's baseline creatinine and its state of decline after a few days of urethral catheter, drainage is useful to delineate further treatment.

Next, renal and bladder ultrasonographies will confirm the grade of ureteral and pelvicalyceal dilatations and document parenchyma morphology. Also well recognized is the importance of assessing bladder wall thickness and whether upper urinary tract dilatation ameliorates with an empty bladder.

Persistent dilatation of the upper tracts with bladder emptying suggests obstruction at the uretero-vesical junction secondary to bladder wall hypertrophy or inadequate ureteric peristalsis.

Once a clinical response is recognized and urine sterility is confirmed by urine culture analyses, VCU under prophylactic antibiotics is obtained. This study documents the existence of PUV showing the outline of the valve membrane in the rounded lower margin of the distended posterior urethra and a distended and thick-walled bladder with or without vesicoureteral reflux. Radioisotopic studies are also useful for providing reliable estimations of differential renal function.

Medical and Surgical Management

Prenatal

Prenatal suspicion of PUV allows, in properly selected cases, *in utero* decompression of the lower urinary tract.

Patients eligible for vesico-amniotic shunt placement include male fetuses (46 XY) with bladder dilatation, bilateral hydroureteronephrosis, decreased amniotic fluid volume, absence of associated congenital anomalies, serially fetal urine electrolyte levels (Na < 100 mmol/L, Cl < 90 mmol/L), and tubular protein (B2 microglobulin < 6 mg/L) below the recommended threshold and osmolality less than 200 mOsm/L.

Freedman and co-workers (1999) applied this selection criteria and reported 60% postnatal survival and 33% incidence of renal failure (nadir creatinine > 1 mg/dL) in fetuses with PUV, detected before 24 weeks of gestation. *In utero* cystoscopy via abdominal-utero-abdominal fetal puncture is another promising alternative method that can provide accurate fetal diagnosis of urethral valves and permit prenatal direct vision valve ablation. This sophisticated procedure will hopefully decrease technical complications of vesico-amniotic shunting and allow early bladder cycling. However, the benefits of this appealing fetal intervention modality should be balanced against the inherent complications of the method.

Postnatal management is aimed at monitoring vital signs, pulmonary and renal functions, rapid intravenous fluid support, and serum electrolyte evaluation. Subsequent decompression of the urinary tract with an indwelling urethral catheter and antibiotic prophylaxis is essential to prevent urinary infection. Surgical treatment recommendations are based on the response of the upper urinary tract in ultrasound examinations and serum creatinine level and its rate of decline after the placement of adequate postnatal bladder drainage with a urethral catheter.

When the neonate or young infant is clinically stable, primary endoscopic valve ablation with direct vision is the preferred postnatal treatment. Controversy exists regarding the most appropriate initial surgical management of neonates and infants whose clinical condition fails to improve and whose upper urinary tract remains dilated after bladder decompression with a urethral catheter. In these circumstances, some authors favor high urinary diversion and delayed valve ablation, while others think that upper tract drainage is irreversible. The advantage of cutaneous drainage is the rapid improvement of the patient's general condition, the control of urinary infection, and fast renal function recovery; however, if renal dysplasia is present, temporary high diversion cannot reverse this unfavorable condition. A further disadvantage for diverted patients is the complications of later urinary tract reconstructive procedures. Supravesical diversion and delayed valve ablation should be reserved for selected cases where despite both satisfactory bladder drainage and medical treatment the upper tracts remain grossly dilated and serum creatinine continues to increase, or when severe urinary tract infection is present and does not respond to antibiotic treatment.

In our practice, we do not perform high diversion in patients whose renal function improves and who remain free of urinary infection in spite of persistence of dilated upper tracts. These patients are managed by transurethral valve ablation.

Cutaneous vesicostomy is another temporary urinary diversion alternative that avoids long periods of bladder defunctionalization. This method is reserved for young infants in whom the urethra is so small that it precludes transurethral valve ablation or in patients with severe reflux complicated with urosepsis and also non-responsive to urethral catheter drainage and aggressive antibiotic treatment. In these cases, delayed valve ablation should be done simultaneously with vesicostomy closure to avoid dry ablation of valves, which may favor the development of a urethral stricture.

Late Outcome

Patients with PUV require long-term follow-up with monitoring of blood pressure, renal function, kidney growth, urinary tract dilatation, bladder function, urinary continence, urinary infections, acid–base balance, and proteinuria. Although renal function recovery is frequently noted after the relief of the urethral obstruction, a number of older children and adolescents develop end-stage renal failure. In a study of 98 children with PUV followed-up for 11 to 22 years, Parkhouse *et al.* (1988) reported a rate of 32% poor renal function outcome, 10% died of renal failure, 15% were on dialysis, and 6% had a glomerular filtration rate <25 ml/min/1.73. Parkhouse *et al.* (1988) also found an incidence of end-stage renal failure in 26% of 50 adolescents with PUV, even though all cases but one had normal renal function in infancy.

As previously stated, the diagnosis of dysfunctional voiding is another important factor that can adversely affect renal function in older children. A poorly complianted bladder associated with persistently high intravesical pressure during filling will cause progressive hydroureteronephrosis. This condition may be enhanced by the high urine output polyuria which is frequently found in patients with tubular renal damage. The urodynamic evaluation of the filling and emptying phase of the lower urinary tract is the best way to investigate the presence and severity of bladder dysfunction. Treatment for detrusor hyperactivity during filling is usually initiated with anticholinergic drugs and related agents. Selective alpha adrenergic blocker therapy or intermittent catheterization is used in patients with voiding detrusor underactivity. Medical treatment should always be carefully monitored with periodic urodynamic studies. Occasionally, bladder augmentation is needed in patients with severely decreased compliance, worsening bilateral hydroureteronephrosis, and the progressive deterioration of renal function, which is non-responsive to medical management.

We compared long-term bladder function in children with PUV treated with initial high diversion and delayed valve ablation with primary valve ablation alone. Altered bladder function occurred more frequently in patients treated with initial supravesical diversion regardless of the level of diversion. Moreover, in a previous publication comparing long-term bladder and renal function outcomes after initial vesicostomy and delayed valve ablation versus valve ablation alone, we drew the same conclusions. Interestingly, in the former study, 64% of the patients who had undergone high diversion were incontinent at a median follow-up of 16 years after undiversion and delayed valve ablation, 28% of whom needed renal replacement therapy, whereas 37% of patients who had valve ablation alone were incontinent at a median follow-up of 12.6 years.

These results confirm the association of wetting with bladder dysfunction and impaired renal function reported previously by other authors.

Conclusions

The survival of patients with PUV has improved significantly in recent years. Previous mortality rates were approximately 40% in young infants presenting PUV before the age of three months, whereas over the last decade, mortality has decreased to 3–5%. A better understanding of the pathophysiology of the intravesical obstruction of the urinary tract and antenatal diagnosis, together with more effective medical and surgical treatments, are responsible for improving the quality of life of these patients.

OTHER URETHRAL ANOMALIES

Congenital posterior urethral polyp is a rare fibromatous benign tumor with a long pedicle arising from the posterior urethral wall, near the verumontanum. Symptoms are related to difficulties in voiding, hematuria, or recurrent urinary tract infection. The VCU shows a filling defect close to the bladder neck or distal to the verumontanum. The removal of the polyp by endoscopic resection is the treatment of choice.

Other urethral lesions occasionally found in the posterior urethra, which are discussed in other chapters, comprise the entrance of differentiated Müllerian structures in patients with abnormalities of sexual development, the presence of a large bowel-urethral stump in patients with imperforate anus after reconstruction, or an ectopic ureteral opening in the urethral lumen. Distension of these structures may compress the urethra and cause voiding obstruction and sometimes urinary tract infections.

ANTERIOR URETHRAL VALVES

Anterior urethral valves are extremely rare congenital lesions observed in male patients. The lesion is often located in the distal bulbar urethra or at the penoscrotal junction. It is considered, by some urologists, an intrinsic urethral defect causing proximal urethral dilatation, on occasion developing a diverticulum; others postulate that the diverticulum is the primary lesion whose distal rim causes bladder outflow obstruction.

Symptoms and signs vary according to the degree of severity of outflow obstruction, the presence of infected urine, and the degree of renal function deterioration. A poor stream or urinary dribbling is commonly noted. Associated bladder enlargement and upper tract dilatation are also frequent findings.

The most useful diagnostic imaging study is an oblique view of a voiding cystourethrography showing urethral dilatation proximal to a rounded linear shadow that represents the valve; although the urethra distal to the valve is not stenotic, it appears collapsed (Figure 17-4). The endoscopic demonstration of anterior urethral valves requires patience

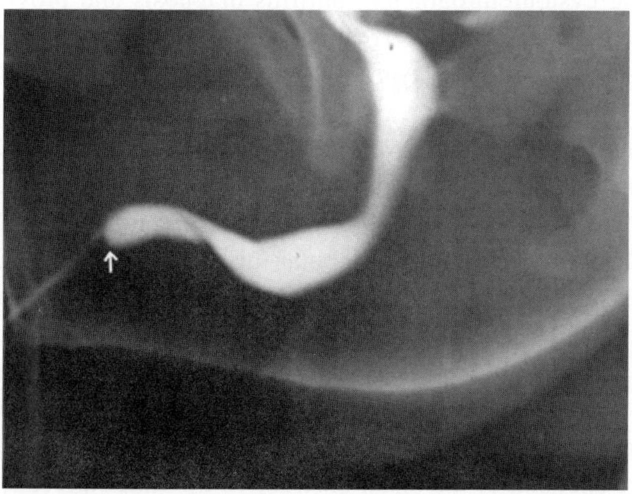

Figure 17-4. VCU depicts a rounded linear defect caused by anterior urethral valve at the penile urethra. Note the dilatation of the proximal urethra and the diminished urethral caliber distal to the obstructive lesion.

and expertise. Valves can be ablated via a transurethral approach with the loop or hook electrode of a neonatal resectoscope.

ANTERIOR URETHRAL DIVERTICULA

Diverticula of the anterior male urethra may be congenital or acquired. The penile urethra, as far as the corona, is formed from the urethral endodermal plate from behind forwards. The corpus spongiosum is also formed from behind forwards by growth of the inner genital folds and midline migration covering the bulbar and penile urethra. Focal deficiencies of the corpus spongiosum may cause out-pouching of urethral epithelium leading to the development of urethral saccules. A further explanation of the embryology of this anomaly is attributed to cystic dilatations of normal or accessory urethral glands. These congenital defects can be divided into three categories: globular, saccular, and megalourethra. In the first type, the rounded body of the diverticulum communicates with the urethra by a wide or a narrow opening. This form of urethral diverticulum is rarely associated with an obstructive valvular distal lip.

Voiding cystourethrography confirms diagnosis and provides diverticular anatomy assessment. Treatment consists of the excision of the diverticula wall with two-layered closure of the opened urethra over a catheter.

In contrast, the saccular diverticula have a distal valve flap obstructing the flow of urine, originated from the common wall between the diverticulum and the urethra (Figure 17-5). This valve action differentiates this type of diverticula from the globular diverticula and megalourethral defects. Its clinical expression is related to bladder outlet obstruction and swelling of the penis during micturition. It usually presents in the first years of life, but occasionally diverticula are detected in adulthood. Diagnosis is established radiographically during VCU examinations.

Treatment depends on the size of the diverticulum. When it is small, endoscopic excision of the distal obstructive lip under direct vision is all that is required, whereas larger defects require an open surgical procedure to excise the obstructive flap valve, remove the redundant wall of the saccule, and perform urethroplasty over a catheter.

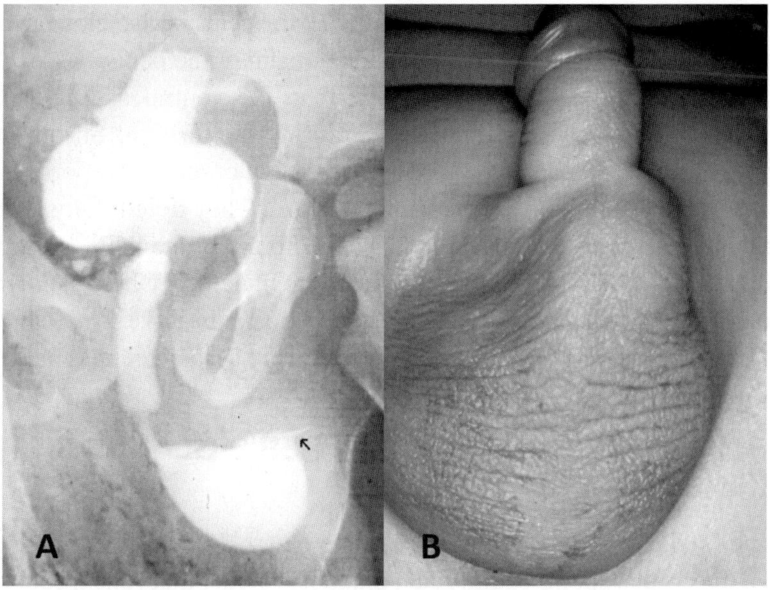

Figure 17-5. **(A)** VCU showing an enlarged diverticulum at the penoscrotal junction. Note the obstructive effect of the distal rim of the diverticula. **(B)** The same patient with swelling at the scrotal region due to the large saccule.

Acquired diverticula may occur because of iatrogenic urethral injury during endoscopy procedures or prolonged bladder drainage with an indwelling urethral catheter. Secondary diverticula may also occur as a complication of hypospadias reconstructive surgery.

Megalourethra

Congenital megalourethra is an enlargement of the pendulous urethra with no evidence of distal valvular obstruction. These uncommon dilatations of the penile urethra may result from an extensive defect of the mesoderm, in the urethral folds that fail to develop the erectile tissue of the corpus spongiosum, alone or in conjunction with both corpora cavernosa. Dorairajan (1963) described two types of megalourethra: fusiform and scaphoid forms. In the former, there is absence of both corpora cavernosa and corpus spongiosum over the penile urethra. The penis is elongated, skin is redundant, and the glands is small. In the scaphoid type, the penis is also elongated but both corpora cavernosa are present in the dorsum of the penis.

The roof of the urethra is shorter than the ventral aspect causing the characteristic scaphoid appearance during micturition. Shrom *et al.* (1981) reviewed 26 cases of patients with megalourethras, reporting that 21 had scaphoid and only five fusiform forms. They noted that scaphoid megalourethras were associated in 19 cases to the prune belly syndrome, the dilatation of the upper tracts, or other system defects whereas only five patients had an isolated anomaly. In contrast, the five patients with fusiform megalourethral defect had more severe associated anomalies.

CYSTS OF THE DUCTS OF COWPER'S GLANDS (SYRINGOCELES)

Cowper's glands are located caudal to the external urethral sphincter and above the corpus spongiosum. Each gland has a duct that runs through the erectile tissue, under the urethral epithelial surface, before opening independently on the floor of the bulbar urethra. The dilatation of the ducts and the gland may create a saccule that bulges and compresses the perineal urethra causing dysuria or even acute urinary retention. Voiding cystourethrography establishes diagnosis by showing a dilated duct in the proximal segment of the bulbar urethra. Treatment comprises identification of the orifice of the dilated duct followed by the endoscopic excision of the common flap between the bulbar urethra and the dilated duct.

COMMENT FROM THE EDITORS

This is a complete review of the topic of urethral obstruction. Despite enormous progress in the last two decades, PUVs continue to present a challenge to the pediatric urologists and are an important cause of renal failure in children. We agree completely with the management proposed by the author, primary valve ablation should be done whenever possible. For the exceptional newborn, in whom after a few day of catheter drainage, the serum creatinine remains above 0.8 mg/dl and the upper urinary tract remains dilated, the use of a high partially diverting ureterostomy, as described by Sober, can provide good drainage to the kidneys avoiding bladder defunctionalization, with the adverse consequences described in the chapter.

FURTHER READING

Atwell JD. Posterior urethral valves in the British Isles: a multicenter B.A.P.S. review. *J Pediatr Surg* 1983; **18**:70–74

Beck AD. The effect of intra-uterine urinary obstruction upon the development of the fetal kidney. *J Urol* 1953; **105**:784–789.

Denes ED, Barthold JS, González R. Early prognostic value of serum creatinine levels in children with posterior urethral valves. *J Urol* 1997; **157**(4): 1441–1443.

Dewan PA, Zappala SM, Ransley PG, Duffy PG. Endoscopic reappraisal of the morphology of congenital obstruction of the posterior urethra. *Br J Urol* 1992; **70**:439–444.

Dorairajan T. Defects of spongy tissue and congenital diverticula of the penile urethra. *Aust NZ J Surg* 1963; **32**:209–214.

Duckett JW. Are "valve bladders" congenital or iatrogenic? *Br J Urol* 1997; **79**: 271–275.

Freedman AL, Johnson MP, Smith CA, González R, Evans MI. Long-term outcome in children after antenatal intervention for obstructive uropathies. *Lancet* 1999; **354**:374–377.

Glick PL, Harrison MR, Adzick NS, *et al.* Correction of congenital hydronephrosis *in utero* IV: *in utero* decompression prevents renal dysplasia. *J Pediatr Surg* 1984; **19**:649–657.

Henneberry MO, Stephens FD. Renal hypoplasia and dysplasia in infants with posterior urethral valves. *J Urol* 1980; **123**:912–915.

Hutton KA, Thomas DF, Arthur RJ, *et al.* Prenatally detected posterior urethral valves: is gestational age at detection a predictor of outcome? *J Urol* 1994; **152**:698–701.

Kelalis PP. Anterior urethra. In: *Clinical Pediatric Urology* (eds.) PP Kelalis, LL King. Philadelphia: WB Saunders, 1979, pp. 328–341.

Kim KM, Kogan BA, Massad CA, *et al.* Collagen and elastin in obstructed fetal bladder. *J Urol* 1991; **146**:528–531.

Mahoney BS, Filly RA, Cullen PW, *et al.* Fetal renal dysplasia sonographic evaluation. *Radiology* 1984; **152**:143–146.

Mitchell ME. Persistent ureteral dilatation following valve resection. *Dial Pediatr Urol* 1982; **5**:8–10.

Parkhouse HF, Barratt TM, Dillon MJ, *et al.* Long-term outcome of boys with posterior urethral valves. *Br J Urol* 1988; **62**:59–62.

Parkhouse HF, Woodhouse CRJ. Long-term status of patients with posterior urethral valves. *Urol Clin North Am* 1990; **17**:373–378.

Peters CA, Bolkier M, Bauer SB, *et al.* The urodynamic consequences of posterior urethral valves. *J Urol* 1990; **144**:122–126.

Peters CA, Vasavada S, Dator D, *et al.* The effect of obstruction on the developing bladder. *J Urol* 1992; **148**:491–496.

Podestá M, Ruarte AC, Gargiulo C, *et al.* Urodynamic findings in boys with posterior urethral valves after treatment with primary valve ablation or vesicostomy and delayed ablation. *J Urol* 2000; **164**:139–144.

Podesta M, Ruarte AC, Gargiulo C, *et al.* Bladder function associated with posterior urethral valves after primary valve ablation or proximal urinary diversion in children and adolescents. *J Urol* 2002; **168**:1830–1835.

Quintero RA, Johnson MP, Romero R, *et al. In utero* percutaneous cystoscopy in the management of fetal lower obstructive uropathy. *Lancet* 1995; **346**: 537–540.

Reinberg Y, De Castano I, González R. Influence of initial therapy on progression of renal failure and body growth in children with posterior urethral valves. *J Urol* 1992; **148**:532–533.

Shrom SH, Cromie WJ, Duckett JW. Megalourethra. *Urology* 1981; **17**:152–156.

Stephens FD. *Congenital Intrinsic Lesions of the Posterior Urethra in Congenital Malformations of the Urinary Tract*. New York: Praeger Publishers, 1983.

Tank ES. Anterior urethral valves resulting from congenital urethral diverticula. *Urology*, 1987; **30**:467–469.

Williams DI, Retik AB. Congenital valves and diverticula of the anterior urethra. *Br J Urol* 1969; **41**:228–234.

Williams DI, Whitaker RH, Barratt TM, *et al.* Urethral valves. *Br J Urol* 1973; **45**:200–210.

Young HH, Frontz WA, Baldwin JC. Congenital obstruction of the posterior urethra. *J Urol* 1919; **3**:289–354.

Chapter 18

Undescended Testes and Development of the Testes

Manuel García Mérida and Carlos Miguélez Lago

INTRODUCTION

The process of foetal migration of the testes from its original location in the abdomen to its definitive position in the scrotum may be abnormal in several ways:

- incomplete descend or testicular maldescent,
- migration to an abnormal location (testicular ectopia), and
- return to a higher position after having descended into the scrotum (testicular ascent).

In all cases, the clinical manifestation is the absence of the testis in the scrotum. This is significant because it may have repercussions on fertility, it carries a greater incidence of testicular tumours and it may have psychological consequences. Extrascrotal testis may also have a greater predisposition to torsion, but evidence for this is lacking.

Testicular maldescent or cryptorchidism (hidden testis) may present as an isolated anomaly or as a sign of certain congenital anomalies (prune belly syndrome), endocrinopathies, chromosomal abnormalities (Carpenter's syndome, Klinefelter's syndrome, and trisomy 13–18, among many others), or it may be a sign of a disorder of sexual differentiation. In this chapter, we discuss isolated cryptorchidism.

EPIDEMIOLOGY

Cryptorchidism is the most frequent anomaly of the genitourinary tract in boys (1%).

Testicular Maldescent

Its incidence is related to the gestational age and weight of the newborn (Table 18-1).

- Sixty per cent of testes not descended at birth will descend between the first and third month of life. Thereafter, the prevalence of cryptorchidism remains at 1% during the first year of life. It is rare to observe spontaneous descent after the third month of life, except in prematurely born babies.
- It is more frequent on the right side (70%).
- It is bilateral in 10–20% of cases.
- The most frequent location for a cryptorchid testis is inguinal (72%), followed by high scrotal (20%), and abdominal (8%).
- In 3% of the cases, the testis is absent.

Testicular Ascent

It has been observed in one-third of children whose testes descended postnatally and in 2–4.5% of children whose testes were in the scrotum at

Table 18-1. Prevalence of empty scrotum according to age.

Testicular maldescent	
• Preterm neonates	30%
• Term neonates	2.5–9%
• 3 months	1–2%
• 12 months	1–2%
Testicular ascent	
• Ascended testis	1–3%
Mean prevalence of empty scrotum	**2.5–5%**

birth, particularly those with retractile testis. Therefore, about 3–4% of children have a unilateral empty scrotum.

CLASSIFICATION AND TERMINOLOGY

We consider that a normal testis is one visible and palpable at the bottom of the scrotum without manipulation. When the testis is not in the scrotum, we are dealing with testicular maldescent. Following physical examination, two groups of patients can be distinguished. They are discussed below.

Non-Palpable Testes

A testis may be non-palpable because it is absent (monorchidism in unilateral cases) or because it is not accessible to palpation (intra-abdominal testis). The testis may be in the groin but may not be palpable because of obesity or the lack of cooperation from the child during examination.

Palpable Maldescended Testes

In this category, we can distinguish the following possibilities.

Palpable Undescended Testis

The testis is located along the path of normal descent. With palpation, it might be manipulated into the scrotum but it does not remain there.

Ectopic Testes

The testis is neither in the scrotum nor along the normal path of descent. It can be femoral, perineal, etc.; however, the most frequent location is in the subcutaneous space between the external oblique aponeurosis and the skin (Brown's pouch).

Retractile Testes

The testis is in the inguinal canal and can be brought down to the scrotum where it remains but goes up again with the cremasteric reflex. It usually stays in the scrotum in the squatting or crossed leg positions. This condition is seen between the ages of one and 14 years.

Ascended Testis (*Acquired Cryptorchidism*)

The testis was in the scrotum in the first few years of life, which became retractile and eventually stayed in the inguinal canal. This condition develops in 3–45% of retractile testes.

The clinical signs of testicular ascent in a child with an empty hemiscrotum in whom the testis was previously in the scrotum include:

- the involved testis is smaller than the contralateral testis,
- immediate retraction into the canal after manipulating it into the scrotum, and
- these manouvers are painful.

A testis can be considered ascended when two of these signs are present.

AETIOLOGY

Normal testicular descent requires:

- adequate function of the hypothalamic-hypophisis-gonadal axis and normal androgen receptors,
- the appropriate genes and their receptors (Insl3 — Insulin like 3, CGRP — calcitonin gen-related peptide, homeobox — HOX10 y 11, GREAT-G — protein coupled receptor affecting testis descent, etc.), and
- the lack of exposure to endocrine disruptors (pesticides, phtalates, etc.) that can inhibit the synthesis of cholesterol and testosterone.

Current thinking suggests that the aetiology of chryptorchidism is complex and multifactorial.

Genetic Predisposition

Although chryptorchidism is not associated with a specific gene, it is seen in many chromosomal anomalies and is present in about 50 different syndromes. There is also familial predisposition so that if a close relative has cryptorchidism, the risk for a child increases 3.6 times.

Non-Genetic Risk Factors

Non-genetic risk factors can be present in the mother, foetus, or environment (Table 18-2).

EMBRYOLOGY

Gonadal development starts in the fourth week of gestation when germinal cells migrate from the yolk sac to the genital crest, which lies next to the mesonephros. At this moment, the gonad is bipotential. By the seventh gestational week if SRY (sex-related gene on the Y chromosome) is present, it begins to develop into a testis and starts secretion of testosterone.

There are two stages of testicular descent, each under the influence of specific genes and hormones.

The first stage takes place between the 8th and 15th weeks. In the past, the initial descent of the testes was attributed to the differential foetal growth, but is now established that Müllerian inhibiting factor (MIF) and Insl3 cause the development of the gubernaculum from the genito-inguinal ligament; the contraction of the gubernaculum causes testicular descent. Foetal androgens also play a role by causing the regression of

Table 18-2. Risk factors for undescended testis.

Maternal	
• Advanced age, obesity, placental insufficiency, twin gestation, and diabetes.	
• Ingestion of caffeine, alcohol.	
Environmental	
• Endocrine disruptors.	
Foetals	
Preterm: <30 weeks	30%
Low birth weight: <900 gm	100%
Hypospadias:	
Proximal	30%
Distal	2.5–5%

the cranial gonadal ligament. Hadziselimovic (2009) insists on the importance of the junction between the gubernaculum to the epididymis, not to the testes. The traction exerted upon it might explain the high incidence of anomalies of the testicular epididymal junction seen in cryptorchidism.

The second stage of descent, the inguinoscrotal phase, takes place between the 25th and 35th gestational weeks. During this phase, the gubernaculum becomes longer and thicker and grows outside the inguinal region migrating to the scrotum. It is believed that this stage is under androgen control and the CGRP gene in the genitofemoral nerve and its neurotransmitters. At this time, a fold of peritoneum adheres to the gubernaculum, which is giving rise to a communication between the abdominal cavity and the scrotum (the processus vaginalis) along which the testes descends. The sympathetic autonomous nervous system may also play an important role.

Abnormalities in the first stage of descent are rare and result in an intra-abdominal testis (10%), while the failures of the second stage are commoner resulting in inguinal and high scrotal testis.

TESTICULAR MATURATION

Four stages of testicular maturation can be recognised. Two of them are prenatal and two are postnatal. The recognition of these stages has led to earlier orchiopexy.

The first stage takes place between the 7th and 11th gestational weeks. Germinal cells become gonocytes. Human chorionic gonadotropin (HCG) causes the development and proliferation of the Leydig cells and testosterone secretion begins. Simultaneously, Sertoli cells develop from support cells that accompanied the gonocytes in their migration. This is followed by the masculinisation of the Wolffian ducts, the development of the epididymis and vas deferens, external genital development, and the regression of the Müllerian structures. In the end, there are two compartments in the testes; one is formed by the seminiferous epithelium and Sertoli cells and the other is constituted by the Leydig cells.

The second stage goes from the 12th week to the end of gestation. In the 12th week, the rete testis and the seminiferous tubules start to develop.

An HCG surge in the 13th week causes an increase in the number of Leydig cell with the consequent increase in the production of testosterone. As a result, the gonocytes migrate to the basal zone of the seminiferous tubules and they become foetal spermatogonia.

The third stage occurs between the second and third months of age under the influence of a surge in the production of LH and FSH, which causes another proliferation of foetal Leydig cells. The germinal cell population in the somniferous tubules, which until now consisted of half gonocytes and half foetal spermatogonia, is transformed into spermatogonia A, which form the seminiferous pool of the adult testes.

By the seventh month of age, sex hormone levels go down, the foetal Leydig cells become inactive juvenile Leydig cells, the spermatogonia A become pale spermatogonia A, and Sertoli cells become Sertoli Sa cells.

The fourth stage begins at five years of age and ends around 14 years. At the age five years, a new rise in gonadotropins causes an increase in juvenile Leydig cells and the pale spermatogonia A become primary spermatocytes. Primary spermatocytes are the cells in the prophase of the first meiotic division.

At the age of 13 or 14, there is a new rise in sex hormones and juvenile Leydig cells become adult Leydig cells and the Sertoli Sa become Sertoli Sb cells. Through the action of testosterone produced by the adult Leydig cells, the primary spermatocytes start division and maturation eventually becoming the spermatozoa that are capable of fertilisation

DIAGNOSIS

The evaluation and management of the patient with testicular maldescent are based on the anamnesis and the physical examination.

Anamnesis

It is important to know the familial history, as well as the gestational age and the weight at birth. It is also important to ask since when the testis has been noticed not to be in the scrotum. If at birth, both testes were in the scrotum; one may be dealing with an ascended testis.

Physical Examination

The following is recommended to perform a correct examination and minimise the cremasteric reflex:

- comfortable room temperature,
- the child should be comfortable and relaxed, and
- the hands of the examiner should be warm and he or she should not be in a hurry.

It is best to perform the initial examination in the neonatal period because at this age, the cremasteric reflex is minimal or absent and there is less subcutaneous fat. The possible areas where the testis can be should be carefully palpated including the inguinal, penopubic, femoral, and perineal areas.

From the physical examination, the following should be recorded: initial position of the testis before manipulation, location to which the testes can be brought down to and whether it remains in this new location. The size of the testes should be recorded (orchidometer) and compared to the other side. The development of the scrotum; for example, in retractile or ascended testes, the scrotum is well developed while in all other cases, it is common to find some degree of scrotal hypoplasia. Several manoeuvre help avoid the cremasteric reflex to distinguish between the undescended and the retractile testes. These include leg crossing, sitting with legs spread apart, and squatting position.

One should also record the characteristics of the spermatic cord (the silk glove sign described in Chapter 8 or thickening of the cord are suspicious for a patent processus vaginalis). The size of the penis and position of the urethral meatus are also important. The association of testicular maldescent and hypospadias or micropenis should raise the suspicion of a disorder of sex differentiation.

Additional Tests

In special cases, such as bilateral non-palpable testis and possible disorders of sex differentiation, the following are helpful:

Hormonal studies are useful between two and three months of age. The determination of testosterone and LH evaluate Leydig cell function.

Inhibin B and MIF evaluate Sertoli cells. In older children, the HCG stimulation test, best done in consultation with a paediatric endocrinologist, may be useful. In cases of anorchia, FSH is elevated; testosterone and inhibin B are low and MIF is undetectable. In anorchia, LH values do not rise till puberty. In addition, necessary in these cases are genetic studies and karyotype, pelvic ultrasonography looking for Müllerian structures, MRI, and laparoscopy.

In the unilateral non-palpable testis, many consider ultrasonography is not routinely needed since it has a lower yield than a good physical examination. However, in obese or uncooperative patients, inguinal ultra-sonography has a high sensitivity (76%) and specificity (100%) for inguinal testes but not for vanished (0–9%) or intra-abdominal testes (0–33%).

Magnetic resonance imaging with the administration of gadolinium with delayed images is useful to identify the vessels of the pampiniform plexus and therefore the anatomical location and morphology of the testis. Despite claims that MRI can even detect vanished testes (sensitivity 67–96%, specificity 90%), it has not replaced laparoscopy. Computerised axial tomography is no longer used for this purpose.

Laparoscopy should be done under general anaesthesia immediately before the planned orchidopexy. It had the advantage of providing an accurate diagnosis and the means to treat the condition.

TREATMENT

A scrotal testis has a lower temperature (2–4°C) than the core body temperature. An extrascrotal testis suffers biochemical and physiologic alterations and has an abnormal maturation.

The objectives of treatment include: improved fertility, prevent malignant degeneration, allowing a normal body image, allowing an easy examination for early diagnosis of malignancy; the risk of which is increased compared to the general population.

Retractile testes require no treatment but the child should be examined annually since they have a risk greater than 30% of becoming ascended testes.

Hormonal Treatment

Hormonal treatment has been used extensively in the past but a met-analysis in 2007 recommended abandoning its use based on low efficacy (20%) and in many cases, the descent is only temporary. The efficacy seems greater with testes in lower locations. The results using HCG or GnRH are similar. In addition, the administration of HCG carries undesirable side effects including penile growth, growth of pubic hair, inguinal pain, painful erections, and behavioural problems. In addition, adverse effects on the testis include temporary inflammatory changes including interstitial oedema and leukocyte infiltration as well as apoptosis and reduction in the number of germinal cells. These effects are more pronounced between the ages of one and three years. Given the effectiveness of surgical treatment, hormonal treatment should be abandoned.

However, some authors still recommend GnRH administration prior or at the time of surgery with the intent of improving fertility.

Surgical Treatment

In the last few years, the recommended age for orchiopexy has decreased in hopes to improve fertility. Many think that the cryptorchidism is a manifestation of an endocrinopathy rather than a simple anatomical problem and recommend to bring the testes down between six and 12 months of age and certainly not after the age of 18 months. This recommendation is based on several premises. First, the testis can descend spontaneously up to the age of three months. Second, the histology of the undescended testis is normal up to six months of age. Third, the assumption that germ cell anomalies are preventable or reversible once the testis is in the correct location. Fourth, better growth of the testis brought down early. Fifth, improved histology, better fertility index, and lower risk of malignancy. Sixth, genital surgery is better tolerated between two and 18 months of age.

Evidence for early surgery comes from animal models. Ten to 20 years must go by before we have the answers in humans.

Operation

The operation varies depending on whether the testis is palpable or not. Palpable testes are approached through a classical inguinal incision or a high scrotal incision (Bianchi approach); those are not palpable laparoscopically.

In bilateral non-palpable testes, preoperative hormonal studies are recommended (see above).

In palpable testis, the operation should include the following steps: the separation of the hernia sac from the cord and its ligation, the sufficient mobilisation of the testis and cord to allow tension-free placement in the scrotum, section of the cremaster, and avoid dissection of the vas from the spermatic vessel to prevent risk of vascular injury. Open the tunica vaginalis to inspect the testis and the testiculo-epididymal junction and to remove testicular appendages, if present. Place the testis in a subdartos pouch. Avoid fixation sutures that penetrate the tunica albuginea. The role of testicular biopsy is debatable.

In cases of malignant degeneration, it should be remembered that orchiopexy changes the lymphatic drainage of the testis from retroperitoneal only to inguinal and retroperitoneal.

If the spermatic vessels are short, the following manoeuvres are useful: (1) Enlarge the internal ring to dissect the spermatic vessels in the retroperitoneum. (2) Bring the spermatic vessels medial to the epigastric vessel. Dividing them or not. (3) If division of the spermatic artery is needed, the technique described by Koff and Sethi (1996) with division near the testis is recommended.

In cases of non-palpable testis, after the child is anaesthetised, the groin is carefully palpated. If the testis is palpable, one precedes with an inguinal orchidopexy, otherwise laparoscopy is performed. The following possibilities arise:

- The vas and vessels are seen entering the internal inguinal ring. If the ring is closed and a preoperative ultrasound showed no inguinal testis, the procedure can be terminated or a testicular prosthesis implanted. If the ring is open or the ultrasound was not done or was equivocal, an inguinal exploration is indicated to perform and orchiopexy, close the hernia sac or remove the atrophic nubbin.

- If the vas and vessels end blindly above the internal ring, we are dealing with an abdominal vanished testis and nothing further is needed or a prosthesis can be implanted.
- If there is an intra-abdominal testis, we proceed with a laparoscopic orchiopexy. When the testis is 2 cm or less from the internal inguinal ring, a one-stage laparoscopic orchiopexy is possible. If the testis is farther away, a planned two-stage procedure is needed, ligating or clipping the spermatic vessels and then proceeding with the orchidopexy in a second stage six months later.
- If neither the vas nor the vessels are seen, the mobilisation of the colon is necessary to explore all possible sites where the testis can be located and if found in a high location, a first stage of the Fowler–Stephens procedure is done. At the end of any laparoscopic exploration, there must be certainty about the presence and location but not the testis.

A laparoscopic orchidopexy consist of the following steps. The division of the gubernaculum followed by the dissection of the vas and vessels from the peritoneum leaving, when possible, a triangle of peritoneum between them to preserve anastomosis between the deferential and spermatic vessels. When the testis can be made to reach the opposite internal inguinal ring, the dissection is considered sufficient to bring it down to the scrotum. A dartos pouch is then created. When the cord is long, it can be brought through the inguinal canal; but in many cases, it is necessary to bring it medial to the epigastric vessels. The testis is then attached to the dartos pouch as in an open orchidopexy.

Some surgeons insert prosthesis when the testis is absent and they recommend changing it at puberty to make it match in size with the other side. This is done for alleged psychological reasons to improve body image but evidence in favour of this practice is lacking. Others prefer to wait till puberty and insert adult site prosthesis if the patient requests it.

RESULTS OF SURGERY AND PROGNOSIS

In experienced hands, morbidity from orchiopexy is low. The most frequent complications include lesions to the vas deferens, the spermatic vessels, and rarely the testis. Surgery is effective to bring down the testis in 95% of palpable testes and 85–90% in non-palpable cases. The Fowler–Stephens technique has success.

Semen Analysis

According to the WHO, oligospermia is a sperm concentration less than 20×10^6 per ml. Virtanen *et al.* (2007) reported better sperm concentration in children with unilateral disease operated on early. The initial location of the testis had no effect on fertility.

Tumour Development

The risk of tumour development in a previously undescended testis is two to six times greater than in the general population. The risk is greater in bilateral cases, intra-abdominal location, and when there are associated genital anomalies.

In non-operated cases, the most frequent tumour is seminoma whereas after orchiopexy, tumours tend to be embryonal and teratomas. There is only one case of tumour reported in a vanished testis.

Long-Term Follow-Up

We follow children after orchiopexy at one, six, and 12 months postoperative and every one or two years thereafter. As the child gets older, teaching self-examination is important. Although the risk of malignancy is low, it is increased, and tumours may develop in the third or fourth decades of life.

COMMENT FROM THE EDITORS

The authors of this chapter have excelled in reviewing in detail the embryology and postnatal maturation of the testes and have reviewed the topic of testicular maldescent in detail. We wish to address some practical points. We recommend an inguinal ultrasound in all non-palpable testes since it may obviate the need for laparoscopy. On the other hand, MRI requires anaesthesia or heavy sedation and is, therefore, cannot replace laparoscopy except when laparoscopy is contraindicated (i.e. multiple previous abdominal operations). All palpable testes can be brought down by inguinal orchiopexy. We discourage the low ligation of the vessels as described by Koff and Sethi (1996) since it is unnecessary and has unknown long-term results. All non-palpable testes not visualised on ultrasonography as clearly inguinal are approached laparoscopically. Except in older children and exceptional circumstances, laparoscopic orchiopexy with the preservation of the spermatic vessels is successful. We also discourage biopsy of the undescended testes and the contralateral one as advocated by some, because it carries some risks to future fertility (i.e. lesion of the contralateral epididymis) and has no proven clinical benefit.

FURTHER READING

Agarwal PK, Diaz M, Elder JS. Retractile testis — is it really a normal variant? *J Urol* 2006; **175**:1496–1499.

Barthold JS, González R. The epidemiology of congenital cryptorchidism, testicular ascent and orchiopexy. *J Urol* 2003; **170**:2396–2401.

Barthold JS. Undescended testis: current theories of etiology. *Curr Opin Urol* 2008; **18**:395–400.

Desireddi NV, Liu DB, Maizels M, Rigsby C, Casey JT, Cheng EY. Magnetic resonance arteriography/venography is not accurate to structure management of the impalpable testis. *J Urol* 2008; **180**:1805–1809.

Elder JS. Ultrasonography is unnecessary in evaluating boys with a nonpalpable testis. *Pediatrics* 2002; **110**(4):748–751.

Gapany C, Frey P, Cachat F, *et al.* Management of cryptorchidism in children: guidelines. *Swiss Med Wkly* 2008; **138**(33–34):492–498.

Hadziselimovic F. Lecture given at the VIII CIPESUR Congress, Chile 2009, held on 25 November 2009.

Hughes IA, Acerini CL. Factor controlling testis descent. *Eur J Endocrinol* 2008; **159**(Suppl 1):S75–S82.

Hutson JM, Hasthorpe S. Testicular descent and cryptorchidism: the state of the art in 2004. *J Pediatr Surg* 2005; **40**:297–302 (Review).

Hutson JM, Clarke MCC. Current management of the undescended testes. *Sem Pediatr Surg* 2007; **16**:64–70.

Koff SA, Sethi PS. Treatment of high undescended testes by low spermatic vessel ligation: an alternative to the Fowler–Stephens technique. *J Urol* 1996; **156**(2):799–803; discussion 803.

Kollin C, Karpe B, Hesser U, Granholm T, Ritzén EM. Surgical treatment of unilaterally undescended testes: testicular growth after randomization to orchidopexy at age 9 months or 3 years. *J Urol* 2007; **178**:1589–1593.

Kolon TF. Cryptorchidism. In: *Kelalis-King-Belman Textbook of Clinical Pediatric Urology*, 5th Edn. (eds.) SG Docimo, DA Canning, AE Khoury. London: Informa Healthcare UK Ltd., 2007, pp. 1295–1307.

Mizuro K, Hayashi Y, Kojima Y, Kurokawa S, Sasaki S, Kohri K. Early orchidopexy improves subsequent testicular development and spermatogenesis in the experimental rat model. *J Urol* 2008; **179**:1195–1199.

Park KH, Lee JH, Han JJ, Lee SD, Song SY. Histological evidences suggest recommending orchidopexy within the first year of life for children with unilateral inguinal cryptorchid testis. *Int J Urol* 2007; **14**:616–621.

Ritzen EM, Bergh A, Bjerknes R, *et al.* Nordic consensus on treatment of undescended testes. *Acta Pediatr* 2007; **96**:638–643.

Ritzen EM. Undescended testes: a consensus on management. *Eur J Endocrinol* 2008; **159**(Suppl 1):S87–S90.

Schewentner C, Oswald J, Kreczy A, Lunacek A, Bartsch G, Deibl M, Radmayr C. Neoadjuvant gonadotropin-releasing hormone therapy before surgery may improve the fertility index in undescended testes: a prospective randomized trial. *J Urol* 2005; **173**:974–977.

Shlegel PN, Ardí M, Goldstein M. Fisiología reproductiva masculina. In: *Campbell-Walsh Urología*, 9ª Edicíon. (eds.) AJ Wein, LR Kavoussi, AC Novick, AW Partin, CA Peters, MP Arce. Buenos Aires: Editorial Panamericana, 2008, Chap. 18, pp. 577–608.

Taghizadeh AK, Thomas DFM. Ascent of the testis revisited: fact not fiction. *BJU Int* 2008; **102**:676–678.

Taran I, Elder JS. Results of orchidopexy for the undescended testis. *World J Urol* 2006; **24**:231–239.

Virtanen HE, Bjerknes R, Cortes D, Jorgensen N, Rajpert-De Meyts E, Thorsson AV, *et al*. Cryptorchidism: classification, prevalence and long-term consequences. *Acta Pediatr* 2007; **96**:611–616.

Wenzler D, Bloom DA, Park JM. What is the rate of spontaneous testicular descent in infants with cryptorchidism? *J Urol* 2004; **171**(2):849–851.

Wood HM, Elder JS. Cryptorchidism and testicular cancer: separating fact from fiction. *J Urol* 2009; **181**(2):452–461.

Chapter 19

Hypospadias

Daniel M. Weber

DEFINITION, CLASSIFICATION, AND INCIDENCE

Hypospadias is a malformation of the penis that is characterised by a urethral opening that lies too proximal and on the ventral side of the penis, which occurs in approximately 1 out of 250 boys. Glanular and coronal forms account for 85% of all hypospadias. It is usually associated with a ventrally split prepuce that looks like a hood on the dorsum of the penis. A ventral curvature of the penis, due to tethers, the so-called chordee, and a hypoplasia of the corpus spongiosum, can be found. An uncommon variation of hypospadias may present with intact foreskin and may be discovered at circumcision.

The classification of hypospadias is based on the position of the meatus that can be located anywhere between the glans of the penis and the scrotum (Figure 19-1). All forms with a meatus between the glans and the corona are called distal hypospadias, whereas other forms are classified as proximal hypospadias. The classification of the hypospadias according to the position of the meatus should be confirmed intraoperatively because a much hypoplastic urethra may mask a more proximal form of hypospadias. Although some authors use the term severe hypospadias as a synonym for proximal hypospadias, the severity depends much more on the degree of the curvature of the penis that is caused by a chordee and hypoplasia of the corpora (Figures 19-2A–19-2B).

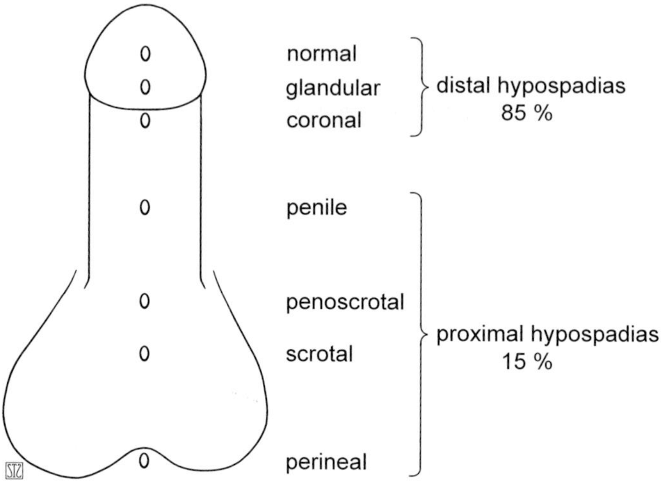

Figure 19-1. Classification of hypospadias is based on the position of the meatus that can be located anywhere between the glans of the penis and the scrotum.

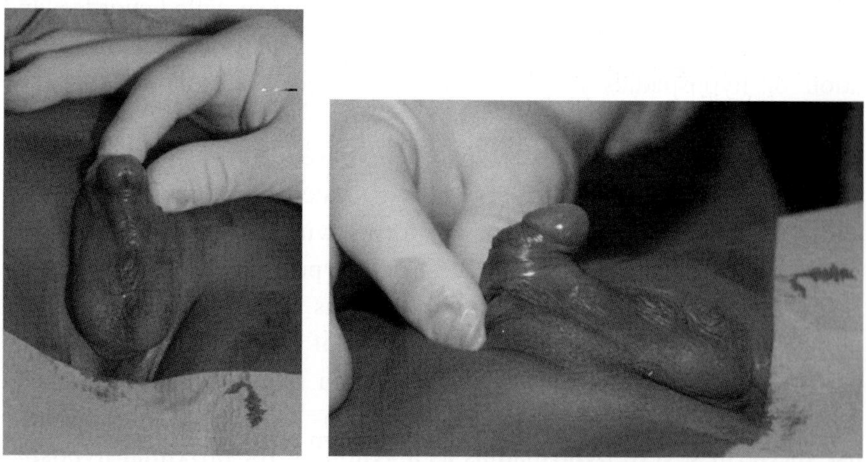

(A) (B)

Figure 19-2. The severity of the hypospadias depends much more on the degree of the curvature of the penis that is caused by a chordee and hypoplasia of the corpora and the ventral skin.

CLINICAL RELEVANCE OF HYPOSPADIAS

Hypospadias may impair normal micturition, sexual function, and insemination. The urinary stream may be deviated due to the ventral position of the meatus and micturition in a standing position can be difficult even in distal hypospadias. However, voiding disorders due to a narrow meatus in uncorrected hypospadias are exceedingly rare and continence is not affected even in proximal forms. Sexual function may be impaired due to the ventral curvature can be found in some distal and most proximal hypospadias. In the most severe forms of hypospadias, the semen ejaculates proximal to the penile shaft and thereby affects fertility. Other forms of hypospadias are not a risk factor for fertility. Nevertheless, hypospadias has an increased association with bilateral cryptorchidism that has got a poor prognosis for fertility.

The vast majority of men with hypospadias do not have any relevant functional impairment regarding micturition or sexual function. The main concern is the impact of the malformation on the psychosexual development and the psychological behaviour of the affected men. Data on the psychological outcome of boys and men with hypospadias are based almost exclusively on patients with corrected hypospadias. Overall, psychosexual development seems not to be affected severely and delayed onset of the first sexual relation was one of the few differences found in comparison with control groups. The only study on the health-related quality of life demonstrates, however, that it is impaired relevantly and significantly in boys after hypospadias repair. In this and in most other studies, the psychological outcome after hypospadias repair does not correlate with the surgical result or the severity of the malformation. However, the coping of the patient and his family with the malformation seem to affect the psychological outcome. No data on the psychological outcome of men with uncorrected hypospadias is available. A recent study of men with uncorrected hypospadias of whom only a minority were dissatisfied with the appearance of their penis is intriguing and challenges the current trend to operate every hypospadias. On the other hand, hypospadias even in its mildest form may have a tremendous pressure on men. This can be illustrated with a historical perspective reminding that men-accepted procedures such as the amputation of their penis distal to the meatus in the hope of cure from hypospadias long before the era of anaesthesia.

AETIOLOGY

In the normal foetal development, indistinguishable male and female genital tubercles can be found at the seventh week of gestation. Just after the differentiation of the male gonads and their production of testosterone in the eighth week, the virilisation of the genitalia can be observed. The phallus elongates and the urethral folds fuse from proximal to distal. Recent evidence supports that the entire urethra is of urogenital sinus origin. It is formed by dorsal growth of the urethral plate into the genital tubercle and the fusion of the urethral folds.

Hypospadias resemble an arrest in the normal penile development caused by undervirilisation of the male genitalia. Aetiologies can be categorised into three groups: hormone synthesis defects, receptor defects, and undervirilisation due to exogenous antiandrogens. Several endocrinopathic factors that are responsible for inadequate foetal dihydrotestosterone levels have been identified, among which 5a-reductase enzyme deficiencies appear to be the most frequent. Numerous receptor defects have been described and in some of them, genetic defects and inheritance have been identified. Exogenous substances, the so-called endocrine disruptors, can inhibit the function of androgens on testosterone receptors and may be responsible for hypospadias. The increase in the incidence of hypospadias in the 1990s may be explained by the substances that are almost ubiquitous in our food and freshwater supply. Baskin (2007) has developed a two hit hypothesis, claiming that environmental exposure to endocrine disruptors in the presence of genetic susceptibility is responsible for hypospadias. This theory could explain the difficulties in identifying inheritance patterns in hypospadias despite a 15% incidence in the first degree relatives of men with hypospadias.

Genitals of females with a prenatal androgen exposure may mimic hypospadias. Therefore, in the absence of testes or other signs of DSD, full investigation in the neonatal period is mandatory.

DIAGNOSTIC METHODS

Distal hypospadias without the association of other malformations do not need anything other than a clinical examination. Although numerous entities such as partial androgen insensitivity can be assessed, their diagnosis is not mandatory since it does not alter the clinical management. Genetic counselling with respective investigations may be advisable for parents wishing further pregnancies. A utriculus seminalis can be found frequently in severe hypospadias. Although it can be visualised by cystoscopy or ultrasound examination, routine investigation is not necessary because only symptomatic patients need treatment.

In children with ambiguous genitalia or in the absence of palpable testes, full investigation for DSD must be performed in the neonatal period. Consultation with an endocrinologist, an ultrasound examination to look for a uterus, the determination of sex chromosomes, and hormone analysis are recommended. In children with DSD, treatment options and sex assignment should be discussed with an interdisciplinary group of specialists and the parents before any hypospadias repair or genital reconstruction is attempted (see Chapter 11).

SURGICAL MANAGEMENT

Severe hypospadias must be repaired so that the patient can achieve a normal micturition and sexual function. However, the vast majority of hypospadias are distal and quite often penile curvature due to a chordee is absent or at least not severe. Although it is common practice to reconstruct every hypospadias, the issue of whether a repair must be attempted at all should be addressed with parents before planning surgery for glanular and coronal forms. It is open to debate, whether all boys with hypospadias must be reconstructed or whether some distal hypospadias may be left untreated or just circumcised to correct at least the particular appearance of the split prepuce. If urologists decide to operate, they must accept that they enter the field of cosmetic surgery and that mere absence of complication is not a sufficient outcome parameter.

The spectrum of hypospadias cannot be corrected with only one technique and every surgeon treating hypospadias must be familiar with several methods. Since the true aspect, as for example, the position of the meatus or the severity of the chordee can be detected only during surgery, the inexperienced surgeon should refrain from operating on hypospadias since presumably "easy cases" can be demanding. Unfortunately, hypospadias surgery has a cumbersome learning curve and trainees and their units must be prepared to accept an elevated complication rate despite expert teaching.

Principles of Surgical Repair

Every hypospadias repair must address all of the following tasks:

- Penis orthoplasty with the resection of the chordee and the eventual correction of the corpora cavernosa for a straight erection.
- The reconstruction of the urethra so that it can reach the tip of the glans.
- The closure of the split glans and the reconstruction of the meatus.
- The circumcision or reconstruction of the foreskin.

Penis Orthoplasty and Artificial Erection

The curvature of the erect penis with a ventral tilt of the glans is often reported by parents. Even without a positive history, curvature must be assessed with an artificial erection under anaesthesia.

Most techniques start with degloving the penis by mobilising the penile shaft skin. This simple release of skin tethers may be sufficient to correct mild curvatures. If a chordee, a scar-like structure on the ventral side of the penis, is visible, it must be resected to the level of the tunica albuginea of the corporeal bodies.

An artificial erection test according to Gittes is performed by introducing a 25-gauge butterfly needle through the glans into one corpora cavernosa and injecting normal saline. A tourniquet may be put proximally onto the penile shaft, however, this tends to masquerade proximal curvatures and a good erection can often be achieved without a tourniquet.

Pharmacologic erections are an alternative to the Gittes technique. Intracorporal injection of prostaglandin E1 (Alprostadil 14 micrograms initial injection with 6 micrograms in reserve as an arterial vasodilator) provokes prolonged erections that allow observation throughout the surgical intervention. Intracavernous injection of 40 micrograms phenylephrine can be given for detumescence.

If curvature persists, the urethral plate must be observed carefully. Further mobilisation, including undermining it from the corporal bodies or even transecting it transversally may be necessary, although this precludes some reconstructive techniques of the urethra (Figures 19-3A–19-3B). If the penis has not been straightened yet, an orthoplasty must be performed. A dorsal plication allows straightening most curvatures, including lateral deviations. We advocate using a modification of the Nesbit dorsal tunica albuginea plication. The formal mobilisation and elevation of the neurovascular bundles avoids injury of this structure. The tunica albuginea is, then, incised in the dorsal midline at the apex of the curvature and the incision is closed transversely with simple interrupted, non-absorbable, and monofilament sutures (Figure 19-4). After the release of the neurovascular bundles, they cover the knots that would otherwise remain palpable under the thin shaft skin. For lateral curvatures, additional longitudinal incisions can be performed laterally on the corpora cavernosa.

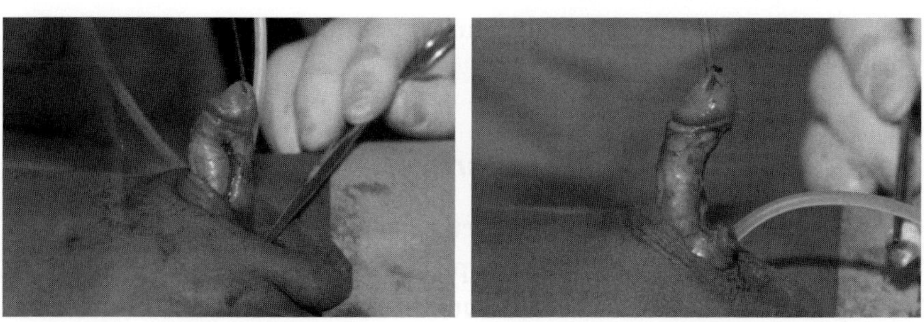

(A) (B)

Figure 19-3. Further mobilisation of the urethral plate, including dissecting it off the corporal bodies or even transecting it transversally may be necessary, although this precludes some reconstructive techniques of the urethra.

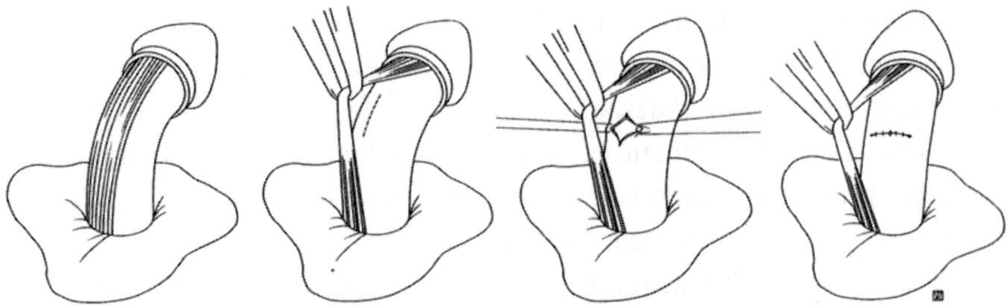

Figure 19-4. The formal mobilisation and elevation of the neurovascular bundles avoids injury of these structures. The tunica albuginea is then incised in the dorsal midline at the apex of the curvature and the incision is closed transversely with simple interrupted, non-absorbable, and monofilament sutures.

Ventral grafting of the penile shaft is an alternative to dorsal plication. A transverse incision is made on the ventral side of the penis at the maximal curvature, either in the midline, or in both corpora. The resulting defect is closed with a graft, be it deepithelialised dermis, tunica vaginalis, or small intestinal submucosa. Proponents of this technique claim that it allows lengthening of the penis in contrast to the dorsal plication that further shortens the corpora. However, there is concern that the dermal graft shrinks or does not grow adequately during puberty. Furthermore, arteriovenous fistulas that endanger erection are a possible complication of this technique. Therefore, if ventral grafting is being used at all, it should be reserved for severe curvatures.

After the correction of the curvature, the erection test must be repeated.

Reconstruction of the Urethra

Tissue is needed to lengthen the urethra in hypospadias. The most obviously available tissue is the urethral plate. However, simple tubularisation usually results in a narrow and sometimes short tube. There are three options to fill the gap to augment the size of the urethra: flaps, skin grafts, and healing by secondary intention. Flaps are tissues that are transferred with a vascular pedicle so that they do not depend on the vascular supply of the recipient site. For hypospadias, they can be sutured on the top of the urethral plate or tubularised so that they can be used as a urethral substitute. Grafts are tissues that are being transferred to a donor area, where they need to be revascularised by the local tissues. For hypospadias, the inner and outer layers of the prepuce, extragenital non-hair bearing skin, or buccal mucosa are used frequently. Tubularisation of a skin graft is not an option because shrinkage is likely to occur. Healing by secondary intention leaves a skin defect that closes by ingrowth of adjacent epithelial cells. This technique is used frequently when incising the narrow urethral plate in the midline before tubularisation (TIP technique). After reconstruction of the urethra, the suture lines and tissues are often covered with additional flaps of subcutaneous tissue to prevent leakage and fistula formation.

Closure of the Glans and Reconstruction of the Meatus

In hypospadias, the glans is often relatively small and split ventrally. The glans must be closed over the neourethra; however, none of the standard techniques allows the augmentation of a small glans. Many urologists pay attention to the shape of the meatus and for most techniques, modifications have been described to allow a vertical orientation of the meatus. Avoidance of meatal strictures is essential, as this is probably the commonest complication in modern hypospadias repair. An important detail in avoiding meatal strictures is to do the urethroplasty "on the short side". Several studies confirm that the shape and position of the meatus correlate poorly with patient satisfaction, so that perfection need not be aimed at and it may be wise to have a wide meatus at the cost of a slightly more proximal opening. Furthermore, the meatus of the neourethra should be anchored to the glans with fine resorbable sutures.

Circumcision or Reconstruction of the Foreskin

There is abundant skin, mainly from the hooded foreskin, to cover the penile shaft even in severe hypospadias. In most distal hypospadias, direct skin closure in the ventral midline after a dorsal relaxing incision of the

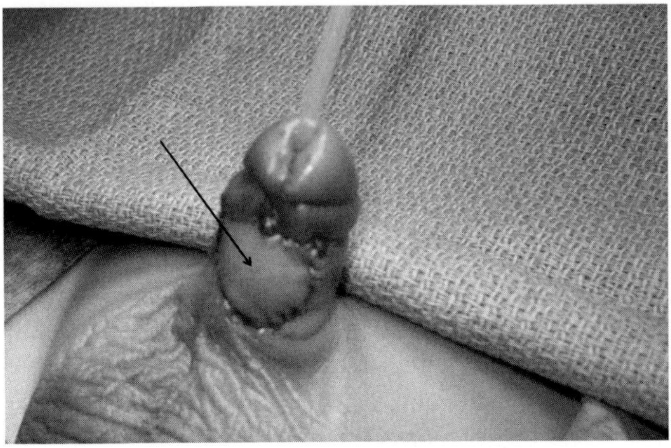

Figure 19-5. A pedicled preputial skin flap is a good alternative to Byar's flaps to cover the ventral skin defect.

shaft skin is possible. Alternatively, the skin flaps from the dorsum can be brought ventrally beyond the midline, one more proximal than the other. These so-called Byar's flaps tend to have a poor venous backflow, so that they may become oedematous with a risk of partial necrosis. A pedicled preputial skin flap is a good alternative (Figure 19-5). In desperate cases with very little skin or after flap necrosis, full thickness skin grafts may be applied to the penile shaft.

Circumcision is performed as an integral part of most hypospadias repair techniques. Although the preservation of the foreskin is technically feasible and has been used in recent years, one must assume that the overall complication rate increases and some secondary circumcisions must be anticipated.

Techniques for Repair of Distal Hypospadias

Usually, techniques are being selected according to the position of the meatus, assuming that standard one-stage techniques are suitable for distal hypospadias. However, it is essential to reassure intraoperatively that straight erections are possible when preserving the urethral plate. Hundreds of techniques and modifications have been described and although many of them have become fashionable during their time, not a single technique has proven to be clearly superior. At present, surgeons have many good alternatives to choose from and low complication rates can be expected in experienced hands. The most popular technique is the tubularised incised plate (TIP) repair that was popularised by W. Snodgrass.

TIP Repair

After insertion of a ch. 8–10 catheter to protect the urethra, a circumferential incision runs 3 mm proximal to the coronal margin, sparing the urethral plate. The shaft skin is degloved and an eventual chordee is resected. An artificial erection according to Gittes is performed. If penile curvature is present, it must be corrected, usually, with a dorsal plication. If only a transection of the urethral plate can prevent persistence of the curvature, an alternative technique must be chosen. Epinephrine 1:200,000 may be injected into the glans for temporary haemostasis, alternatively, a tourniquet may be applied. The urethral plate is demarcated with longitudinal incisions on each side of the urethral plate and a dorsal midline incision runs from the hypospadiac meatus to approximately 3 mm proximal of the tip of the glans, allowing tension-free tubularisation. The glans is incised deeply onto the two corpora, so that the resulting glanular wings can be closed tension free. The neourethra is then tubularised with running single layer 7-0 resorbable monofilament sutures. A very thin dorsal tunica dartos flap is raised, incised at its base, and brought ventrally onto the neourethra, where it is sutured in place. A U-stitch should incorporate the glans, the neourethra, and the tunica dartos flap to avoid meatal stenosis. The glans is closed with resorbable sutures in two layers. The foreskin is trimmed in the dorsal midline, so that some of it can be brought ventrally and closed together with the shaft skin in the ventral midline and sutured in place with resorbable sutures (Figure 19-6).

Modified Thiersch–Duplay Repair

An excellent alternative to the TIP repair is based on Thiersch's and Duplay's principles: in patients with a wide urethral plate, the tubularisation

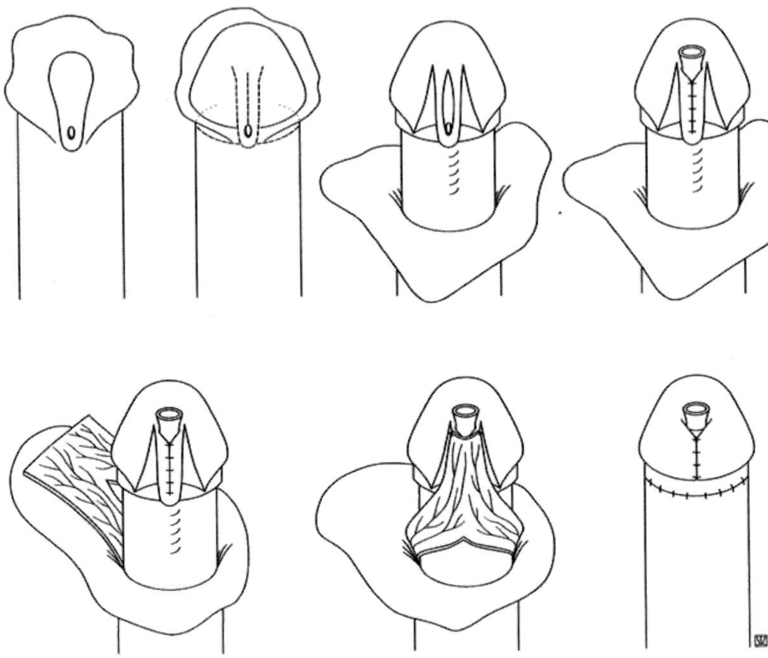

Figure 19-6. TIP repair. Please refer to text in Section "TIP repair".

of the urethral plate does not necessitate dorsal incision, thereby avoiding potential scarring and stenosis. In contrast to Duplay's original description, we recommend the application of the tunica dartos flap as described above for the TIP repair.

Urethral Advancement Techniques and Meatal-Based Flap Techniques

Distal hypospadias with mobile urethras and no penile curvatures can be treated with urethral advancement techniques. Meatal-based flaps as, for example, the Mathieu flap is suitable for distal hypospadias. With recent modifications, a slit-like meatus can be achieved and combination with a tunica dartos flap lowers the fistula rate, so that complications and results are similar as those of a TIP repair.

Techniques for Repair of Proximal Hypospadias

The position of the meatus is not crucial for the choice of the surgical technique. If the penile curvature can be corrected without transecting the urethral plate, even proximal penile hypospadias can be corrected with a tubularisation technique, for example, the TIP. Due to the increasing risk for urethral stenosis in long TIP reconstructions, some authors recommend a dorsal skin graft to fill the gap of the urethral plate after incision of the urethral plate and call it "Snodgraft-technique". An alternative is to avoid the dorsal incision of the narrow urethral plate and to augment it with an island onlay flap.

Difficulties arise if the urethral plate must be incised transversely to straighten the penis, resulting in a gap. No consensus has been found to whether these patients should be operated with a one-staged or a two-staged repair. Proponents of two-staged repairs claim that they can reliably achieve good cosmetic and functional results for all hypospadias including the most severe forms.

Those choosing one-stage reconstructions, for example, the double-onlay preputial flap, point out, however, that they often achieve a good result after their first and only step. They point out that they are entitled to high complication rates and on an average still need fewer operations per patient than those going for planned staged repairs.

Two-Stage Repair (Bracka)

The planned two-stage repair allows, in the first step, a radical resection of the chordee and the short urethral plate. A dorsal plication and, if one favours the technique, a ventral dermal graft onto the corpora can be combined to straighten the penis. Distal to the meatus, a large skin graft from the preputial skin can be secured with a tie-over technique to substitute the urethral plate. The preputial and the shaft skin are incised in the dorsal midline, so that they can be brought ventrally and be attached to the substituted urethral plate. Six months later, during the second stage of the repair, the "neourethral plate" can be tubularised. The neourethra is protected with a second subcutaneous layer before the abundant shaft skin and the glans are closed on top of the neourethra (Figure 19-7).

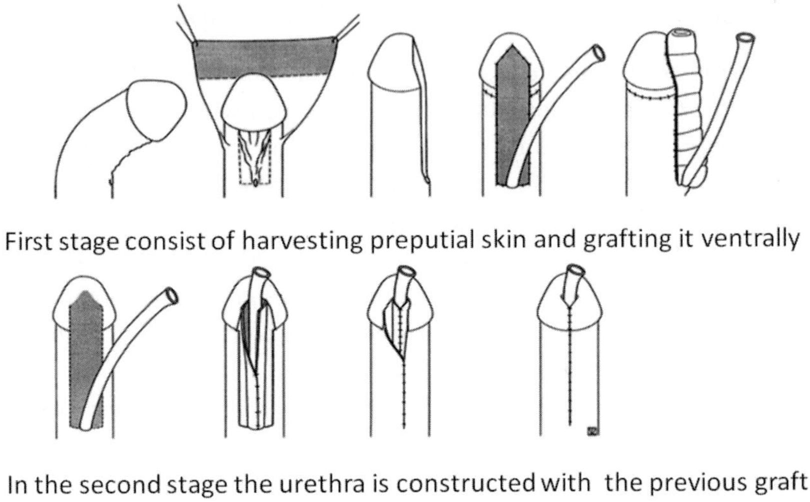

Figure 19-7. Two-stage repair (Bracka). Please refer to text in Section "Two-stage repair (Bracka)".

Preputial Island Flap Repairs

The preputial island flap is probably the most versatile flap in hypospadiology. It consists of inner and/or outer preputial skin that is pedicled dorsally on the tunica dartos (Figure 19-8A). When brought ventrally, it not only provides skin for the urethra but also provides a very good vascular supply to the ventral aspect of the penis too. It is a very reliable flap with several modifications. When used as an onlay flap, it can augment a thin urethral plate that is particularly useful for proximal hypospadias. A further evolution is the double-onlay preputial flap described by González. The vascular pedicle is split and, therefore, it is possible to use it as two separate skin flaps, one onto the urethral plate and the other to supplement the ventral skin defect of the penis in severe hypospadias. Back in 1980, Duckett has popularised the use of a tubularised pedicled preputial flap to replace a urethral segment. Finally, most of these techniques can be combined with each other. One of the promising evolutions is the use of the flap as an onlay flap onto the preserved urethral plate proximally and to tubularise it distally to bridge a gap to reach the tip of the penis (Figure 19-8).

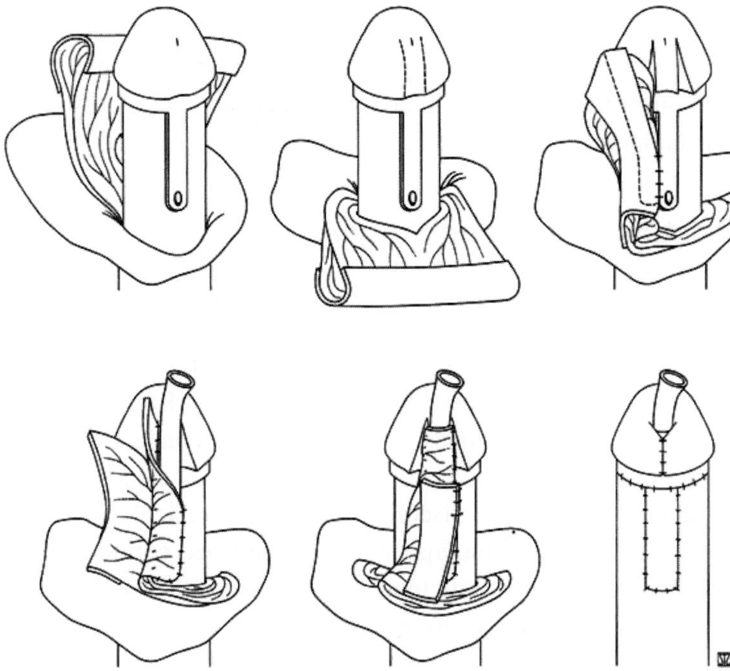

Figure 19-8. Preputial island flap repairs. The drawings illustrate the steps used in creating a total preputial flap for an eventual double face onlay preputial flap (DOPF). Please refer to text in Section "Preputial island flap repairs".

To discuss all aspects of this flap is beyond the scope of this text. However, it should be pointed out that long tubularised flaps have a high risk of late stenosis, so that many urologists have abandoned this technique.

Onlay island flap repair

After degloving the penis, the elevation of the glandular wings and orthoplasty, an erection test must confirm the straightness of the penis. A skin area according to the length of the urethral defect is incised superficially on the dorsal preputial skin and a wide vascular pedicle is dissected. The base of the pedicle is incised and the flap brought ventrally onto the urethral plate. The width of the flap is trimmed, so that the neourethra can accommodate a Charrière 10 catheter. Anastomosis is performed with fine resorbable running sutures. The vascular pedicle can be advanced to provide a second layer over the neourethra. At the meatus, the preputial flap with the neourethra must be anchored to the glans with the skin suture. The glans and shaft skin can be closed as in previously mentioned techniques.

Complications and Redo Surgery

The commonest early complications of hypospadias surgery are urethral stenosis, urethrocutaneous fistulas, postoperative haemorrhage, breakdown of the repair, and cosmetic imperfection. Late complications include recurrent penile curvature and Lichen Sclerosus (Balanitis Xerotica Obliterans BXO), an inflammatory reaction with secondary scarring and retraction of unknown origin. Reoperation for urethral stenosis is mandatory, as patients may be at discomfort and infravesical obstruction is harmful to the bladder and the upper tracts. Published complication rates vary widely, but one must anticipate complication rates around 7% for anterior and 15% for posterior hypospadias.

Scars must mature for at least six months before secondary procedures should be attempted. The principles of these repairs are the same as those for primary repairs. The first intraoperative step is to reassure a straight artificial erection and an adequate width of the entire urethra. If these prerequisites are fulfilled, fistulas can be excised and closed directly with at least two flaps to protect it. If erection is insufficient or stenosis is present, the resection of the neourethra and possibly two-stage reconstructions must be considered.

Long-Term Outcome of Hypospadias Repair

Several studies confirm that most men are satisfied with the cosmetic result after hypospadias repair and sexual function as well as fertility are similar to that of control groups. However, scars remain visible, chordee may persist, and voiding may be impaired. Men with corrected hypospadias are at risk to have lower maximum urine flow, particularly after proximal hypospadias. Voiding dysfunction and spraying of urine are common after hypospadias repair than in control groups. Furthermore, no true long-term outcome studies are available on the newer techniques such as the TIP repair. We, therefore, advocate that all men with hypospadias should be followed by the treating urologists until adulthood. This not only allows clinical examination but reassurance with education that may be beneficial to patients and parents during important developmental periods.

Special Technical Considerations

Timing of Surgery

The American Academy of Pediatrics recommends surgery between the age of six and 12 months without providing scientific evidence for this recommendation. Psychological developmental theories postulate that genital corrections should be performed before the age of 18 months. It appears reasonable to do hypospadias repair around the child's first birthday. However, centres treating hypospadias must be aware of the elevated anaesthesia risks within the first year of life. Genital surgery between the age of 18 months and four years should be avoided and the age around the fifth birthday may be a good alternative to very early surgery.

Preoperative Androgen Stimulation

A very small phallus may be stimulated with preoperative androgen stimulation. However, it should be used very restrictively, as it may have an adverse effect on wound healing. Recommended application forms for children > 12 months of age:

- Intramuscular injection testosterone enanthate intramuscularly (2 mg/kg/dose, maximum 25 mg/dose) five and eventually two weeks prior to surgery.
- Topical application: daily application of dihydrotestosterone cream on the penis, starting four weeks prior to surgery.

Loupe Magnification

2.5–3.5× loupe magnification is a standard for safe and relaxed surgery. Use of an operating microscope is an alternative according to a surgeon's preference.

Tourniquet

Many surgeons like to use a tourniquet at the base of the penis for temporary haemostasis. As an alternative, diluted epinephrine 1:200,000 may be injected into the glans. The use of local anaesthetics with vasoconstrictive agents avoids dilution errors of epinephrine.

Catheters and Dressings

Most authors recommend insertion of an indwelling Silastic tube for five to seven days. This protects the neourethra and avoids traumatic postoperative catheterisation for urinary retention. Postoperative success depends neither on whether any dressing is used at all nor the type of dressing. Therefore, inexpensive dressings that are easy to apply should be chosen according to the surgeon's preference.

Antibiotics

Perioperative antibiotics until two days after catheter removal can be recommended. This regime has been proven effective with cephalexin, however, inexpensive alternatives, for example, cotrimoxazole may be used according to surgeon's preference.

COMMENT FROM THE EDITORS

This excellent chapter highlights the complexities of the treatment of one of the commonest operations performed by paediatric urologists. Despite enormous progress made in the last three decades in the surgical techniques available, controversy still exists evens for the treatment of the commonest forms of distal hypospadias. We personally prefer to do a simple tubularisation of the urethral plate (Thiersch–Duplay) when it is wide and to augment it with a skin flap when narrow. It is not yet proving that incising the plate dorsally will increase its final calibre in the long term. For proximal hypospadias, we prefer one-stage techniques with preservation of the urethral plate and the use of a total preputial flap whenever possible. In our experience, dividing the plate increases the complexity of the repair and the number of operation ultimately required to solve the problem and rarely helps make the penis straight. Nevertheless, the surgeon must use techniques that are reliable and have low complication rate in her/his own hands.

FURTHER READING

Baskin LS. Can we prevent hypospadias? *J Pediatr Urol* 2007; **3**(6):420–425.

Baskin LS, Ebbers MB. Hypospadias: anatomy, etiology, and technique. *J Pediatr Surg* 2006; **41**(3):463–472.

Baskin LS, Duckett JW. Dorsal tunica albuginea plication for hypospadias curvature. *J Urol* 1994; **151**(6):1668–1671.

Dodds PR, Batter SJ, Shield DE, Serels SR, Garafalo FA, Maloney PK. Adaptation of adults to uncorrected hypospadias. *Urology* 2008; **71**(4):682–685; discussion 5.

Duckett JW, Jr. Transverse preputial island flap technique for repair of severe hypospadias. *Urol Clin North Am* 1980; **7**(2):423–430.

González R, Smith C, Denes ED. Double onlay preputial flap for proximal hypospadias repair. *J Urol* 1996; **156**(2 Pt 2):832–834; discussion 4–5.

Kogan BA. Intraoperative pharmacological erection as an aid to pediatric hypospadias repair. *J Urol* 2000; **164**(6):2058–2061.

Kropp BP, Cheng EY, Pope JCt, Brock JW, 3rd, Koyle MA, Furness PD, 3rd, *et al.* Use of small intestinal submucosa for corporal body grafting in cases of severe penile curvature. *J Urol* 2002; **168**(4 Pt 2):1742–1745; discussion 5.

Manzoni G, Bracka A, Palminteri E, Marrocco G. Hypospadias surgery: when, what and by whom? *BJU Int* 2004; **94**(8):1188–1195.

Rynja SP, Wouters GA, Van Schaijk M, Kok ET, De Jong TP, De Kort LM. Long-term followup of hypospadias: functional and cosmetic results. *J Urol* 2009; **182**(4 Suppl):1736–1743.

Schonbucher VB, Landolt MA, Gobet R, Weber DM. Health-related quality of life and psychological adjustment of children and adolescents with hypospadias. *J Pediatr* 2008; **152**(6):865–872.

Wang MH, Baskin LS. Endocrine disruptors, genital development, and hypospadias. *J Androl* 2008; **29**(5):499–505.

Weber DM, Schonbucher VB, Gobet R, Gerber A, Landolt MA. Is there an ideal age for hypospadias repair? A pilot study. *J Pediatr Urol* 2009; 5(5):345–350.

Chapter 20

Urogenital Tumors in Children

Francisco I. P. deBadiola and Pablo A. Lobos

INTRODUCTION

The annual incidence of cancer in children under 15 years of age is considered to be between 100 and 160 per million. Regarding anatomical sites, recent reports on international registries have shown that when leukemias are excluded, about 50% of childhood tumors are originated in the urogenital tract.

This chapter reviews the epidemiology, clinical presentation and diagnosis, treatment strategies and controversies, and long-term outcomes and prognosis for a heterogeneous group of tumors involving the genitourinary tract.

Different types of tumors will be presented first regarding the varied clinical presentations and later an overview of every histological type will be given.

CLINICAL PRESENTATION OF PEDIATRIC GENITOURINARY TUMORS

Palpable Abdominal Mass

An asymptomatic abdominal tumor is the most frequent presentation of both renal and adrenal tumors in children. Typically, an enlarged abdomen is found by the parents or on routine pediatric examination. In order of frequency, nephroblastoma, adrenal neuroblastoma (NB), and retroperitoneal rhabdomyosarcomas (RMSs) are the commonest tumors that present in this way.

Age is a useful diagnostic criterion for differentiating underlying diagnosis. NB presents more frequently within the first two years of life. Wilms' tumor (WT) usually affects children between two and four years of age. RMS patients are often aged between two and six years, with a second incidence peak at 12 to 14 years. Ovarian tumors often present as a silent abdominal distension in adolescent females.

General clinical status is another clue that can be of help. WT patients are often apparently healthy babies, with no associated clinical features. On the other hand, toddlers affected by NB are ill appearing, usually pale, with significant weight loss and generalized pain.

Hypertension can be a common feature between NB, WT, and pheochromocytoma. Hematuria is not usually described in adrenal or retroperitoneal tumors, as it is described in renal tumors.

Diagnostic imaging allows differential diagnosis in most cases. Usually, ultrasound (US) is enough to differentiate renal from adrenal or retroperitoneal involvement, although sometimes more advanced methods are needed. Complex tumors, i.e. solid-cystic structures, in females are often related to an adnexal origin.

Non-genitourinary oncological conditions can present as an abdominal mass, including appendiceal abscess, urinary retention, vascular malformations, severe constipation, ascitis, trauma, parasitic cysts, etc.

Prenatal Diagnosis

Although an US scan in the third trimester of pregnancy is not routinely performed, some people advocate that it could be useful for detecting gastrointestinal and genitourinary anomalies that are usually not detectable on earlier studies.

Intra-abdominal cysts are a frequent finding, and a formidable list of potential etiologies can be made. Possible diagnoses range from duodenal atresia to enlarged bladder or choledochal cyst. Ovarian cysts are the commonest cystic lesions seen in female fetuses; most of them will be follicular cysts, produced by the hypothalamic-pituitary-ovarian endocrine axis stimulation.

One-fifth of all NB are diagnosed either antenatally or in the first three months of life. The typical presentation is a cystic or solid mass detected on fetal US, being the solid lesions more likely to grow either pre- or postnatally. Cystic NB must be differentiated from adrenal hemorrhage, which is the commonest cause of adrenal mass in the newborn, and usually appear early in pregnancy, and from subdiaphragmatic extralobar pulmonary sequestrations.

Renal tumors can also be detected prenatally. Most of them are congenital mesoblastic nephromas (CMNs), which presents with polyhydramnios in 70% of cases because of excessive urine output.

Hematuria

About 30% of patients with WT present with macroscopic hematuria, although it is less frequent than in renal cell carcinoma (RCC). This rare presentation was also described in other types of renal tumors such as CMN, malignant rhabdoid tumors, and anaplastic sarcoma.

Bladder tumors often present with hematuria, whenever infiltration of the mucosa is present. RMS is the most frequent etiology involved in this clinical setting, especially when the bladder roof is affected; occasionally, hematuria can be associated with urinary retention, when the floor is compromised.

Hypertension

Twenty-five of WT patients will have hypertension on physical examination. Besides renal tumors, severe hypertension is typical of pheochromocytoma, because of oversecretion of catecholamines. Hypertension can be sustained or paroxysmal, and it can be associated with headaches, palpitations, and tachycardia.

Hypertension can also appear secondary to surgical procedures, especially in cases of extensive retroperitoneal NB, because of renal parenchymal or vascular damage.

Scrotal Mass

Scrotal enlargement is one of the commonest consults in the pediatric surgical office. Hydrocele, inguinal hernia, varicocele, testicular torsion, and traumatic hematoma are the most frequent diagnosis (see Chapter 8).

Testicular tumors (TTs) can present at any age, being more frequent in adolescence. Paratesticular RMS presents at a younger age. Usually, clinical examination and US imaging are enough to decide therapeutic approach.

RENAL TUMORS

Wilms' Tumor

Nephroblastoma represents 85% of pediatric renal tumors with a peak incidence under five years of age. It accounts for 6% of all childhood malignancies, being the second commonest intra-abdominal cancer in this group.

Presentation

The commonest presenting feature in WT is a palpable abdominal mass. Typically, the mass is an incidental finding in an otherwise healthy child. Other presenting symptoms include hypertension, hematuria, and abdominal pain. Prenatal diagnosis is rare.

WT is associated with several congenital syndromes in just under 10% of cases (Table 20-1).

Genetic abnormalities have been described in relation to WT. The deletions of chromosome 11, known as WT1 and WT2, are the most important genetic abnormalities. Familial cases of WT accounts for 1–2% of all cases and have not been related to the associated clinical syndromes.

Table 20-1. Congenital syndromes associated with WT.

- Sporadic aniridia.
- Isolated hemihypertrophy.
- Denys–Drash syndrome: nephropathy, renal failure, male pseudohermaphroditism, and WT.
- Beckwith–Wiedemann syndrome: visceromegaly, macroglossia, omphalocele, and hyperinsulinemic hypoglycemia in infancy.
- WAGR complex: WT with aniridia, genitourinary malformations and mental retardation.

Pathology

The presence of nephrogenic rests (NRs) has been associated with the occurrence of WT. NRs are persistent metanephric tissue that develops in the kidney after 36th week of gestation. The incidence of NR is significantly higher in patients with WT, ranging from 40% in unilateral cases to almost 100% in children with synchronous bilateral WT (BWT).

WT is characterized as a triphasic embryonal neoplasm with blastemal, stromal, and epithelial components. Each of these components can express different patterns of differentiation, which define the histological subgroups of WT. Anaplastic tumors are characterized by large, pleomorphic, and hyperchromatic nuclei with abnormal mitotic figures. Patients who present with anaplasia have a poor prognosis.

Approximately, 1% of children with unilateral WT will develop contralateral disease. Between 5 and 8% present initially with bilateral tumors.

Diagnostic Methods

Careful palpation of the abdomen must be done. Blood pressure determination should not be omitted. Lymph node palpation is important, especially in the supraclavicular area (nodal metastasis there suggest NB). A thorough search for congenital anomalies, genitourinary in particular, and coagulopathy signs must be made.

At minimum, the patient should have a complete blood count, urinalysis, renal function tests, chest X-ray, and an abdominal US. US is useful for assigning a possible renal origin to the tumor, identifying normal renal parenchyma displaced by the mass, the evaluation of the contralateral kidney, and the identification of nodal involvement. Doppler US is mandatory to rule out intravenous tumor thrombi at the renal vessels and inferior vena cava.

Sometimes, differentiating WT from non-Wilms' renal tumors is not easy by US. Contrast-enhanced computed tomography (CT) is useful for further anatomical details and it also shows contralateral kidney's adequate excretion (Figure 20-1).

Depending on the treatment protocol used (see later), initial chemotherapy may be given, based on clinical features, laboratory studies,

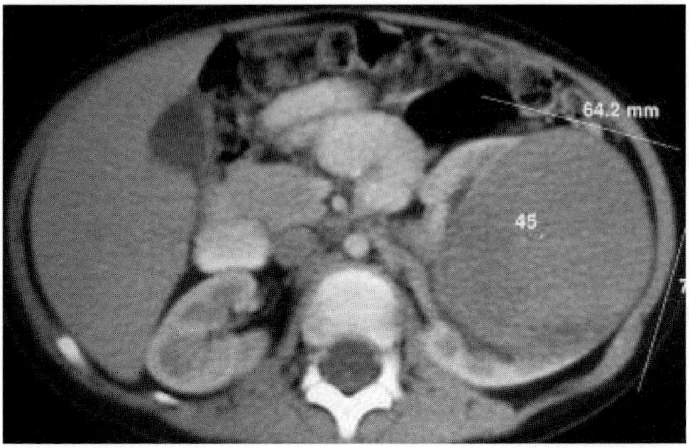

Figure 20-1. Unilateral WT. Note the peripheral rim of renal parenchyma displaced by the tumor.

and imaging. Definitive diagnosis is ultimately made at the time of nephrectomy. Preoperative differential diagnosis may be difficult, especially with NB; another very common intra-abdominal malignancy that can rarely be involved is the renal parenchyma (see Table 20-2 for some differentiating features).

Table 20-2. Differential diagnosis between WT and NB.

	Wilms'	Neuroblastoma
Age (> incidence)	6 months to 6 years	<2 years
General health status	Usually good	Usually poor
Pain	Rare	Frequent
Metastasis	Lymph nodes and lung	Bone marrow, lymph nodes, and skeletal
Calcifications	Rare	Frequent
Elevated catecholamines	Never	Very frequent
Relation with vessels	Displace	Encase
Renal involvement	Intraparenchymal distortion of normal figure	Indentation of the kidney from outside
Overall prognosis	Good	Poor

Needle biopsies may differentiate WT from non-WTs, but are not useful for classifying WT. The violation of renal capsule also implies an upstaging of the tumor.

Therapy

Based on the development of large cooperative multicenter studies, very good long-term results have been achieved in the last decades. Actual protocols include the combination of surgery and chemotherapy, with or without radiotherapy (RT). Chemotherapy agents include vincristine and actinomycin-D, with the addition of doxorubicin in advanced cases.

Treatment is dependent upon staging, which is done using a combination of diagnostic imaging, surgery, pathology, and, more recently, biological markers such as loss of heterozygosity (LOH) at chromosomes 1p and 16q.

> As with all pediatric oncology treatments, patients should be treated according to the established protocols, recognizing that protocols may need to be modified according to local conditions.

Optimal chemotherapy regimens have been established by a series of well-designed randomized studies primarily performed by the National Wilms' Tumor Study Group (NWTSG) in USA and Canada and by the International Society of Pediatric Oncology (SIOP) in Europe (see Table 20-3). Despite advances in chemotherapy, surgery continues to play a critical role in the treatment of WT. Accurate staging and safe and complete resection of the tumor are the key elements in achieving cure. Local control is rarely achieved by chemotherapy and RT alone.

Radiographic imaging is critical prior to the resection of a renal tumor. The presence of two functioning kidneys, contralateral tumor, and the evidence of intravascular invasion of the tumor must be carefully assessed. Pulmonary metastases must be ruled out by chest X-ray or CT scan.

Table 20-3. Summary of stage and therapy in the NWTS and SIOP studies for favorable histology WT.

	NWTS-5		SIOP93-01	
Stage	**Chemotherapy**	**Radiation therapy**	**Postoperative chemotherapy**	**Radiation therapy**
I: Tumor limited to kidney, completely resected, vessel of renal sinus not involved	VA × 18 weeks	—	VA × 4 weeks	—
II: Tumor beyond the kidney but completely resected	VA × 18 weeks	—	VDA × 27 weeks	Node negative: None Node positive: 15 Gy
III: Residual non-hematogenous tumor (+) lymph nodes, biopsy, local rupture	VA × 24 weeks	10.8 Gy	VDA × 27 weeks	15 Gy
IV: Hematogenous metastases (lung, liver, bone, etc.)	VA × 24 weeks	12 Gy lung (if metastasis) 10.8 Gy flank (if local stage III)	CR after 9 weeks: VDA × 27 weeks No CR after 9 weeks: ICED × 34 weeks	None if lung lesions disappear by week 9, otherwise 12 Gy
V: Bilateral	Individualized			

Note: V, vincristine; A, actinomycin-D; D, doxorubicin.

Renal tumors must be resected through a large transverse or subcostal laparotomy, to avoid tumor rupture (Figure 20-2). A flank incision should be avoided in pediatric renal tumors. The contralateral kidney and the inferior vena cava should be palpated to exclude tumor extension.

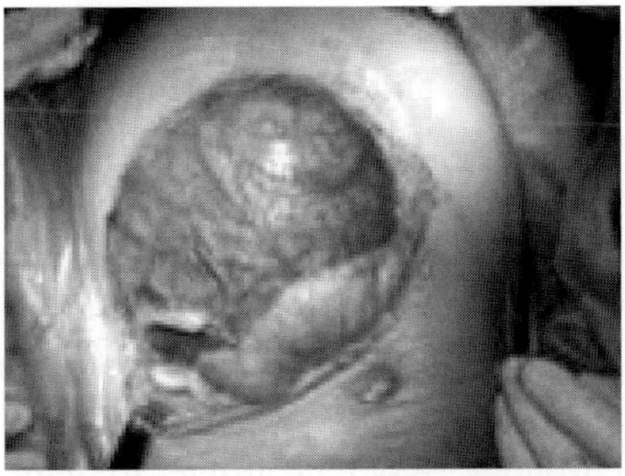

Figure 20-2. Wide transverse anterior laparotomy for a big right WT.

Complete resection of the tumor must be achieved, preserving an intact capsule to avoid tumor spillage. Initial vascular control is not necessary and may be dangerous in large tumors.

Lymph node sampling must be carefully done in the renal hilum and along the vena cava or aorta, as it is critical for adequate staging. It will determine whether or not abdominal RT will be utilized.

Nephron-sparing surgery and laparoscopic nephrectomy had been proposed recently in selected cases, although this is a highly controversial issue, not included yet in the current protocols.

Children presenting with BWT are generally younger than unilateral cases, accounting for about 5% of all WT. The preservation of renal parenchyma is a critical issue for these children and the challenge is to achieve high cure rates maintaining adequate long-term renal function. Combined individualized approaches using needle biopsy, preoperative chemotherapy, and nephron-sparing surgery have shown good results.

Prognosis and Late Complications

Disease-free survival using either the SIOP or the NWTS protocols is approximately 95% for favorable histology stage I and 75% for stages II–IV. Prognosis in low-income countries is 10–20% less because of later presentation, more advanced stage at diagnosis, bulky disease, and the lack of experienced surgeons and pathologists.

About 75% of relapses will occur within the first 12 months. Nevertheless, close follow-up is mandatory for at least the first five years.

Long-term complications are mainly related to the treatment. Surgical complications most commonly reported are bowel obstruction (5%) and more rarely, major vascular lesions and major bleeding. Renal failure is infrequent for unilateral WT, but is significant when dealing with synchronous or metachronous BWT. Cardiac toxicity is a well-known complication of doxorubicin and other anthracyclinic agents, and cardiac function must be monitored for many years after treatment. The complications of radiation therapy include renal failure, growth impairment, and infertility. Second malignancies have been described, especially in irradiated patients.

Current Controversies

NWTSG and SIOP studies began more than three decades ago. Since the beginning, there has been a philosophical difference of opinions about the use of preoperative chemotherapy. The NWTSG and its successor, the Children's Oncology Group (COG), advocate up-front resection of the primary tumor before chemotherapy is given. In contrast, SIOP recommends the administration of chemotherapy before surgery. Both approaches yield excellent clinical outcomes, yet a great debate and controversy continues about the relative merit of each approach (see Table 20-4 for the pros and cons of each one).

Some authors have advocated that in low-income countries where patients tend to present later, with bigger tumors and less-experienced surgical teams, should embrace preoperative chemotherapy, although this issue is still under debate.

According to SIOP protocols, in most patients, the histological confirmation is not required before initiating the therapy. The potential risk of this approach is to treat patients with a benign disease or mistreat patients with a different type of cancer. Despite modern imaging techniques, diagnostic error as high as 5% has been reported.

Table 20-4. Controversial issues between NWTSG and SIOP protocols.

	Pros (+)	Cons (−)
NWTSG	• Certain pretreatment histological diagnosis. • Adequate lymph node status. • Less number of patients treated with doxorubicin (less cardiac toxicity).	• More tumor rupture. • More number of patients treated with RT. • Need for more experienced surgeons.
SIOP	• Easier surgical resection (smaller tumor burden). • Less tumor rupture (<RT). • Recommended for low-income countries.	• Diagnostic error (chemotherapy without biopsy). • Difficulty in staging because of postchemotherapy changes. • More doxorubicin (more than in stage III): More cardiac toxicity.

Preoperative chemotherapy is always given for bilateral tumors, unilateral tumors arising on a solitary or horseshoe kidney, intracaval extensive tumoral thrombus that reaches above the hepatic veins, or very bad general condition of the patient. In our opinion, this should always be performed after an adequate biopsy.

Conversely, there is agreement from both sides of the Atlantic that cystic renal tumors should be submitted to upfront resection without preoperative chemotherapy, as the incidence of benign disease is higher.

Non-Wilms' Renal Tumors

Although WT is the most frequent renal tumor in children, both NWTSG and SIOP studies have demonstrated an incidence of almost 10% of other diagnosis in their series.

We will briefly review the differential diagnosis of the WT. Final diagnosis is most commonly confirmed by the pathologist, but some of them have clinical and imaging distinguishing features.

Renal Cell Carcinoma

Two to six percent of malignant renal childhood tumors. It is, typically, present in older children, being the mean age at diagnosis 15 years. Classical presentation triad of palpable mass, hematuria, and flank pain described in adults may not always be present. Pediatric RCCs have association with the prior history of irradiation for hepatoblastoma or NB and with tuberous sclerosis or the family history of von Hippel Lindau Syndrome. Surgery remains the mainstay of treatment, and prognosis is dependent on stage at diagnosis.

Congenital Mesoblastic Nephroma

It is the commonest renal tumor identified in the neonatal period and in almost all patients present under the age of six months. CMN is usually present as a palpable mass and it is the most probable diagnosis when a renal tumor is observed in prenatal US. CMN generally presents a solid appearance on US scan (Figure 20-3). A characteristic chromosomal translocation, t(12; 15)(p13; q25), has been described for the cellular variant of CMN, which is present also in the cases of infantile fibrosarcoma, suggesting a probable common origin. Surgery is the treatment of choice, and most patients will be cured with surgery alone. Transabdominal nephrectomy with clear margins must be performed, giving special attention to the hilar region, as the tumor may invade this area. The cellular

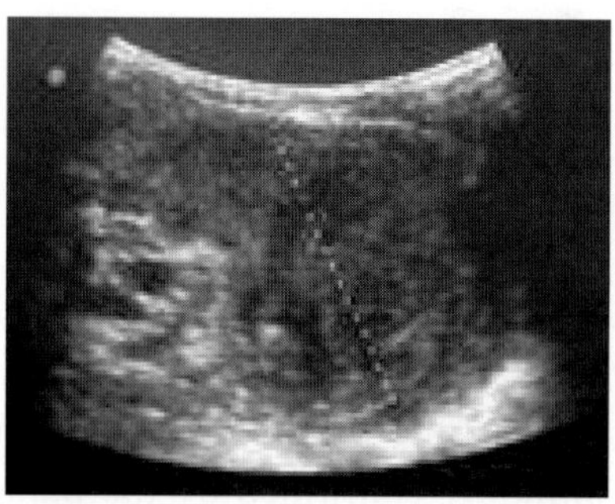

Figure 20-3. US scan of a left CMN in a three-month-old boy. Note the heterogeneous solid structure involving the inferior renal pole.

variant may recur, especially over the age of three months, so close follow-up is necessary, at least during the first year. Patients with recurrent or unresectable disease do respond to chemotherapy.

Cystic Nephroma (CN)

It is a benign tumor, which is clinically and radiographically indistinguishable from the malignant cystic partially differentiated nephroblastoma (CPDN) and cystic nephroblastoma (Figure 20-4). Distinction between these entities must be made by the pathologist, as treatment varies significantly. Although CN has been described as primarily affecting adult patients, actually, it is present with a bimodal distribution, with a proportion of cases occurring under four years of age. CN has been associated with pleuropulmonary blastoma. Chest roentgenogram or CT should be made in patients with known CN.

Clear Cell Sarcoma of the Kidney (CCSK)

It is a highly malignant tumor with an unusual proclivity to produce *bony metastasis*. CCSK, typically, invades the surrounding renal parenchyma, rather than forming a pseudocapsule as WT. In addition to skeletal metastasis, CCSK also has a high incidence of *brain metastasis*. Even in stages I–II, the addition of doxorubicin to standard therapy has dramatically improved the results. ICE chemotherapy with radiation

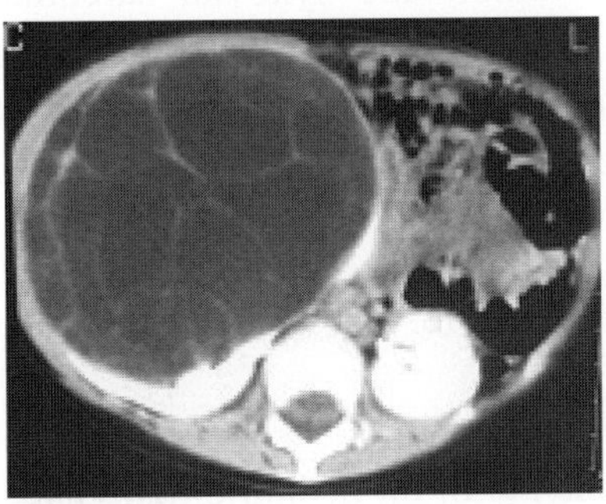

Figure 20-4. Image of a well-circumscribed CN. The normal renal parenchyma is displaced by the tumor.

therapy and surgery is effective for salvage of brain metastasis. Late recurrence has been reported, with 30% of relapses occurring after two years of diagnosis.

Malignant Rhabdoid Tumors (MRT)

They occur in young infants, with 85% of cases presenting under two years of age, and account for 1.5 to 4% of all pediatric renal tumors, being the most aggressive tumor in this group. They are notable for the occurrence of second primary neuroglial tumors in the midline of the brain resembling medulloblastoma. MRT is more aggressive than WT, with a marked poorer prognosis, and early recurrence is the rule. Gross total resection of the primary tumor is a condition for survival, and patients who recur cannot be rescued. Age at diagnosis could be a prognosis factor, being the younger age as a sign of poor results.

Other Tumors

Recently, a subgroup of renal tumors have been characterized by unique common histological features. The *anaplastic sarcoma of the kidney* is a highly aggressive tumor, histologically related to the pleuropulmonary blastoma and the undifferentiated sarcoma of the liver. They are usually treated with the same regimens as anaplastic WT, but the prognosis remains dismal. Lymphoma, NB, teratoma, angiomyolipoma, desmoplastic small round cell tumor, and synovial sarcoma are rare diagnosis occasionally found in the kidney. *Primitive neuroectodermal tumor (PNET)* may have renal involvement (Figure 20-5), usually appearing in older children, especially adolescents.

Adrenal Tumors

Neuroblastoma

NB accounts for about 7% of all pediatric malignancies and it is responsible for about 15% of all pediatric deaths for cancer. It is the most common extracranial solid tumor presenting in children. It is an embryonal

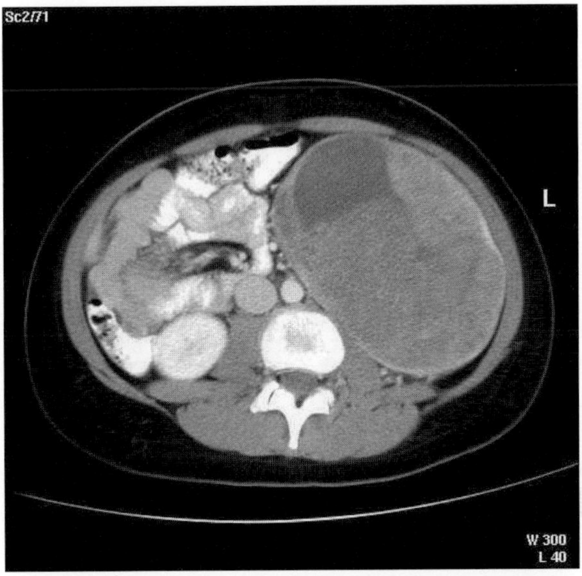

Figure 20-5. Abdominal CT scan showing a large left renal PNET in a 14-year-old boy. At surgical exploration, a thrombus at the left renal vein was resected.

tumor, and the median age at diagnosis is two years; 90% of cases are diagnosed in children aging less than five years.

NB origins in neural crest cells appearing anywhere along the distribution of the sympathetic nervous system. This origin explains the clinical presentation of NB, which may appear at the adrenal site, and all along the paravertebral area, from the neck to the pelvis; it also explains the uptake of metaiodobenzylguanidine (MIBG), a radiopharmaceutical agent analogous to the catecholamine precursors, and the release of catecholamines or adrenergic immature precursors.

Histopathology

Histologic and molecular analyses are very important for diagnosis and treatment planning. An open biopsy is usually recommended to obtain enough material for different determinations.

Histologically, NB is characterized by a proliferation of small round blue cells with hyperchromatic nuclei and a scant amount of cytoplasm

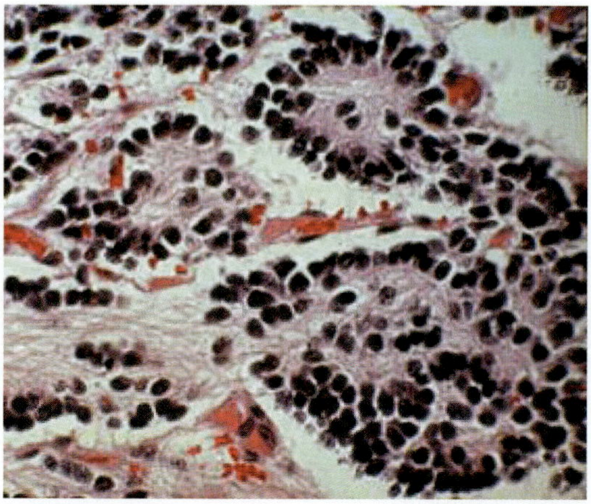

Figure 20-6. Histological image of an NB. See the small round blue cells with large hyperchromatic nuclei and the formation of pseudorosettes.

(Figure 20-6). They must be differentiated with other tumors that also present with small round blue cells as the lymphoma, RMS, and Ewing sarcoma.

The *Shimada system* of histological classification divides NB patients in favorable and unfavorable histologies. These groupings are based on age of the patient, the mitotic-karyorrhexis index, the amount of Schwann cells, and the degree of cellular differentiation.

The *DNA index* (*DNA ploidy*) has been identified as an important indicator of disease responsiveness. It is measured by flow cytometry or cytogenetic analysis. Hyperdiploidy (DNA index >1) correlates with a lower stage at presentation, better response to chemotherapy, and improved overall outcome. Conversely, the opposite is true for diploid tumor specimens.

The oncogenic transcription factor MYCN, located in chromosome 2, is considered the most critical oncogene of primary NB and is amplified in 25% of patients. Amplification of MYCN is associated with advanced-stage disease, rapid tumor progression, and poor overall clinical outcome. Deletion of chromosome 1p has also been linked to bad prognosis.

> Shimada classification, DNA index and MYCN amplification have all been found to be independent prognostic variables in disease progression and outcome.

Clinical presentation

Most NBs are found in children less than one year of age, and can be seen in prenatal US during the third trimester. 65% of all NBs arise at the adrenal gland, but this number raises to 90% for NB diagnosed perinatally. The second most frequent location is the organ of Zuckerkandl, located at the retroperitoneal area around the aortic bifurcation.

Adrenal tumors usually presents with a large abdominal palpable mass, associated frequently with generalized pain, irritability, anorexia, and fever. This occurs because nearly half of NB presents with metastasis, especially to bone and bone marrow. Paraspinal tumors can invade the vertebral channel through the neural foramina, occasionally presenting with neurological symptoms.

Skin compromise can be seen as bluish, non-tender subcutaneous nodules. When they present in young infants, with infiltration of the liver and the bone marrow only, patients are staged as 4S and generally have a very good prognosis.

When presenting as a large abdominal mass, sometimes it may be difficult to differentiate NB from WT. Differentiation is very important before initiating treatment, to avoid unnecessary nephrectomies or incorrect chemotherapy regimens. The presence of an ill-appearing child, usually at a young age, and imaging signs, as vascular encasement or intratumoral calcifications, should raise the diagnostic suspicion of NB. Preoperative catecholamine dosage must be done in order to avoid misdiagnosis (see Table 20-2).

Diagnostic work-up

Diagnosis of NB is established by demonstrating unequivocally the presence of tumor tissue by histological analysis. However, the international consensus accepts a diagnosis made by demonstrating the presence of

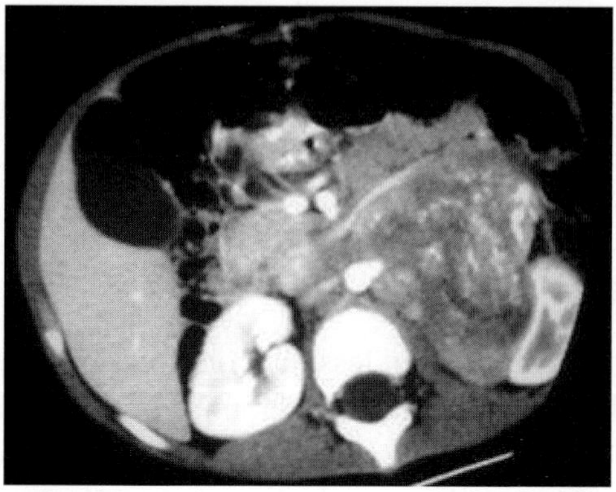

Figure 20-7. CT image of a large left adrenal NB. Note the diffuse calcifications, vascular encasement, and lateral displacement of the kidney.

tumor cells in the bone marrow aspirate, together with increased urinary or plasma catecholamine levels.

Laboratory studies must include a complete blood count, the determination of catecholamine metabolites (VMA and HVA), ferritin, and LDH. CT is the preferred imaging method to evaluate abdominal masses, which may also extend to the thorax and pelvis. Calcification of soft tissues is characteristic of NB and it is very rare in other intra-abdominal malignancies (Figure 20-7). MRI is useful for the evaluation of the vertebral channel, especially for paraspinal locations. Total body bone scan is useful to search for osseous metastasis, but MIBG scan is far more sensitive and specific for the detection of NB foci. Bone marrow disease should be assessed via bilateral bone marrow aspirates and biopsies, and standard histological analyses should be done to determine extent of the disease.

Staging and risk stratification

Recently, an International Neuroblastoma Risk Group Task Force was formed by experts from both sides of the Atlantic. A new classification was built, based on primary tumor stage, age, histologic category, grade of tumor differentiation, MYCN status, presence/absence of 11q aberrations, and tumor cell ploidy. Based on this schema, 16 different groups were identified and stratified from very low to high risk (Table 20-5).

Table 20-5. International Neuroblastoma Risk Group (INRG) consensus pretreatment classification.

INRG stage	Age (months)	Histologic category	Grade of tumor differentiation	MYCN	11q Aberration	Ploidy	Pretreatment risk group
L1/L2		GN maturing; GN intermixed					A Very low
L1		Any, except GN maturing or GN intermixed		NA			B Very low
				Amp			K High
L2	<18	Any, except GN maturing or GN intermixed		NA	No		D Low
					Yes		G Intermediate
	≥18	GNB nodular; NB	Differentiating	NA	No		E Low
					Yes		
			Poorly differentiated or undifferentiated	NA			H Intermediate
				Amp			N High

(*Continued*)

Table 20-5. (Continued)

INRG stage	Age (months)	Histologic category	Grade of tumor differentiation	MYCN	11q Aberration	Ploidy	Pretreatment risk group
M	<18			NA		Hyperdiploid	F Low
	<12			NA		Diploid	I Intermediate
	12 to <18			NA		Diploid	J Intermediate
	<18			Amp			O High
	≥ 18						P High
MS	<18			NA	No		C Very low
					Yes		Q High
				Amp			R High

Note: Pretreatment risk group H has two entries. 12 months: 365 days; 18 months: 547 days; blank field: "any"; diploid (DNA index: 1.0); hyperdiploid (DNA index: 1.0 and includes near-triploid and near-tetraploid tumors); very low risk (five-year EFS: 85%); low risk (five-year EFS: 75 to 85%); intermediate risk (five-year EFS: 50 to 75%); high risk (five-year EFS: 50%). GN, ganglioneuroma; GNB, ganglioneuroblastoma; Amp, amplified; NA, not amplified; L1, localized tumor confined to one body compartment and with the absence of image-defined risk factors (IDRFs); L2, locoregional tumor with the presence of one or more IDRFs; M, distant metastatic disease (except stage MS); MS, metastatic disease confined to skin, liver, and/or bone marrow in children <18 months of age; EFS, event free survival.

Therapy

The planning and treatment of the NB patient is closely linked with the stage and prognosis of the patient's disease. All patients should have baseline urinary catecholamine metabolites and MIBG scan performed before initiating the therapy. They will act as the markers of treatment success. NBs diagnosed prenatally are most of the times located in the adrenal gland. They usually do not produce symptoms either in the fetus or in the mother.

> After birth, observation can be done safely in tumors less than 5 cm, which do not grow under US surveillance. In larger or growing tumors, surgical treatment is recommended, as stage I is frequently achieved.

Low-risk patients with localized tumors are managed with initial surgery. Chemotherapy is reserved for patients in whom $<50\%$ of the tumor has been resected or in patients who have organ-/life-threatening symptoms. Chemotherapy agents are carboplatin, cyclophosphamide, doxorubicin, and etoposide. Stage 4s patients are usually managed with surgery of the primary tumor alone, as metastases are expected to regress.

Intermediate risk tumors are frequently unresectable initially, but after adequate biopsy and staging, chemotherapy is indicated to reduce tumor volume and permit further resection. Radiation is reserved for cases not amenable to complete resection.

High-risk patients must be treated with chemotherapy, surgery, and RT. Induction chemotherapy with cyclophosphamide, ifosfamide, carboplatin, doxorubicin, vincristine, and etoposide is directed to reduce tumor burden and clear bone marrow for harvesting cells for autologous transplantation. Consolidation myeloablative therapy with bone marrow transplantation is the next step, after surgical resection when possible.

Surgery is the mainstay of treatment in localized NB. It is usually indicated after an initial period of chemotherapy. The goal to achieve is the removal of all gross visible disease. Thoracoabdominal or large transverse incision is recommended for large adrenal primaries. Laparoscopic adrenalectomy has been used for small and well-encapsulated tumors. Aggressive surgery has been shown to improve survival in stage 4 patients.

NB is a radiosensitive tumor, so all high-risk patients must be submitted to RT after surgery, regardless of the presence of gross or microscopic residue, to reduce the incidence of local relapse. Retinoic acid has been increasingly used for maintenance therapy to obtain long-term progression-free survival.

Prognosis

NB is usually "bad news". Although NB has a remarkable propensity to regress or differentiate, final prognosis is determined by local control and biological features. Survival figures are >90% for low-risk patients and 70–90% for intermediate risk. Long-term outcome for high-risk patients continues to be poor, despite aggressive therapies with long-term survival of 10–30%.

Other Adrenal Tumors

Pheochromocytoma

They have the potential for oversecretion of catecholamines, presenting frequently with hypertension. 90% of them are benign, 10% bilateral and 10% extra-adrenal (known as paragangliomas). Affected patients may also present with flushing, headaches, palpitations, tachycardia, and nervousness. Ten percent of cases can be associated with hereditary syndromes such as multiple endocrine neoplasias (MEN) type 2A and 2B, von-Hippel Lindau disease, Sturge–Weber Syndrome, and von Recklinghausen's disease. Surgical re-section, even laparoscopical, can be curative in most localized cases.

Cortical adrenal tumors

The majority of cases are female and under five years of age. These tumors can be benign adenomas or malignant carcinomas. Symptoms are related to excessive hormonal secretion, such as virilization, hypertension, and hypercortisolism. Infrequently, high incidence has been reported in certain areas such as Brazil. Treatment of these tumors is dependent on complete surgical resection, being prognosis poorer in cases of big tumors and older children.

Rhabdomyosarcoma

RMS is a primary malignancy in children and adolescence that arises from embryonic mesenchyme with the potential to differentiate to skeletal muscle. It is the commonest soft tissue sarcoma in children.

RMS has a bimodal age distribution, with peaks between two and four years and between 12 and 16 years of age. The genitourinary tract is the second most frequent site of appearance of RMS, after the head and neck region.

Genitourinary RMS (26% of all primary sites) are:

- bladder/prostate tumors (10%), and
- non-bladder/prostate tumors (16%): paratesticular, vagina, perineum, vulva, and uterus.

Clinical Presentation

It will depend on the site of the primary tumor, the age of the patient, and the presence or the absence of metastatic disease.

- Paratesticular: painless scrotal swelling, mimicking and inguinal hernia or hydrocele; particular predilection of lymph node spread to the retroperitoneum.
- Bladder: hematuria and urinary obstruction.
- Prostate: large pelvic masses, causing constipation/urinary frequency.
- Vagina: very young girls with a perineal mass or vaginal bleeding or discharge.
- Uterus: older girls, present with pelvic mass, usually advanced disease.

Approximately 15% of patients present with metastatic disease (group IV).

Diagnosis

RMS is usually diagnosed by direct open biopsy. The type of biopsy, open or core-needle, does not affect the stage. Embryonal histology is more frequent than alveolar presentation in genitourinary tumors and it has a better prognosis. There are no known tumor markers. Imaging studies must include CT or MRI for exact anatomic localization and measurement of the tumor (Figure 20-8). For bladder/prostate location, cystoscopy is advised for evaluation of mucosal extent. Staging is completed by bone marrow aspiration/biopsy, bone scan, and chest X-ray/CT.

Staging and Clinical Grouping

Besides site, size is a prognostic factor. It is determined preoperatively by imaging. If diagnosis of RMS is performed after surgery, adequate negative margins must be confirmed. If not, primary re-excision is advisable when possible. Initial staging is not changed during treatment. Lymph node sampling must be done to histologically confirm clinically or radiographically suspected enlarged nodes. The presence of distant metastasis is another very important prognosis indicator.

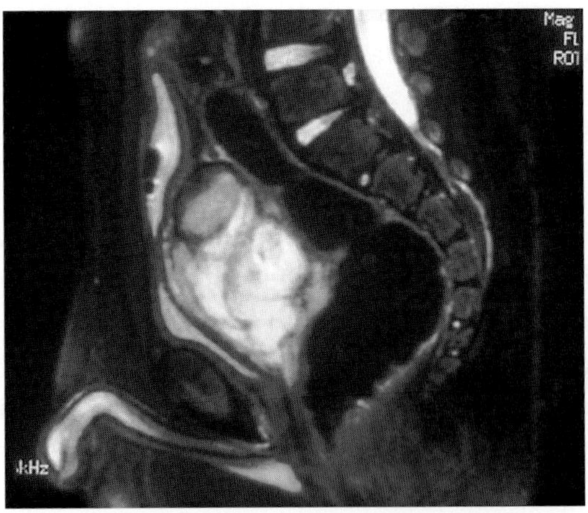

Figure 20-8. MRI image of a prostate RMS. In large tumors, it may be difficult to distinguish bladder and prostate origin.

The Intergroup Rhabdomyosarcoma Study Group (IRS) has defined four clinical groups, combining pretreatment and operative outcomes. Combination of pretreatment staging and clinical grouping divides affected children from low to high risk.

Treatment

Because of the rarity of RMS, all patients should be placed under a protocol-driven therapy. Several multi-institutional studies have shown good results using multimodal therapy for RMS. Briefly, local control must be achieved by surgery and/or RT; systemic therapy with chemotherapy will be helpful not only for treating distant disease but also for reducing primary tumor burden.

The basic principle of surgical care for RMS is a complete resection of the primary tumor, with a 0.5 cm margin of normal tissue and lymph node sampling of the regional basin. In addition, given the overall good survival for RMS patients, resections that would require destruction of vital structures with possible loss of function or cosmetically unacceptable results should be avoided.

> For bladder/prostate tumors, the preservation of the bladder without adversely impacting survival is a principal goal of therapy. Radical resection procedures are delayed as long as there is evidence of response to therapy. However, if the tumor can be completely resected with the preservation of the bladder and urethral function, it should be removed.

The basis of chemotherapy and RT regimens is the risk group assignment. The VAC regimen (vincristine, actinomycin D, and cyclophosphamide) has been used for low-risk patients. Intermediate-risk patients also receive VAC, with cyclophosphamide dose intensification for certain situations, including irinotecan. High-risk patients have a poor prognosis, and ifosfamide and etoposide have been added to VAC.

Radiation therapy is guided by the primary site and the magnitude of disease following operative resection. Group I patients with embryonal tumors may not receive RT. All alveolar tumors must be treated with RT. Treating volume is determined before surgical resection, which includes a 2 cm margin.

Prognosis and Complications

Low-risk patients have greater than 90% of five-year survival, intermediate-risk ranging from 55 to 70% of five-year survival, and high risk is less than 50% of five-year survival. Bladder-preservation rates reported are about 60%, although normal bladder function is significantly less. Significant bladder dysfunction, associated with urinary incontinence and voiding problems, is important sequelae of this disease and requires expertise for functional reconstruction. RT complications as growing problems, scoliosis and second malignancies have also been frequently reported.

Current Controversies

For bladder/prostate tumors, a long-term controversy has been running, regarding the balance between surgical and radiation therapies for local control. Although widely used initially, IRS studies have shown a marked reduction of radical resective procedures in favor of conservative surgery after initial chemotherapy. Some authors have preferred the use of RT as the only treatment, to avoid surgery-related bladder/urethral dysfunction, especially with the recent advances in intensity-modulated radiation therapy (IMRT) and brachytherapy. On the other hands, acute and long-term bladder dysfunctions related to irradiation have been widely documented. At this time, insufficient data are available to recommend the omission of RT in patients with bladder/prostate RMS.

Another controversy is about the timing of continent reconstruction after extirpating surgery, for the patients who do require total or near-total cystectomy. Although some have advocated that complex reconstructive procedures can be done at the same operative time as the resection of the primary tumor, it seems to be a safer approach to confirm the adequacy of the local control obtained, before proceeding to function restorative techniques.

Testicular Tumors

Although rare in children, having an estimated incidence of 0.5 to 2.0 per 100,000, they are especially important for the pediatric urologist and surgeon, as management is strongly dependent on them.

Differential diagnosis is summarized in Table 20-6. TT almost always present as a painless scrotal mass. Of course, most of the time, this finding is related to a benign disease.

The most frequent solid tumors in children are yolk sac tumors and teratoma, being 85% of TT of germ cell histology. Most of teratomas are mature, although malignant components must be ruled out. For males with undescended testis, orchiopexy before puberty has shown to decrease the incidence of cancer later in life.

Table 20-6. Differential diagnosis of TTs.

1. Benign diseases:
   - Hernia
   - Hydrocele
   - Varicocele
   - Traumatic hematoma
   - Mature teratoma
   - Testicular torsion
   - Orchiepididymitis
2. Malignant tumors:
   - Paratesticular RMS
   - GCT:
     - Yolk sac tumor (endodermal sinus)
     - Embryonal CA
     - Malignant teratoma
     - Seminoma (germinoma)
   - Gonadoblastoma
   - Leydig/Sertoli cell tumor
   - Leukemia

Diagnosis

Most TT present with a palpable mass incidentally found by the patient, the parents, or the pediatrician (Figure 20-9). A thorough physical examination will rule out virilization signs, palpable lymph nodes, or the other signs of metastatic disease. US is a useful method to determine macroscopical aspects of the tumor. Benign tumors are usually well circumscribed and often have a cystic predominance. If malignancy is suspected, abdominal and pelvic CT should be performed to exclude retroperitoneal lymphadenopathy, and chest X-ray/CT to rule out pulmonary metastases.

> Serum tumor markers are very useful for the differential diagnosis of testis tumors and should be determined prior to surgery. Alfa fetoprotein (AFP) is present in 90% of yolk sac tumors, which is clearly the most frequent malignant tumor in children. β-Human chorionic gonadotropin must also be determined, although it is not so useful in children as in the adult population.

When stromal tumors present in childhood, they are usually benign. Leydig cell tumors and juvenile granulosa cell tumors are universally benign in children.

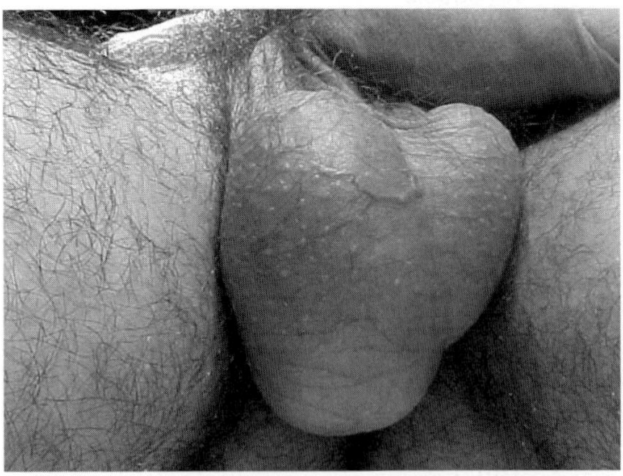

Figure 20-9. Clinical aspect of a right TT in an adolescent boy. After surgery, a seminoma was confirmed.

Treatment and Prognosis

Whenever a TT is suspected, and after the initial evaluation described above, surgical exploration must be performed.

For malignant tumors, an inguinal radical orchiectomy is the indicated method, with early clamping of the inguinal cord. Scrotal approach is not advised, as it has been associated with greater local relapse.

Although the majority of yolk sac disease is clinical stage I, this tumor can spread by both blood and lymphatics. Due to low rates of nodal involvement in children, retroperitoneal lymph node dissection is reserved for the cases with persistently elevated tumor markers or persistent retroperitoneal lymphadenopathy following radical inguinal orchiectomy and chemotherapy.

For children in whom chemotherapy is indicated, germ cell tumors (GCTs) are usually very sensitive to many agents. Platinum-based therapy is indicated.

The survival of children affected by GCT is almost 100%.

Paratesticular RMS should be treated through the same guidelines as other RMS sites (see above).

Current Controversies

In the past, most TTs in children have been treated by orchiectomy, by using the same approach as in adult patients. As most tumors in the pediatric age are benign, testis-sparing surgery has been proposed for selected patients. Preoperative evaluation must include negative serum tumor markers and a US evaluation with well-defined limit between the tumor and normal testicular tissues. Through a standard inguinal approach, inguinal cord is clamped and the tunica vaginalis opened; the tumor is

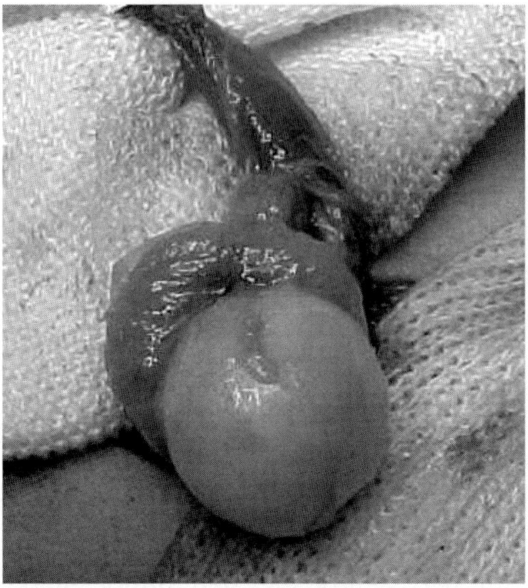

Figure 20-10. Testicular teratoma in a two-year-old boy. Tumorectomy is being performed; note the remaining normal testicular remnant.

then enucleated (see Figure 20-10) and sent for frozen section analysis. Once a benign tumor is confirmed, remnant testis can be reconstructed and preserved. If diagnosis is not clear, orchiectomy must be performed. Although the described approach is still questioned, the initial evidence suggests that it is safe, providing that missed malignant tumors can be safely rescued by chemotherapy.

Ovarian Tumors

Of all ovarian masses, most (80%) are benign, often with predominantly cystic components. Symptoms include pain, abdominal distention, or the presence of a palpable mass. Occasionally, an acute abdomen secondary to ovarian torsion or tumor rupture and precocious puberty or virilization can be seen.

Although a perinatal finding of a cystic ovarian mass is frequent, malignancy at this age is very rare and minimally invasive management should be used. Almost all of these lesions are follicular cysts, produced by maternal hormonal influence.

Table 20-7. Classification of ovarian tumors in children.

GCTs	
• Germinoma	Most primitive GCM. Markers (–)
• Embryonal carcinoma	
• Yolk sac tumor	The commonest ovarian malignancy in children. AFP (+)
• Choriocarcinoma	Resembles placental tissue. β-HCG (+)
• Gonadoblastoma	Features of dysgenetic gonadal tissues
• Teratomas and TeratoCA	Three distinct cell fetal lines represented
Stromal tumors	
• Granulosa-Thecal tumor	Estrogen production, isosexual precocity
• Androblastoma	Testosterone production, virilization
Epithelial tumors	
• Serous cystadenoma/CA	Usually large, cystic lesions
• Mucinous cystadenoma/CA	May have peritoneal mucinous implants

Table 20-7 summarizes the different types of ovarian tumors and the most prominent clinical features. GCTs are the commonest neoplasms of the ovary in childhood and adolescence, representing 67–87% of pediatric ovarian tumors. If the neonatal group is excluded, the risk of GCT malignancy in pediatric and adolescent ovarian neoplasms is 20%. This relatively high incidence means that all pediatric ovarian tumors should be approached with the possibility of cancer in mind.

The preoperative finding of AFP or β-HCG confirms malignancy, but tumors with pure germinoma or embryonal carcinoma have normal markrs. In addition, for girls presenting with acute abdomen, serum markers will not be available to aid in decision-making. Most of the remaining tumors are benign, mostly teratomas and some epithelial tumors, as cystadenomas.

Diagnosis

Most ovarian tumors are diagnosed by US. US characterizes an adnexal mass as cystic, solid, or mixed and demonstrates the anatomic relationship to other pelvic structures. The presence of solid components, free intraperitoneal fluid, or peritoneal nodes should raise the suspicion on malignancy, although the absence of these signs does not exclude a malignant tumor. Sometimes, a plain X-ray may show calcifications, which may be related to a mature teratoma.

Whenever possible, tumor markers must be determined, especially AFP, β-HCG, and CA 19-9.

Chest and abdominal CT is recommended for preoperative staging. Most of the time, staging is made by the intraoperative evaluation of extension of disease and tumor pathology.

Therapy

Simple cystic lesions can be diagnosed at the perinatal period or after puberty. A conservative approach should be used for lesions that are <5 cm. In larger cysts, the risk of torsion justifies surgical treatment. The preservation of normal ovarian tissue should always be attempted.

Solid ovarian lesions must be completely removed, avoiding tumor spillage within the peritoneal cavity. This is especially important as stage I GCT can be treated with surgery alone. The incorrect management of the tumor may convert it to stage II, which will require chemotherapy. Any structure that is adherent to the tumor, as Fallopian tubes or omentum, must be removed. Careful attention must be given to the exploration of the contralateral gonad, as GCT can be bilateral in 10% of cases.

Intraoperative staging consists of:

- Collection of ascites fluid or peritoneal washings for cytology.
- Examination of peritoneal and liver surface for lesions, excise if present.
- Unilateral oophorectomy.
- Inspection of contralateral ovary and wedge biopsy only if suspicious.
- Omental inspection and removal only if adherent to the tumor or present nodules.
- Biopsy of suspicious or enlarged lymph nodes.

When extensive pelvic involvment is observed, a biopsy and post-chemotherapy excision are recommended. Extensive initial surgery must be avoided as ovarian tumors are chemosensitive.

Platinum-based chemotherapy has proved to be very effective in the treatment of GCT. In recurrent or refractory cases, VAC regimen may also be used.

Prognosis and Complications

Results of multimodal therapy for malignant ovarian neoplasms have been reported to be over 90% for survival, even for stage IV patients. Present efforts are directed to reduce treatment toxicity. Infertility is a rare complication, so ovarian GCT should be treated always thinking in the possibility of a second tumor in the contralateral gland.

Current Controversies

Many patients present with predominantly cystic lesions. Laparoscopy has been widely used for the management of ovarian cysts in children and adults (see Figure 20-11).

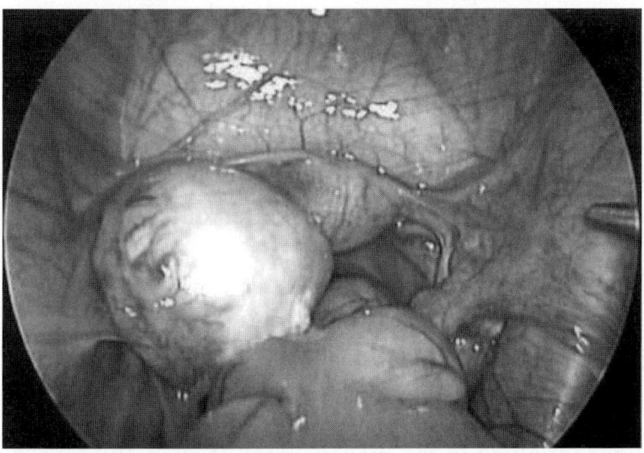

Figure 20-11. Laparoscopic view of a left ovarian teratoma. Macroscopic appearance does not rule out malignancy.

The main controversy surrounds the ability to perform a cancer type procedure in cases where the exact tumor histology (benign vs. malignant) cannot be determined preoperatively.

> If the lesion is primarily solid or if the serum markers are elevated, an open surgical approach should be used.

If the serum markers are normal and the lesion is primarily cystic, a less invasive technique may be considered. Efforts must be made to avoid fluid spillage within the abdominal cavity, by introducing the ovary in a plastic bag or evacuating fluid through an open incision. Intraoperative staging may be performed laparoscopically.

SUMMARY

Genitourinary tumors include a complex and heterogeneous group of diseases, with a significant incidence among the pediatric population.

Many of these patients will primarily present to the pediatric urologist/surgeon's office and we must be aware of the basic principles of their management. Knowledge of clinical aspects, diagnostic methods, and surgical guidelines is unavoidable.

As with every oncological disease, a team approach is recommended. All patients should be treated under a protocol-driven therapeutic approach, to gather information in a collaborative effort. Close interaction between pediatric oncologists, surgeons, and radiation therapists is necessary to obtain better outcomes for the affected children.

COMMENT FROM THE EDITORS

This extensive review of pediatric GU tumors should be an excellent guide to those involved in the management of such children. A multidisciplinary approach, since the onset of the diagnosis and treatment, is the standard of care.

FURTHER READING

Billmire DF. Germ cell tumors. *Surg Clin N Am* 2006; **86**:489–503.

Castellino SM, Martinez-Borges AR, McLean TW. Pediatric genitourinary tumors. *Curr Opin Oncol* 2009; **21**:271–283.

Cohn SL, Pearson AD, London WB, *et al.* The international neuroblastoma risk group (INRG) classification system: an INRG task force report. *J Clin Oncol* 2008; **27**:289–297.

Davidoff AM. Wilms' tumor. *Curr Opin Pediatr* 2009; **21**:357–364.

Metzger ML, Domme JS. Current therapy for Wilms' tumor. *Oncologist* 2005; **10**:815–826.

Ferrer FA, Isakoff M, Koyle MA. Bladder/prostate rhabdomyosarcoma: past, present and future. *J Urol* 2006; **176**:1283–1291.

Glick DR, Hicks MJ, Nuchtern JG, *et al.* Renal tumors in infants less than six months of age. *J Pediatr Surg* 2004; **39**:522–525.

Hayes-Jordan A, Andrassy R. Rhabdomyosarcoma in children. *Curr Opin Pediatr* 2009; **21**:373–378.

Hyett J. Intra-abdominal masses: prenatal differential diagnosis and management. *Prenat Diagn* 2008; **28**:645–655.

Kalapurakal JA, Dome JS, Perlman EJ, *et al.* Management of Wilms' tumour: current practice and future goals. *Lancet Oncol* 2004; **5**:37–46.

Luithle T, Szavay P, Furtwängler R, *et al.* Treatment of cystic nephroma and cystic partially differentiated nephroblastoma — a report from the SIOP/GPOH group. *J Urol* 2007; **177**:294–296.

La Quaglia MP, Rutigliano DN. Neuroblastoma and other adrenal tumors. In: *The Surgery of Childhood Tumors*, 2nd Edn. (eds.) R Carachi, J Grosfeld, A Azmy. Berlin, Heidelberg: Springer-Verlag, 2008.

Miniati D, Gay AN, Parks KV, *et al.* Imaging accuracy and incidence of Wilms' and non-Wilms' renal tumors in children. *J Pediatr Surg* 2008; **43**:1301–1307.

Maris JM, Hogarty MD, Bagatell R, *et al.* Neuroblastoma. *Lancet* 2007; **369**:2106–2120.

Monclair T, Brodeur GM, Ambros PF, *et al.* The International Neuroblastoma Risk Group (INRG) staging system: an INRG task force report. *J Clin Oncol* 2008; **27**:298–303.

Rescorla F. Malignant germ cell tumors. In: *The Surgery of Childhood Tumors*, 2nd Edn. (eds.) R Carachi, J Grosfeld, A Azmy. Berlin, Heidelberg: Springer-Verlag, 2008.

Rodeberg D, Paidas C. Childhood rhabdomyosarcoma. *Semin Pediatr Surg* 2006; **15**:57–62.

Ross JH. Prepubertal testicular tumors. *Urology* 2009; **74**(1):94–99.

Shamberger R. Renal tumors. In: *The Surgery of Childhood Tumors*, 2nd Edn. (eds.) R Carachi, J Grosfeld, A Azmy. Berlin, Heidelberg: Springer-Verlag, 2008.

Williams J, Metzger M, Kaste S, *et al.* Wilms' tumor. www.oncopedia.org. Last updated 10-02-2009.

Chapter 21

Neuropathic Bladder

Maya Horst

DEFINITION

Neuropathic bladder refers to the dysfunction of the urinary bladder due to the disease of the central or peripheral nervous system involved in the control of micturition. Various types of lesions of the nervous system can present with neuropathic bladder disease (NBD), in which the bladder partially or completely loses the ability to store and release urine at low pressure. NBD in children is frequently seen in patients with myelomeningocele (MMC). This disorder carries a high risk for renal damage and renal failure and in pediatric urology, more than one-fourth of clinical problems related to lower urinary tract function are the result of neurologic lesions.

ETIOLOGY

Neuropathic bladder dysfunction can develop from a lesion at any level in the nervous system, including the cerebral cortex, spinal cord, or peripheral nervous system. Predominantly, NBD develops in children with congenital neural tube defect including MMC, lipomeningocele, sacral agenesis, and occult lesions causing tethered cord. Other conditions involving the spinal cord, such as tumors and traumatic lesions, are less frequent. Cerebral palsy, brain tumors, sacrococcygeal teratoma, and tethered spinal cord associated with imperfortate anus can also result in abnormal innervation of the bladder, sphincter, or both.

MMC is one of the commonest major congenital malformations induced by closure defects of the neural tube. It is the most frequent cause of NBD in children; therefore the vast majority of knowledge about NBD comes from long-term experience with this condition. Today, early closure of the primary spinal defect with improved neurosurgical techniques and ventricular peritoneal shunting significantly increases the survival rate of children with MMC and shifts the main causes of morbidity and mortality from central nervous system infection and hydrocephalus to long-term urological complications such as pyelonephritis, hypertension, and chronic renal failure.

NEUROANATOMY AND PHYSIOLOGY OF THE BLADDER

Normal voiding mainly is a spinal reflex, modulated by the central nervous system (brain, brain stem, and spinal cord), which coordinates the functions of bladder and urethra. Bladder and urethra are innervated by three sets of peripheral nerves: from the autonomic nervous system (ANS) including sacral parasympathetic (pelvic nerve) and sympathetic nerves (hypogastric nerves and sympathetic chain) and from the somatic nervous system (SNS) primarily the pudendal nerve (Figure 21-1).

The micturition control center is located in the frontal lobe of the brain. The primary activity of this area is to send topically inhibitory signals to the detrusor muscle to prevent the bladder from contracting; furthermore, it controls the activity of the micturition center in the brain stem.

The pontine micturition center (PMC) is located in the brain stem. It works as a relay switch in the voiding pathway. During bladder filling, neurons within the PMC are turned off, but at a critical level of bladder distention, afferent activity arises from mechanoreceptors in the bladder wall switching the PMC on and enhancing its activity. This activation results in the relaxation of the urethra and the contraction of the bladder due to simultaneous stimulation of parasympathetic and inhibition of sympathetic stimuli to the bladder, as well as the removal of somatic activation of the external urethral sphincter. The brain is able to control PMC activity. Gaining this control is part of the social training children experience during development and most children are toilet trained at 3–4 years of age.

The spinal cord provides communication between brainstem and sacral spinal cord. The sacral spinal cord is the terminal portion of the spinal cord,

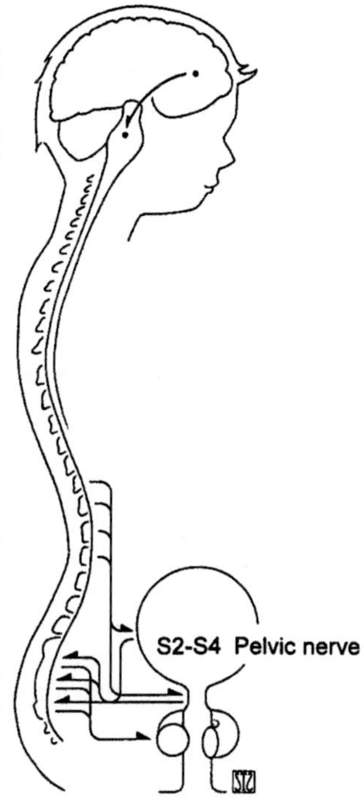

Figure 21-1. Innervation of bladder, urethra, and pelvic floor.

which is known as the spinal reflex center. It is responsible for bladder contractions and works under normal conditions as the primitive voiding center in infants, as long as the control center is not mature enough to command the bladder. When urine fills the infant bladder, an excitatory signal is sent to the sacral cord automatically triggering the detrusor to contract. The result is involuntary detrusor contractions with coordinated voiding. As the child's brain matures, it gradually dominates the control of the bladder and the urinary sphincters to inhibit involuntary voiding.

The peripheral nerves arising from the ANS innervate bladder and internal urethral sphincter. When the sympathetic nervous system is active, it causes detrusor relaxation and stimulation of the internal urinary sphincter to remain tightly closed. The parasympathetic nervous system functions in an opposite manner and stimulates the detrusor to contract. The SNS regulates the action of the muscles under voluntary control. Activation of the pudendal nerve causes the contraction of the external sphincter and the pelvic floor muscles.

During the course of a day, an average person will void approximately 4–8 times. The normal micturition cycle consists of two phases — filling and emptying — and requires urinary bladder and internal and external urethral sphincters that function as a synergistic unit.

Filling Phase

During urinary storage, the bladder acts as a low-pressure reservoir, accumulating increasing volumes of urine while the pressure inside the bladder remains low. Bladder filling is primarily a passive event depending on the compliance of the bladder wall and the ANS activity. Sympathetic nerves are constantly active during bladder filling:

- directly causing relaxation and expansion of the detrusor muscle,
- inhibiting the parasympathetic nerves from triggering bladder contractions, and
- closing the bladder neck by constricting the internal urethral sphincter.

In healthy bladders, the change in bladder pressure between empty and full is minimal (less than 10–15 cm H_2O) and stays below the urethral pressure. As the bladder fills, the urinary sphincter remains contracted to keep the bladder outlet closed. In addition, the pudendal nerve becomes excited, contracting the external urethral sphincter with increasing abdominal pressure. Therefore, outlet resistance remains higher than normal bladder pressure and urinary continence is ensured. If the intra-abdominal pressure rises sharply, for example, during physical activities and with coughing, sneezing, or laughing and the pressure transmitted to the bladder is greater than the outlet resistance and urine will leak out.

Emptying Phase

During micturition, the bladder contracts to expel urine while the urinary sphincter opens to allow urine outflow. The emptying phase can be induced either involuntarily or voluntarily. Involuntary reflex voiding occurs in infants. When the bladder is full, an excitatory signal is sent to the sacral cord, which automatically triggers a detrusor contraction. After maturation, this primitive voiding reflex becomes suppressed and the brain dominates with the bladder function. The individual senses the activation of the mechanoreceptors as the bladder being full, which signals a need to void. Bladder emptying can now be triggered by the individual via PMC and parasympathetic nerve stimulation:

- directly inducing detrusor contraction,
- suppressing sympathetic nerves, and
- causing the relaxation of the internal sphincter.

In addition, the pudendal nerve will be deactivated, relaxing the external sphincter.

If voiding needs to be delayed, the brain sends inhibitory signals to the PMC to prevent detrusor contractions. Furthermore, the levator muscle may actively be contracted to keep the external sphincter closed or initiate distracting techniques to suppress urination.

PATHOPHYSIOLOGY

The urinary bladder and urethra form a functional unit. If any part of the nervous system is affected, including brain, pons, spinal cord, sacral cord, and peripheral nerves, the entire voiding cycle is affected. This chapter will focus on bladder dysfunction caused by MMC, which is the commonest pathology in the pediatric age group. At the level of the lesion, efferent as well as afferent inputs are interrupted or impeded. Below the level of the lesion, intact spinal cord segments will function without supraspinal control and coordination. According to the level and extent of the lesion, myelodysplasia may cause either an atonic or a hypertonic pelvic floor and either an areflexia or hyperreflexia of the detrusor muscle, leading to four classic combinations (see Table 21-1). The four patterns represent the clinical expressions of the primary neurological lesion in MMC and it has become evident that children with this condition can be categorized into high- and low-risk groups for secondary damage from a neurogenic bladder based on intravesical pressure.

Hypertonic sphincter in combination with detrusor hyperactivity leads to the most dangerous pattern of neuropathic bladder, referred to as the "unsafe" bladder. It causes either decompensation of the detrusor with vesicoureteric reflux or deterioration of the bladder wall with hypertrophy and stiffness resulting in vesicoureteric obstruction. The subsequent

Table 21-1. Classification of the neurogenic bladder, with four subtypes according to the dysfunctional activities of sphincter and detrusor. For each subtype, clinical implications if untreated and the principles of management are summarized.

Dysfunction			
Sphincter	Detrusor	Consequences	Management
Overactivity	Underactivity	Unsafe, leaking, and infections	Safe and dry with CIC
Overactivity	Overactivity	Unsafe from birth and DSD (VUR, infections, and renal damage)	Safe and dry with CIC + oxybutynin
Underactivity	Underactivity	Safe but wet	Safe and dry with CIC + outlet surgery. Cave detrusor instability after outlet surgery
Underactivity	Overactivity	Wet and unsafe	Safe and dry with CIC + oxybutynin outlet surgery

insufficient drainage of the upper urinary tract leads to the decompensation of the ureters and the development of reflux and hydronephrosis. The elevation of bladder pressure above 40 cm H_2O leads to renal tubular injury and finally chronic renal disease, persisting even if hydronephrosis is reversed. This process is accelerated by urinary infections.

Intermittent elevation of bladder pressure may occur from detrusor hypertonia or hyperreflexia, especially, if the external sphincter acts reflexively and tightens rather than relaxes. This uncoordinated interplay is called detrusor sphincter dyssynergia (DSD) leading to functional infravesical obstruction. Bladder outlet obstruction may result in chronically overdistended detrusor (areflexia from myogenic failure) or in detrusor hypertrophy with associated trabeculation and subsequent diverticula formation. These pathophysiologic changes affect the elastic properties of the bladder and also result in mechanical vesicoureteral junction obstruction. Finally, recurrent urinary tract infections (UTIs) due to bladder residue may aggravate damage to the neurogenic bladder through the processes of transmural inflammation and fibrosis. Together with high-intravesical pressures and/or vesicoureteral reflux, these lower UTIs will lead to the episodes of acute pyelonephritis and irreversible renal damage.

DIAGNOSTIC METHODS

Early and targeted assessments as well as regular follow-up investigations are essential in patients with NBD in order to avoid the deterioration of bladder and kidney function.

In the newborn, the need for closure of the MMC determines the initial management. Nevertheless, the renal ultrasound (US) and the measurement of residual urine are performed as early as possible after birth. Urodynamic studies are delayed until it is safe to perform the investigation postoperatively.

PostVoid Residual Urine

Normal bladder capacity in the newborn period is 10 to 15 ml; therefore, a residual urine volume of less than 5 ml is acceptable. If the residual volume is high, the bladder may be hypoactive or the bladder outlet may be obstructed. Both of these conditions will cause urinary retention with overflow incontinence.

Renal and Bladder Ultrasonography (US)

This is performed to detect hydronephrosis, resulting from VUR or active obstruction of the bladder outlet, and to monitor renal growth. Measurement of bladder wall thickness is also important.

Urodynamics

The goal of urodynamic assessment is to characterize compliance and contractility of the bladder and function of the bladder outlet including bladder neck and external sphincter. This test evaluates bladder pressure, sphincter activity, and emptying ability.

The findings allow differentiating between patients with relatively low- and high-risk for upper urinary tract deterioration.

If the US reveal hydronephrosis or the urodynamic studies suggest outlet obstruction, vesicoureteral reflux (VUR) should be ruled out with a VCUG.

Voiding Cystourethrogram (VCUG)

VCUG enables us to investigate lower urinary tract anatomy including bladder diverticulum and to detect VUR; whenever possible, it can be combined with the urodynamic study (videourodynamics).

To complete baseline investigations, the measurement of serum creatinine after the seventh day of life is recommended. Urinalysis and culture may be performed only if the child is symptomatic for a UTI.

These investigations help to identify infants at risk for urinary tract deterioration because of a poorly compliant or overactive detrusor or outflow obstruction from DSD. In the literature, it has been documented that about 45% of children with MMC show sphincter overactivity, 34% combined sphincter and detrusor overactivity, and 11% detrusor underactivity. 50% of children present with DSD. These initial investigations provide baseline information about the radiologic and functional appearance of the upper and lower urinary tracts that can be compared with findings on follow-up assessments, in order to detect early signs of the deterioration of urinary tract function and drainage, or of progressive neurologic denervation.

Regular follow-up investigations are recommended not only for patients with pathologic findings but also for patients under treatment. Even if the initial assessment is normal, about 30% of patients will show neuro-urological deterioration in the first years of life, mainly due to tethering of the spinal cord. In patients under therapy, adequate follow-up is required, with adjustment if needed (CIC frequency, medication dosing, and administration route). Typically, urinalysis and US are performed at all visits. Urodynamics and VCUG are performed periodically to verify that under treatment, the volumes are age appropriate and stored under safe pressure conditions and to reassess the upper urinary tract. Further investigations such as blood serum analysis or scintigraphy are dependent on the clinical course.

With early instituted and optimal treatment, most of the patients can be adequately controlled without antireflux surgery or surgical bladder augmentation.

MANAGEMENT

The guiding principles for the management of NBD are similar irrespective of the different underlying pathologies. The goal of NBD management in the pediatric age group is to prevent bladder wall alterations, to avoid deterioration of the upper urinary tract and kidney function, as well as to achieve social urinary continence. The key principles to warrant a healthy environment for the kidneys include insurance and maintenance of an adequate sized and compliant reservoir that stores and evacuates urine completely, at a relatively low pressure. There is growing evidence that with early adequate treatment, kidneys are saved and normal bladder growth can be achieved in children; therefore, they might no longer need surgical bladder augmentation to achieve safe urinary continence in adolescence and adulthood. Crucial for long-term prognosis of these patients is an early start of the management, before the consequences of bladder dysfunction become apparent. The urodynamics investigation plays a central role in evaluating the patients and in planning the individually adapted therapy for each patient.

In clinical practice, based on urodynamic findings, four major subtypes can be used to describe NBD (Figure 21-2).

Sphincter Overactivity + Detrusor Underactivity

It is easy to treat. It requires early treatment because of urine retention with high filling pressure and continuous leaking. CIC alone is effective and sufficient and will make the bladder safe and infection free, and the patient will be dry in between.

Sphincter Overactivity + Detrusor Overactivity

High filling and high voiding pressure, being very unsafe from birth onward due to DSD. The act of voiding has to be prevented. With oxybutynin, the

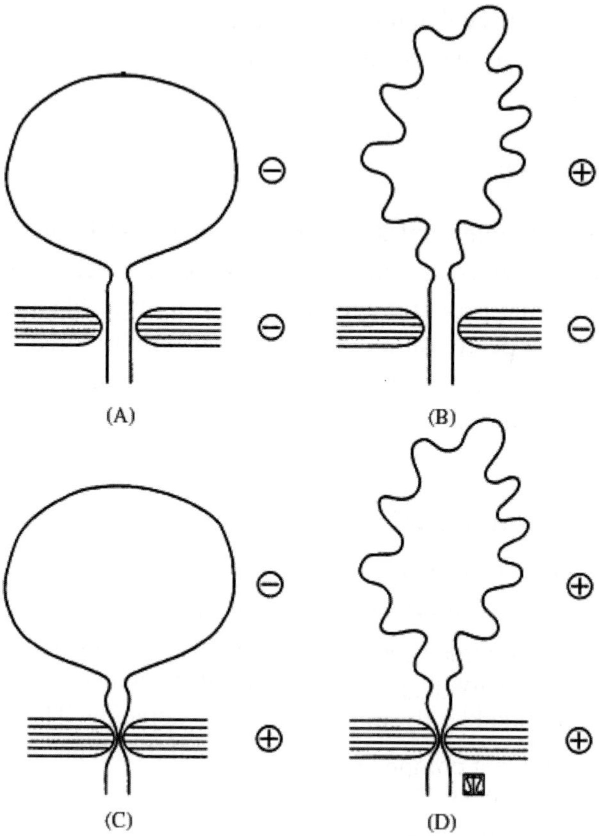

Figure 21-2. Grouping of neuropathic bladders according to the urodynamic findings. (After González R, Guzmán JM. *Pediatría* (*Buenos Aires*) 1981; **5**:29.) Management of incontinence in group A requires a procedure to enhance bladder outlet resistance. In group B, in addition to a procedure to enhance bladder outlet resistance, anticholinergics, Botox, or bladder augmentation is needed. Group C will become continent with regular bladder emptying by intermittent catheterization. In group D, anticholinergics, Botox, or bladder augmentation is also needed.

overactive detrusor can be "pharmacologically converted" to an inactive reservoir, which has to be emptied with CIC.

Sphincter Underactivity + Detrusor Underactivity

CIC reduces the degree of incontinence and offers much better control over UTIs. To achieve continence, patients with this type of dysfunction will at a later age need surgical interventions on the sphincter (e.g. artificial sphincter, slings or injection of bulking substances). An important caveat here is that detrusor instability may emerge only after surgical improvement of outlet resistance. "Wet but safe" to "dry but unsafe".

Sphincter Underactivity + Detrusor Overactivity

The bladder leaks due to detrusor instability and gradually becomes unsafe due to secondary bladder-wall changes with detrusor hypertrophy and the loss of bladder compliance. Therefore, treatment consists of CIC combined with oxybutynin and at a later age, bladder-outlet surgery with or without bladder augmentation.

MEDICAL TREATMENT

Newborn children with NBD and sphincter detrusor dyssynergia, elevated detrusor pressure (> 40 cm H_2O), and/or VUR grade 3 or higher are at high risk for the deterioration of the upper urinary tract. These infants are immediately started on clean intermittent catheterization (CIC) alone or in combination with anticholinergic drugs. Early institution of this standard treatment can prevent complications.

Clean Intermittent Catheterization

The introduction of CIC in 1972 by Lapides meant a milestone in the management of NBD in children, making medical management a successful treatment option. Early administration of CIC has been shown to be effective in preventing renal deterioration and poor bladder compliance and therefore postponing or avoiding the subsequent need for bladder augmentation. Likewise as important as early administration is the fact that it is much easier for the parents and the child to adapt to the routine of CIC than when the child is older. Parents or caregivers carry out CIC in the first years of life. From experience, when children are around six years old and show sufficient dexterity, they usually take over catheterization. CIC is usually started at a frequency of every three hours throughout the day. Additional catheterization once during nighttime is also frequently recommended. The frequency of catheterization can be determined by the bladder capacity at 30 cm H_2O, which is measured during urodynamic evaluations. The goal is to keep the bladder volume within "safe" range.

Anticholinergic Drugs

Oxybutynin is the standard treatment for the pharmaceutical therapy of neuropathic detrusor overactivity and is best started as early as possible together with CIC. It is a tertiary amine with a well-documented therapeutic effect on detrusor hyperactivity. Oxybutynin acts on a combination of anticholinergic, spasmolytic, local anesthetic, and calcium-channel-blocking activities. Several studies have shown its efficacy for decreasing filling pressure, increasing the capacity of the neurogenic bladder, and preserving renal function.

The potential side effects of all anticholinergic agents include blurred vision, dry mouth, heart palpitations, drowsiness, and facial flushing. In children with insufficient response or significant systemic side effects to oral oxybutynin or patients with insufficient suppression of detrusor overactivity despite the maximal dosage of oral oxybutynin, intravesical administration has been shown to be a highly efficacious, reliable, and well-tolerated alternative for children who would otherwise require surgical therapy. Compared to oral oxybutynin, intravesical oxybutynin has more potent and longer-acting detrusor suppressive effects with good tolerance and should be used prior to considering surgical therapies.

Recommended Dose of Oxybutynin

- Oral oxybutynin: 0.2–0.6 mg/kg per day in three doses.
- Intravesical oxybutynin: 0.2–0.6 mg/kg per day in two doses.

Infection Prophylaxis

In principle, all patients with upper urinary tract changes or VUR are put on low-dose chemoprophylaxis, mostly trimethoprim. In case of breakthrough infections, nitrofurantoin of ciprofloxacin can be used. Febrile UTIs should be treated intravenously with amoxicillin/clavulanic acid and gentamycin until the result for bacterial culture is known. Many centers stop prophylaxis after the age of one year, and approximately 50% of patients seem to do well without prophylaxis. Scientific proof is lacking on this subject.

Recommended Dose for Chemoprophylaxis

- Trimethoprim 2 mg/kg per day.

Botulinum A Toxin (BTX)

In about 10–15% of patients, CIC and anticholinergic therapy fails or causes severe systemic side effects. For these patients, intradetrusor injection of BTX has been developed as a second-line treatment option. BTX is a potent neurotoxin produced by the Gram-positive anaerobic bacterium *Clostridium botulinum*. The use of botulinum toxin subtype A is well documented for the treatment of cerebral palsy especially in children. BTX injections into the detrusor muscle under cystoscopic control have been showed to have beneficial effects both on clinical and on urodynamics variables. The effect of BTX injection lasts for six to eight months and can be repeated.

The incidence of side effects is recognized to be less than 10% and the events are usually mild and transient in nature. Despite all the promising reports, well-designed and randomized controlled trials are necessary to confirm the efficacy and safety of this therapy.

Commonly Used Dose of BTX

- Botox® (Allegan, Irvine CA, USA) 10 U/kg with a maximal dose of 300 U.

SURGICAL MANAGEMENT

Surgical bladder enlargement continues to be a standard procedure for patients with hyperactive small bladders with poor compliance and resistant to medical treatment. In patients with insufficient sphincter activity, continence achievement will require bladder outlet surgery in addition to medical treatment.

Bladder Augmentation

When children with neurogenic bladder fail conservative management bladder augmentation, a surgical enlargement of the bladder is the therapy of choice to achieve adequate low-pressure capacity, to improve continence, and to protect the upper urinary tract. Various methods, therefore, have been described.

Currently, the most commonly performed procedure for bladder augmentation is enterocystoplasty. It has become part in the management of NBD with the intention to increase detrusor compliance and lower bladder storage pressure that may place the upper tract at risk for deterioration. Enterocystoplasty involves isolating a full-thickness segment of intestine on its vascular pedicle, which is reconfigured to create a semi-spherical structure that is sutured to the wide open bladder. Small intestine, stomach, and large intestine have all been used as the reconstructing segment, but prevalent ileocystoplasty and sigmoidcystoplasty are the most commonly performed procedures.

Complications of Enterocystoplasty

Despite the fact that enterocystoplasty has been shown to be an efficient treatment option for NBD refractory to conservative treatment, the procedure can result in significant morbidity. The complications are mainly generated by structural and physiological interactions between bowel mucosa and urine. The specific, often intermediate or late, presenting complications of enterocystoplasty include metabolic disturbance, mucus production, stone formation, spontaneous bladder perforation, bacteriuria, and malignancy.

Metabolic Disturbances

The unphysiologic exposure of intestinal mucosa to urine can results in metabolic disturbances because of the absorption or secretion of electrolytes. With ileum and colon, hyperchloremic metabolic acidosis is common and with stomach, hypochloremic, hyperchloremic metabolic alkalosis can occur. Usually, the metabolic imbalance is not severe enough to require electrolyte substitution, but serum electrolytes, including bicarbonate, should be checked annually or as needed. There is some evidence that the absorptive properties of the augmented segment may decrease over time.

Mucus Production and Stone Formation

The lining of the bowel, when incorporated into the bladder, continues to produce mucus. Mucus can cause bladder outlet obstruction and the blockage of the catheters and it is also involved in the formation of calculi. The amount of mucus produced, however, usually diminishes with time.

Lower urinary tract stones are common in augmented bladders, which may occur in 30–52% of patients. It is widely accepted that the combination of different factors are responsible for stone formation; poor patient's mobility, urinary stasis, increased mucus production, recurrence of chronic infections, and abnormalities in urine composition. Stones within the bladder can cause irritation, bleeding, and encourage infection. Therefore, the management after enterocystoplasty should attempt to prevent stone formation. Regular bladder irrigation has been shown to decrease bladder lithiasis from 43 to 7%.

Spontaneous Bladder Perforation

This uncommon but serious complication has been described to occur in 6–13% of augmented patients. Several etiologic mechanisms such as traumatic catheterization, chronic infection, ischemic necrosis of the intestinal segment and increased intravesical pressure are discussed as possible causes. In a large series published by Metcalfe *et al.* (2006) the risk for perforation was decreased by the presence of a continent catheterizable channel, probably because this makes compliance with CIC easier.

Bacteriuria

Asymptomatic bacteriuria in patients who underwent enterocystoplasty is nearly universal. It is generally of no clinical relevance and should not be treated with antibiotics.

Malignancy

Long-term follow-up studies of patients after bladder augmentation have shown that the risk to develop a malignant tumor is of concern. Recent studies revealed an incidence of 1.2–3%. The etiology seems to be multifactorial involving chronic inflammation and different carcinogens (nitrosamines and growth factors). The commonest malignancy identified was adenocarcinoma but others have also been reported. Most of the tumors occurred about ten years after augmentation, but there are some reports on malignancies that appeared as soon as five year after the operation. For early recognition, it is recommended to perform annual cystoscopy and urine analysis, beginning five to ten years after enterocystoplasty.

Because of the significant complications of enterocystoplasty, a number of alternative methods for bladder augmentation have been described, primarily ureterocystoplasty, autoaugmentation, and seromuscular colocystoplasty lined with urothelium. The common principle of these methods is to ensure urothelial continuity within the neobladder. Ureterocystoplasty utilizes the otherwise ineffective megaureter in patients with chronic unilateral hydroureteronephrosis in association with neuropathic bladder. The megaureter is detubularized and reconfigured to be incorporated into the bladder, similar to enterocystoplasty. For autoaugmentation, a detrusorectomy is performed to produce an iatrogenic bladder diverticulum that can increase capacity and compliance. The technique of seromuscular colocystoplasty lined with urothelium also involves detrusorectomy, but in contrast to autoaugmentation, the exposed bladder mucosa is covered with a reconfigured seromuscular segment of sigmoid colon.

All these methods avoid incorporating intestinal mucosa into the urinary tract, although autoaugmentation has questionable long-term results in the neuropathic bladder and ureterocystoplasty is largely limited to a small number of selected patients with megaureter and ipsilateral nonfunctioning kidney.

Recently, the field of tissue engineering and regenerative medicine has offered new approaches to replace lost or deficient tissue, especially in the urogenital tract. Bladder tissue engineering uses the principle of autologous smooth muscle and urothelial cells seeded on a biodegradable scaffold *in vitro* used for bladder augmentation. A small pilot study of seven patients was reported in 2006, showed that bio-engineered bladders increased compliance and bladder capacity and decreased detrusor pressure. Although these first results are promising, further experimental and clinical work is mandatory.

EXTERNAL URETHRAL SPHINCTER DILATATION

Urethral dilatation has been mentioned in the literature as an option when CIC and anticholinergic therapy fail. The dilatation of the external sphincter, normally under general anesthesia, lowers the outlet resistance and leads to the improvement of compliance, the continence, and consecutively of upper tract dilatation and VUR in about 66% of patients. However, this alternative has not been widely practiced and critics believe that dilating the urethra eventually damages the sphincter and leads to urinary incontinence. Further prospective investigations are needed to validate the promising findings of this method.

CONTINENT CATHETERIZABLE STOMAS

After augmentation of the neuropathic urinary bladder catheterization is nearly always required to assure complete drainage. Catheterization may be physically challenging especially when patients are wheelchair-bound or have severe scoliosis/lordosis. Other patients are not able to catheterize because they cannot see or reach the urethra. Creating a continent catheterizable stoma may facilitate catheterization leading potentially to independency regarding bladder management.

The standard procedure is appendicovesicostomy or stoma formation with an ileal tube (Yang–Monti procedure). This procedure can be performed together or in combination with bladder augmentation or other surgical procedures, such as bladder neck interventions.

VESICOSTOMY

Incontinent cutaneous diversion can be considered an option to maintain low-pressure drainage when conservative management fails. Especially, in young children whom are not yet suitable for lower urinary tract reconstruction, vesicostomy may effectively postpone definitive therapy. It can also be useful as a permanent therapy in selected patients, particularly adults who cannot self-catheterize. The procedure is simple and reliable, well tolerated, and easily reversible.

INCONTINENCE SURGERY

Patients with sphincter underactivity show incontinence, especially in combination with detrusor overactivity. The treatment of neurogenic urinary incontinence in children remains challenging. Initial attempts to achieve continence include CIC and drug therapy designed to maintain low-intravesical pressure and a reasonable level of urethral resistance. If this conservative therapy fails, incontinence surgery is indicated. A wide variety of surgical options to increase bladder outlet resistance have been proposed, from minimally invasive injection of bulking agents to complex surgeries such as artificial sphincter implantation, facial sling procedures, and bladder neck reconstructions. In some of the most severe cases, bladder neck closure with a continent stoma is the final option for attaining dryness.

Artificial Urinary Sphincter (AUS)

The artificial sphincter consists of a pressure reservoir implanted in the abdomen, a pump that is placed in the scrotum or labium, and a cuff surgically inserted around the urethra in the area of the normal sphincter. The fluid-filled cuff increases bladder outlet resistance and enhances the patient's ability to retain urine and stay dry. By manipulation of the palpable pump, the cuff can temporarily be emptied, decreasing outlet resistance and enabling micturition or catheterization. Therefore, it is a favorable therapeutic alternative for males and females capable of spontaneous voiding.

Fascial Sling Procedure

In principle, the techniques involve suspension of the bladder neck with a rectangular strip mostly of rectus abdominis fascia. This sling is secured with permanent sutures and anchored suprapubically to the rectus fascia with gentle traction. The mechanism of continence of the sling involves permanent increase in static urethral compression, reinforced during abdominal straining, and the elevation of the functional urethra to the level of the bladder neck and the proximal urethra. Because of the fixed increase in outlet resistance, spontaneous voiding is generally not possible and almost all patients require CIC. The rectus fascia sling is a relatively simple procedure, primarily used in girls with a limited complication rate. Success rates in achieving continence are reported as high as 85%, especially in combination with bladder augmentation.

Bladder Neck Reconstruction

A wide range of bladder neck reconstruction techniques have been proposed for the treatment of sphincter incompetence, with final results between 60 and 90%. In principle, bladder neck reconstruction includes narrowing of the bladder neck region and lengthening the proximal urethra, which is improving bladder outlet resistance. However, a decrease in bladder capacity is the natural consequence of this kind of surgery, leaving it for only a small group of well-selected patients, unless augmentation is performed during the same session.

Kryger *et al.* (2000) compared the different methods comprehensively according to the publications available between 1966 and 2000. Obviously, there is no "gold standard" technique, but they concluded that the best continence rates are obtained not only by AUSs in male and female but also by facial sling procedures, especially in girls appear to be a good option. However, endoscopic treatment with dextranomer-based implants (Deflux®) has shown to be effective especially in the short and medium terms. Although very costly, given its relative simplicity, this treatment can be proposed to manage major incontinence in children as a primary procedure.

MANAGEMENT OF VUR

VUR plays an important role in the development of renal damage in infants and children with NBD. VUR occurs in 3–5% of newborns with MMC, usually in association with poor detrusor compliance, detrusor overactivity, or DSD. If left untreated, the incidence of reflux in these infants increases and by the age of five years, 30–40% are affected. In children with sphincter inactivity, VUR tends to be low-grade with a high rate of spontaneous resolution.

In NBD, there is a clear correlation between VUR and the incidence of renal scars. Early detection and treatment of functional obstruction is important to prevent the progressive scarring of reflux nephropathy. Early lowering of the detrusor pressure with CIC and anticholinergic agents has been shown to significantly reduce the incidence of reflux and its complications.

The indications for antireflux surgery are not very different from those applicable to children with normal bladder function. They include recurrent symptomatic urinary tract infections, persisting hydroureteronephrosis, and severe reflux with an anatomic abnormality at the UVJ while receiving adequate antibiotic prophylaxis and appropriate catheterization technique. Although endoscopic injection of Deflux® is also applied in patients with NBD and VUR, the reimplantation of the ureters is the standard surgical procedure in these patients.

LATEX SENSITIZATION AND ALLERGY

Children with MMC have a high degree of exposure to latex products after mucosal exposure to latex devices or through repeated surgical procedures. The number of surgical procedures is directly correlated with the sensitization and the allergy. The prevalence of sensitization to latex among children with MMC is 29–72% and it is considered the highest prevalence in the general population. In addition to MMC, other children requiring multiple surgeries are also at risk of sensitization to latex. Consequent avoidance of latex from birth at hospital and at home is felt to be the cornerstone for the primary prevention of latex sensitization and therefore to prevent latex allergy including severe anaphylactic reactions.

CONCLUSION

In children with NBD, the preservation of kidney function and the establishment of early urinary dryness as well as the independence regarding the bladder management are important factors for the optimal quality of life. Urodynamics and radiological imaging play an essential role in ascertaining the nature of urological involvement. Based on these investigations, treatment plans are individualized for each patient starting with the most conservative measures first, then advancing as necessary to achieve the goals desired. Early intervention and patient education help to guarantee the most successful outcome.

However, pediatric urologists continue to face many challenges in the management of children with NBD. The most recent literature attempts to identify predictors of upper urinary tract deterioration, to find efficacious strategies to avoid bladder augmentation, and for long-term care. Further prospective studies with adequate follow-up will improve our understanding of this disease and help to choose the best strategies to achieve continence and preserve renal function by minimizing surgical interventions in this patient group.

COMMENT FROM THE EDITORS

Neuropathic bladder has been a challenge for pediatric urologists for many decades. The concerns have changed over time. Initially, we were concerned mostly with survival and later with preservation of renal function. In the developed world, for the last three decades, the focus has been on the quality of life, providing the means to live independently within the possibilities of each individual.

What made many of these changes possible was the acceptance of CIC either urethrally or though continent stomas. The first challenge for the developing world is to introduce programs for CIC to prevent renal failure. The reader should keep in mind that major upper tract damage or renal insufficiency in a child with neuropathic bladder represents a failure of medical management, family education, or cultural biases. The role of the pediatric urologists in these circumstances is crucial to protect the children.

FURTHER READING

Atala A. Bioengineered tissues for urogenital repair in children. *Pediatr Res* 2008; **63**(5):569–575.

Bauer SB. Neurogenic bladder: etiology and assessment. *Pediatr Nephrol* 2008; **23**(4):541–551.

Dave S, Salle JL. Current status of bladder neck reconstruction. *Curr Opin Urol* 2008; **18**(4):419–424.

de Jong TP, Chrzan R, Klijn AJ, Dik P. Treatment of the neurogenic bladder in spina bifida. *Pediatr Nephrol* 2008; **23**(6):889–896.

De Queiroz M, Combet S, Berard J, Pouyau A, Genest H, Mouriquand P, Chassard D. Latex allergy in children: modalities and prevention. *Paediatr Anaesth* 2009; **19**(4):313–319.

Edelstein RA, Bauer SB, Kelly MD, Darbey MM, Peters CA, Atala A, Mandell J, Colodny AH, Retik AB. The long-term urological response of neonates with myelodysplasia treated proactively with intermittent catheterization and anticholinergic therapy. *J Urol* 1995; **154**(4):1500–1504.

Game X, Mouracade P, Chartier-Kastler E, Viehweger E, Moog R, Amarenco GX, Denys P, De Seze M, Haab F, Karsenty G, Kerdraon J, Perrouin-Verbe B, Ruffion A, Soler JM, Saussine C. Botulinum toxin-A (Botox) intradetrusor injections in children with neurogenic detrusor overactivity/neurogenic overactive bladder: a systematic literature review. *J Pediatr Urol* 2009; **5**(3):156–164.

González R, Ludwikowski B, Horst M. Determinants of success and failure of seromuscular colocystoplasty lined with urothelium. *J Urol* 2009; **182**(4 Suppl):1781–1784.

Kiddoo DA, Canning DA, Snyder HM 3rd, Carr MC. Urethral dilation as treatment for neurogenic bladder. *J Urol* 2006; **176**(4 Pt 2):1831–1833; discussion 1834.

Kryger JV, González R, Barthold JS. Surgical management of urinary incontinence in children with neurogenic sphincteric incompetence. *J Urol* 2000; **163**(1):256–263.

Lapides J, Diokno AC, Silber SJ, Lowe BS. Clean, intermittent self-catheterization in the treatment of urinary tract disease. *J Urol* 1972; **107**(3):458–461.

Lopez Pereira P, Moreno Valle JA, Espinosa L, Alonso Dorrego JM, Burgos Lucena L, Martinez Urrutia MJ, Lobato Romera R, Luz Picazo M, Viguer JM, Jaureguizar Monereo E. Enterocystoplasty in children with neuropathic bladders: long-term follow-up. *J Pediatr Urol* 2008; **4**(1):27–31.

Lottmann HB, Margaryan M, Lortat-Jacob S, Bernuy M, Lackgren G. Long-term effects of dextranomer endoscopic injections for the treatment of urinary incontinence: an update of a prospective study of 61 patients. *J Urol* 2006; **176**(4 Pt 2):1762–1766.

MacLellan DL. Management of pediatric neurogenic bladder. *Curr Opin Urol* 2009; **19**(4):407–411.

McGuire EJ, Woodside JR, Borden TA, Weiss RM. Prognostic value of urodynamic testing in myelodysplastic patients. *J Urol* 1981; **126**(2):205–209.

Metcalfe PD, Casale AJ, Kaefer MA, Misseri R, Dussinger AM, Meldrum KK, Cain MP, Rink RC. Spontaneous bladder perforations: a report of 500 augmentations in children and analysis of risk. *J Urol* 2006; **175**(4):1466–1470; discussion 1470–1471.

Morrisroe SN, O'Connor RC, Nanigian DK, Kurzrock EA, Stone AR. Vesicostomy revisited: the best treatment for the hostile bladder in myelodysplastic children? *BJU Int* 2005; **96**(3):397–400.

Park JM, McGuire EJ, Koo HP, Schwartz AC, Garwood CK, Bloom DA. External urethral sphincter dilation for the management of high risk myelomeningocele: 15-year experience. *J Urol* 2001; **165**(6 Pt 2):2383–2388.

Tekgul S, Oge O, Bal K, Erkan I, Bakkaloglu M. Ureterocystoplasty: an alternative reconstructive procedure to enterocystoplasty in suitable cases. *J Pediatr Surg* 2000; **35**(4):577–579.

van Gool JD, Dick P, de Jong TP. Bladder-sphincter dysfunction in myelomeningocele. *Eur J Pediatr* 2001; **160**(7):414–420.

Verpoorten C, Buyse GM. The neurogenic bladder: medical treatment. *Pediatr Nephrol* 2008; **23**(5):717–725.

Chapter 22

Urolithiasis in Children

Erica J. Traxel and Paul H. Noh

DEFINITION OF THE DISEASE

Paediatric urolithiasis, similar to adult urolithiasis, is the occurrence of calculi, more commonly referred to as stones, within the urinary tract. At present, these calculi most often are encountered within the upper tracts, such as renal pelvis and ureter, but can also be found within the bladder and urethra, which were more common sites of stone disease in the past. Historically, the incidence of urolithiasis in children in the Western world was quite low as compared with adults. In 1951, Lattimer *et al.* did not cite any instances of urolithiasis among 21,835 patients seen at Babies Hospital in New York. However, recently, the incidence has increased dramatically. In 1989, Stapleton attributed between 1 per 1000 and 1 per 7600 admissions to paediatric centres to stone disease. This shift is ascribed to changes in the modern diet as well as the increasing prevalence of obesity. As the disease becomes more widespread, it is incumbent upon practitioners, both medical and surgical alike, to familiarise themselves with its presentation, diagnosis, management, and prevention.

AETIOLOGY

The formation of urinary calculi relates to the simple chemical principles of solubility and saturation. A solution consists of solutes dissolved within a solvent. As more of the solute is dissolved within the solution, the saturation level progressively increases until the solution reaches a point of equilibrium referred to as the solubility product, beyond which the addition of more solute will cause the solute to precipitate out of solution in the form of crystals. Certain metabolic conditions, such as hypercalciuria, hyperoxaluria, hyperuricosuria, and cystinuria, lead to an increased solute concentration within urine, thereby causing increased saturation and crystal formation, predisposing to stone formation.

The pH of the urine can affect the solubility of certain substances. Calcium phosphate is more soluble above a pH of 6.0. Uric acid is most soluble between a pH of 6.0 and 7.0. Cystine is soluble above a pH of 7.4. Consequently, altering the acid–base balance of the urine through medical therapy can help with stone dissolution and prevention.

Because urine contains substances to inhibit crystallisation, such as magnesium, citrate, pyrophosphate, glycosaminoglycans, nephrolcalcin, Tamm-Horsfall protein, and uropontin, among others, it is possible for a greater concentration of salts and solutes to remain dissolved within the urine than would otherwise be expected. Thus, urine is typically in a state of supersaturation. A lack of these inhibitors will predispose to stone formation.

Eventually, even these inhibitors can no longer keep the solutes dissolved in the urine, and the formation product is reached. At this point, spontaneous nucleation occurs as crystals begin to form. In a homogenous solution, this nucleation would occur in a uniform fashion. However, in urine and within the collecting system, there are variable factors that allow nucleation to occur in a microcosmic fashion, while it is still prevented in other areas of the collecting system. For instance, particles such as cellular debris can serve as the nidus for crystallisation. Additionally, crystals of one type can serve as the focus for additional crystallisation of another type, a process referred to as heterogeneous nucleation. This perpetuation of crystallisation is known as epitaxy. For this reason, not uncommonly, analysis of kidney stones usually will reveal multiple different components within a single calculus.

The formation of crystals within the urine is not sufficient for calculus formation. These crystals must be retained within the collecting system long enough to allow for continued crystal deposition until the aggregate is of sufficient size to be recognised as a calculus. In order for this to occur, other underlying abnormalities must be present. Most importantly, if a high urine flow rate is maintained, then crystals cannot be retained and instead will wash out regularly along the urinary tract. A high urine flow rate can be sustained with a high fluid intake. Conversely, anatomic abnormalities, such as medullary sponge kidney, congenital ureteropelvic junction (UPJ) obstruction, or vesicoureteral reflux, will alter the drainage of urine, thereby promoting stone formation. Additionally, urinary tract infections (UTIs) can predispose to urolithiasis, as nanobacteria can produce carbonate apatite on their cell walls, serving as a nidus for stone formation. Other genetic factors may also alter the composition of urine, making an individual inherently more likely to form stones.

PRESENTATION

Paediatric patients, just like adults, with urolithiasis can present with flank and/or abdominal pain (see Chapter 4), haematuria (gross or microscopic) (see Chapter 3), UTI (see Chapter 2), and lower urinary tract symptoms, such as frequency, urgency, and dysuria. About one-half of children with urolithiasis will present with pain. Classic renal colic is severe, intermittent, cramp-like flank, and abdominal pain of sudden onset, with radiation to the groin and associated nausea and vomiting. However, the younger the child, the less likely they are to present with classic renal colic. These younger children, particularly under the age of five years, are more likely to present with a UTI or an incidental radiologic finding.

Often, the presenting symptoms will suggest the location of the calculus. Pain that is limited to the flank suggests a stone is still within the renal calyces or pelvis or perhaps at the UPJ. As the stone is passes distally down the ureter, the pain will radiate around the flank towards the lower abdomen and into the groin, even into the testicle or labia. Once the stone reaches the ureterovesicular junction (UVJ) and bladder, the patient will experience urgency, frequency, and dysuria.

UTI is often intimately associated with urolithiasis. Bacteria within the urinary tract can lead to the formation of stones, and these same bacteria can lead to a UTI. Young children will commonly present with a UTI and on further evaluation, they are found to have a stone. When a patient presents with fever in the setting of an obstructing calculus, suggesting pyelonephritis, it warrants urgent evaluation and intervention, as the risk of sepsis is high.

When evaluating a child with urolithiasis, the history-taking should inquire not only as to the common acute symptoms of a stone, but should also investigate potential underlying predisposing factors. One should ask about a history of recurrent UTIs, particularly with urea-splitting organisms such as *Proteus* sp. Additionally, past medical conditions should be addressed, including premature birth (especially if given diuretics as a newborn), malabsorptive gastrointestinal disorders, cystic fibrosis, myelodysplasia, and recent immobilisation. Past surgical history such as prior urologic procedures should be ascertained. Patients with a neurogenic bladder related to myelodysplasia or spinal cord injury or exstrophy–epispadias complex, especially those who have undergone bladder reconstruction with augmentation and who depend upon clean intermittent catheterization, are at increased risk of stone formation. Dietary factors, such as vitamin D intake, enteral or parenteral nutritional formulas high in calcium and phosphorus, or a ketogenic diet designed to treat epilepsy, can influence stone formation. Certain medications, such as chemotherapy drugs, diuretics, antacids, and steroids, are associated with urolithiasis. Family history of urolithiasis must be addressed as upwards of one-third of children with stone disease in the United States have a family history of stones.

Physical examination should begin with the vital signs. Fever can indicate a serious infection. Septic individuals may be tachycardic and hypotensive. Patients with underlying renal disease may be hypertensive. The clinician should then evaluate the general appearance of the patient. Children experiencing acute renal colic will look quite uncomfortable. Costovertebral angle or abdominal tenderness may be present. Laboratory assessment can begin with a urinalysis. Up to 90% of the patients with urolithiasis will have some degree of haematuria. If the urine appears infected (positive for nitrites and leukocyte esterase), a urine culture should be obtained. A complete blood cell count should be obtained when the infection is suspected. Additionally, the presence of anaemia can suggest long-standing underlying renal disorder or insufficiency. A renal profile can evaluate basic renal function. Patients who are dehydrated due to emesis may have significantly elevated blood urea nitrogen along with other electrolyte disturbances. Once a diagnosis of urolithiasis has been established, further future laboratory testing is indicated to help determine the aetiology for stone formation and direct future preventive therapy.

DIAGNOSTIC METHODS

Initial diagnosis of urolithiasis can be determined via multiple imaging modalities. Often in paediatrics, ultrasound is the first-line imaging study, due to its inexpensive and non-invasive nature. In addition, there is no radiation exposure and in keeping with the ALARA (as low as reasonably achievable) principle, it has the least amount of radiation exposure with the potential to gain the most information about the urinary tract in one study. Calculi present within the renal pelvis and calyces can be seen as areas of increased echogenicity. Traditionally, there is a component of acoustic shadowing behind calculi, but with current ultrasound probe technology, this is not always the case. Although the calculus may appear to have blood flow on Doppler examination, this represents an artefact ("twinkle" artefact). Other information to be gathered from an ultrasound includes the size of the kidneys and the overall appearance of the parenchyma to suggest if there is underlying intrinsic renal disease, such as underlying renal mass, dysplasia, or scarring. If a stone is impeding the flow of urine, then proximal to the level of obstruction there should be dilatation. If there is dilatation of the collecting system, an attempt should be made to follow the dilatation as far distally as possible, down into the ureter. Unfortunately, ultrasound does not provide good evaluation of the more distal ureter, until the portion of the ureter just behind the bladder is reached. At the level of the bladder, the wall thickness should be assessed and the evidence of intra-vesical abnormalities (such as ureterocele or other stones) should be determined. In addition, the presence or absence of bilateral ureteral jets can be verified within the bladder, and if seen, suggest that at the least there is not high-grade ureteral obstruction. The sensitivity of ultrasonography in the detection of urolithiasis varies widely from 19 to 93% and is dependent upon the operator as well as the location of the stone, but it seems to be a fairly specific study, with specificity rates of over 90% (Figure 22-1).

The most sensitive study (well over 90%) to diagnose urolithiasis is the non-contrast CT scan of the abdomen and pelvis using 3–5 mm slices. Spiral CT can obtain images rapidly enough that sedation is not necessary. In addition to assessing for urolithiasis, a CT scan can evaluate for the presence or absence of other intra-abdominal and intra-pelvic pathology, as it can often be difficult to parse out the nuances of paediatric abdominal

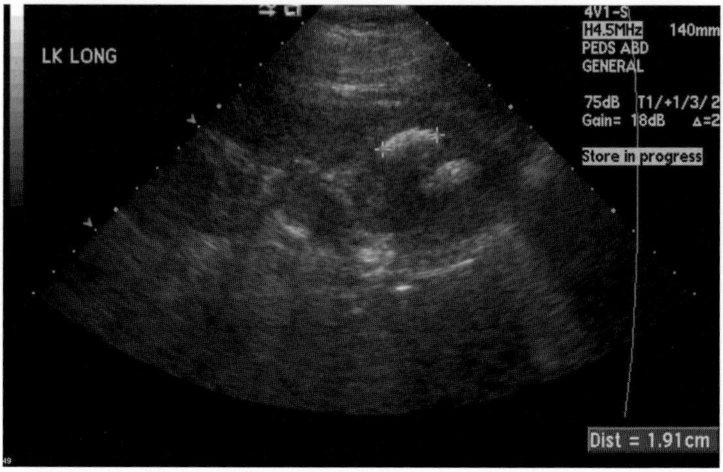

Figure 22-1. Renal ultrasound showing calculus on lower pole.

pain simply via history-taking, in order to determine if a child has urolithiasis versus appendicitis or gastroenteritis or some other pathology. The greatest disadvantage of CT is its radiation exposure. As paediatric stone formers are likely to experience recurrent stone disease, perhaps many times more over their lifetime, it is not feasible to perform a CT every time a child is suspected of having a stone. Another negative feature is the lack of availability, as not every medical centre has a CT scanner, but most will have access to ultrasonography. Of note, not every type of stone is universally visualised on CT as indinavir (antiviral protease inhibitor used in the treatment of HIV) is not visible on CT (Figures 22-2 and 22-3).

Plain X-ray of the abdomen and pelvis, while not sensitive in detecting stones, is important in aiding management decisions. Certain treatment modalities, such as extra-corporeal shock wave lithotripsy (ESWL), depend upon the ability to see the radio-opaque stone using plain film or fluoroscopy. Radiolucent stone types, including uric acid, sodium urate, ammonium urate, xanthine, matrix, triamterene, Indinavir, and silica stones, cannot be seen on traditional plain X-ray. Plain X-ray is also a fairly inexpensive way to follow the passage of a stone if one has elected for observation over intervention or if treatment has been rendered and one would like to follow the passage of residual stone fragments.

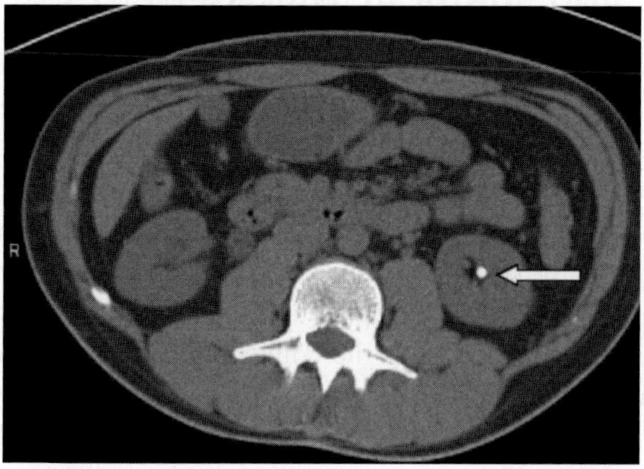

Figure 22-2. CT scan of the abdomen without contrast showing renal calculus.

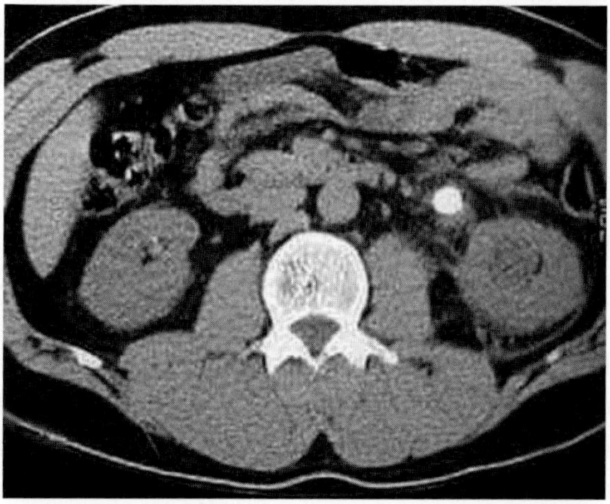

Figure 22-3. CT scan of the abdomen without contrast showing calculus in proximal ureter.

In very rare instances, imaging cannot make a definitive diagnosis of urolithiasis. In a patient with all the clinical features of urolithiasis, but without an obvious stone, surgical intervention may be necessary to make the diagnosis. Endoscopy with direct visualisation may identify the rare stone that was missed on imaging.

MEDICAL AND SURGICAL MANAGEMENTS

The surgical management of urolithiasis will address more acute issues, but the medical management is critical to the prevention of future stones. When managing the acute stone crisis, several options exist. The first option to consider is observation. Stones < 3 mm in size will almost uniformly pass spontaneously, and of those < 5 mm in size, about 70% will pass. In addition, the more distal the stone at presentation, the more likely it is to pass. Almost 50% of proximal ureteral stones will pass versus 80% of stones at the UVJ. Just as in the adult population, a trial of expectant management is a consideration in the absence of severe pain with emesis, infection, immunocompromise, or underlying urologic abnormalities (such as renal insufficiency or a solitary kidney). The use of alpha-adrenergic blockers has been shown in adults to facilitate stone passage via the relaxation of smooth muscle within the ureteral wall distal to the stone. While this has not been proven in children, it seems empirically to be applicable. If a patient with an obstructing stone develops the signs of sepsis, then emergent intervention, either ureteral stenting or percutaneous nephrostomy tube placement, is necessary to relieve the obstruction.

In the paediatric population, due to the likelihood of stone growth with time and the high rate of an underlying metabolic or anatomic abnormality, active surgical intervention for known stones with a goal of rendering the patient stone-free is a commonly accepted approach. The same surgical options are available for children as for adults. When managing the non-emergent stone, the best surgical option is decided based on several factors, including stone size, type, location, and underlying anatomy. In the modern era of stone management, almost never is open stone surgery required for the upper tracts. Table 22-1 lists typical paediatric urology practice patterns, and which surgical techniques are applied to particular stone scenarios.

ESWL is an ideal form of treatment, as it is entirely non-invasive and well tolerated. The principle of ESWL involves a lithotripter where a shock wave is generated, either via electromagnetic or piezoelectric mechanisms, and the energy, then, focused at the stone, the location of which is referred to as the F2. Fluoroscopy or ultrasound is used to

Table 22-1. Treatment options as determined by stone location and size.

Stone location/size	ESWL	Ureteroscopy	PCNL
Renal			
< 1 cm	Most common	Optional	Optional
1–2 cm	Most common	Optional	Optional
>2 cm	Optional	Rare	Most common
Lower pole			
< 1 cm	Most common	Optional	Optional
> 1 cm	Optional	Optional	Most common
Ureteral			
Proximal	Most common	Optional	Occasional
Distal	Optional	Most common	Rare

visualise the stone and help direct the shock waves. The shock waves via a combination of shearing, cavitation, spalling, and other mechanical principles help to break the calculus into smaller fragments, which will, then, pass downstream in the urine. Children seem to tolerate ESWL extremely well and even have a higher stone fragment clearance rate than adults (95% versus 79% for stones over 10 mm in size). Ather and Noor (2003) reported a stone-free rate of 95% following ESWL in children under the age of 14 years, with 5% requiring adjuvant treatment, even in stones up to 30 mm in size. Situations for which ESWL may not be the primary answer include large lower pole stones, cystine and calcium oxalate monohydrate stones that are very hard, and lower ureteral stones, as there is a theoretical concern for damage to reproductive structures in the pelvis. When using ESWL in children, several precautions should be considered. The energy used should be a lower setting (17–20 kV) and the number of shocks should be limited (around 2000). There exists a risk for pulmonary contusion as the lung fields on excursion extend further caudally in children than in adults; therefore, an additional Styrofoam sheet or foam tape can be used to protect the lungs. There is a risk for perinephric haematoma, but this seems to be clinically significant in a very small minority of instances. It is fully expected that the child will experience transient gross haematuria post-operatively, as well as flank pain and some contusions. Some studies have expressed theoretical concern for long-term complications stemming from ESWL, such as hypertension, renal insufficiency, and hyperfiltration. Short-term studies, thus far, have dismissed these worries. At present, ESWL is considered first-line therapy for stones up to 20 mm in size within the kidney and proximal ureter.

Another surgical option is endoscopic management, which has become much more practical in children with advances in fibre optics and miniaturisation of instruments as small as 7 French in size. Such an approach requires access to a significant amount of specialised equipment, including a fluid warmer, a pressure irrigation system, an array of endoscopes, a large selection of wires, fluoroscopy, laser fibres and laser generator, stone baskets, and ureteral stents. Endoscopic access begins via the urethra into the bladder, where the ureteral orifice is cannulated. Fluoroscopic guidance aids in the retrograde passage of a wire first along the ureter and into the renal pelvis, to act as a safety and guidewire. The ureteroscope can, then, similarly be passed retrograde either alongside or over the wire up the ureter to the level of the stone. In small children with delicate ureters, it may be necessary to first leave an indwelling stent for one to two weeks to dilate passively the collecting system before a ureteroscope can be safely passed up the ureter in a subsequent operative setting. Semirigid ureteroscopes are best reserved for more distal ureteral stones below the iliac crest, but flexible ureteroscopes can pass safely into the renal pelvis and even deflect into lower pole calyces. Please refer to Figure 22-4 depicting a ureteroscope and Figure 22-5 showing the direct visualisation of a calculus within the ureter, as seen through a ureteroscope. Once the stone is seen, if it is very small in size, it can be grasped under direct vision using a basket that has been passed through the working channel of the ureteroscope, as seen in Figure 22-6. If the stone is too large to basket out safely, then lithotripsy *in situ* can be performed with the assistance of a laser. Flexible laser fibres as small as 200 microns can be passed within the working channel of paediatric flexible ureteroscopes.

The holmium:YAG laser is preferred by most, as it has a penetration of only 0.4 mm, rendering it very safe to use within the ureter. Laser lithotripsy breaks the calculus into smaller fragments that can then either pass in the urine or be retrieved with a basket. These fragments can then be sent for stone chemical analysis to later aid in stone prevention

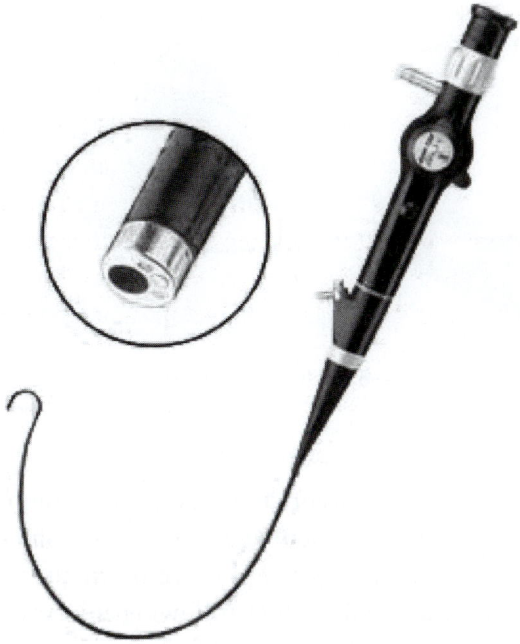

Figure 22-4. Flexible ureteroscope.

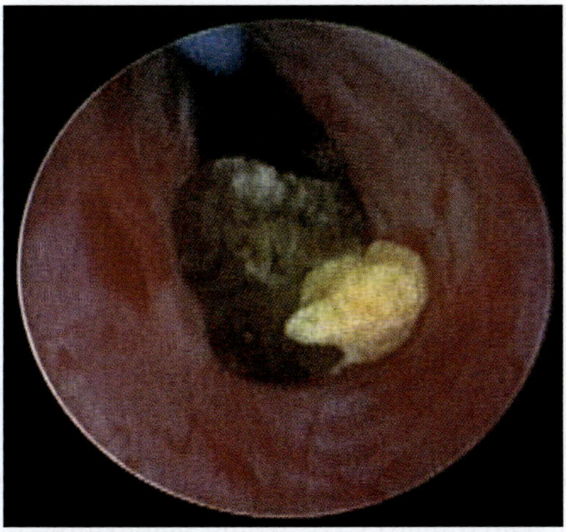

Figure 22-5. Endoscopic view of the ureter showing a guide wire (on top) and two ureteral calculi.

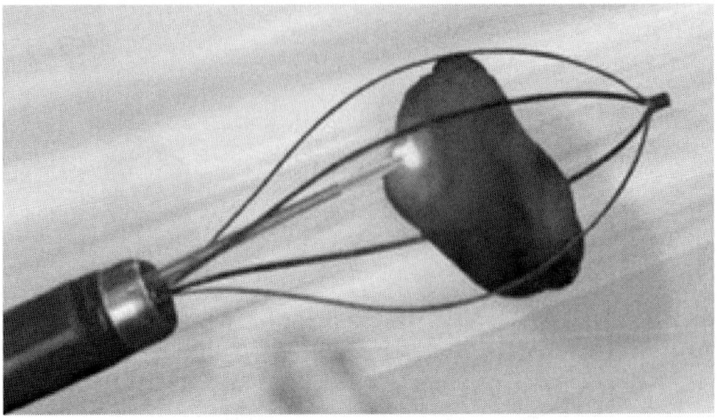

Figure 22-6. Ureteral basket with stone.

strategies. Once lithotripsy and/or stone removal is complete, many will choose to leave an indwelling double-J ureteral stent for a week or two post-operatively to facilitate drainage of urine in the face of ureteral oedema and to aid in ureteral healing following injury. The stent can be removed either endoscopically under a different anaesthetic or externally by pulling a string attached to the distal end of the stent, either by the patient/parent at home or by the physician in the office. This surgical option is very effective for ureteral calculi with 90% stone-free rates following a single procedure. There exists the concern for post-ureteroscopy ureteral stricture formation; however, with careful endoscope and laser manipulation under direct vision, this is a very remote risk. There exists also the theoretical concern for post-ureteroscopy vesicoureteral reflux, but this has not borne out to be clinically of significance. At present, ureteroscopy with or without laser lithotripsy is the treatment of choice for distal ureteral stones.

Percutaneous nephrolithotomy (PCNL), while more invasive, is a very effective form of surgical treatment, particularly for large renal stones in the lower pole or in the setting of anatomic abnormalities that impede fragment clearance (such as UPJ obstruction). This allows direct access to the stone burden while bypassing the delicate paediatric ureter. Originally, many feared that PCNL would damage the paediatric kidney, but, similar to the advent of smaller ureteroscopes, paediatric centres have developed smaller instrumentation to gain percutaneous access. The crucial step to successful PCNL lies in the initial percutaneous access. Some centres will perform this in interventional radiology a day or two before the actual nephrolithotomy, while others will perform this in the same operative setting as the nephrolithotomy in the operating room. Ideal access will give immediate and direct visualisation of the calculi. If the stone is limited to a specific calyx, then access directly into that calyx and onto that stone may be desired. If the stone burden lies in multiple calyces, then access through a posterior calyx will give the best access to many calyces while minimising the degree of torque that must be applied to the scope to deal with all the stones. The patient is laid supine on the operating table. Initial cystoscopy and catheterisation of the ipsilateral ureter may help facilitate percutaneous access, as air can be injected into the collecting system that will then rise to a posterior calyx when the patient is prone. Under fluoroscopic guidance, a finder needle is passed into the desired calyx, through which a wire can then be advanced into the renal pelvis and down the ureter. Then, this tract can be serially dilated, either using a balloon dilator or an Amplatz dilator set. With the smaller paediatric nephroscopes available, it is not necessary to extensively dilate the tract, thereby minimising the risk of bleeding. With a safety guidewire in place, the nephroscope can then be passed into the collecting system and under direct vision, the stone can be fragmented using either the holmium:YAG laser or the ultrasonic lithotripter, and the fragments then grasped and removed. The paediatric patient can easily become hypothermic; therefore, it is important to monitor body temperature, to cover the child appropriately with warming blankets, to drape using an impermeable adherent drape with a fluid-collection sac, to warm the irrigant, and to perform the surgery expeditiously.

After all visible fragments have been cleared, standard practice is to leave an indwelling percutaneous nephrostomy tube or nephroureteral stent for a few days, to help with haemostasis and passage of residual fragments, but with the aid of smaller tracts and fibrin sealants, some centres have begun practicing “tubeless PCNL”. PCNL can provide stone-free rates of 80–90% after a single procedure. Complications are rare and include haemorrhage requiring transfusion, perforation of the collecting system, and sepsis. These complications can be avoided with experience and sometimes with a staged approach between percutaneous access and lithotripsy, as in cases without hydronephrosis and those with known infection or large stone burden. There has been concern that PCNL could damage the paediatric kidney, but post-PCNL studies have shown stabilisation or improvement of GFR and no scarring on DMSA. Currently, PCNL is the treatment option of choice for renal stones over 2 cm, lower pole stones over 1 cm, renal stones in the setting of anatomic abnormalities such as UPJ obstruction, stones that failed management with ESWL or ureteroscopy, or very hard stones such as cystine.

As paediatric centres become more facile with laparoscopic surgery, some have applied it to stone disease. This typically has been the case for large stone burdens in the setting of a UPJ obstruction, where laparoscopic pyelolithotomy can be performed in the same surgical setting as laparoscopic pyeloplasty. The laparoscopic approach has also been used in the setting of failed percutaneous management without significant complications. This modality will likely evolve as a more widely viable option in the future.

The management of bladder stones can be particularly complicated in the paediatric population, due to the small size of the paediatric urethra and as they tend to occur in patients following complex reconstruction, such as bladder augmentation, bladder neck reconstruction, and creation of a continent and catheterisable stoma. Endoscopic access through the native urethra or catheterisable channel is often not practical, leaving percutaneous or open cystolithotomy as an alternative. It is possible to approach bladder stones percutaneously, going through a former suprapubic site, as this is likely the safest point of access. This point of access can then be dilated to allow the basketing and extraction of stones. For stones requiring lithotripsy, it is helpful first to basket the stone or to place it in a lap sac, so that stone fragments are not lost in the bladder, which may be quite capacious or redundant in the setting of prior reconstruction. For particularly large bladder stones, it may be most efficient to remove them in their entirety via an open approach. Following either percutaneous or open bladder surgery for stones, a Foley should be left indwelling for a short period to aid in the healing of the cystotomy and avoid ongoing urine extravasation or the development of a vesicocutaneous fistula. The greatest risk of such surgery is leaving behind the fragments that lead to future stone formation. Additional risks, particularly in the setting of prior reconstruction, especially augmentation, include bladder perforation necessitating laparotomy and repair, and injury to other intra-abdominal organs (especially bowel); however, this is very rare. Counselling patients on preventive measures, especially regular catheterisation and bladder irrigation in the case of neurogenic and augmented bladders, is essential in avoiding the need for multiple surgeries for recurrent bladder stones.

The medical management of stones that are already present within the urinary tract is limited to dissolution therapy, which is only effective for certain stone types. Otherwise, medical management is of paramount importance in the prevention of the development and recurrence of the stones. The dissolution of stones depends upon altering the acid–base balance of the urine. Uric acid stones will dissolve in urine with a pH of ≥ 6.5. Cystine stones will dissolve in urine with a pH of ≥ 7.5. The urine can be alkalinised with the agents such as potassium citrate. Struvite stones can be dissolved by acidifying the urine using either Suby's G solution or Renacidin. This is done via a percutaneous nephrostomy tube, but one must ensure that there is no extravasation or infection prior to initiating the instillation. The irrigation should be done under low pressure (< 25 cm of water) with a rate not to exceed 120 mL/hour. The acidifying solutions (Suby's G and Renacidin) contain a large concentration of magnesium; therefore, magnesium levels should be monitored during dissolution therapy and the irrigation is stopped if magnesium levels are too high or the patient exhibits the signs of toxicity, such as drowsiness, confusion, coma, paralysis, nausea/vomiting, hypotension, and prolonged QT interval. In addition to stopping the irrigation, the patient should be hydrated and given furosemide, and, if symptomatic, calcium gluconate. In severe cases, haemodialysis may be required.

Seventy-five percent of children with nephrolithiasis have a fundamental predisposition to stone formation and 50% are related to metabolic disorders. Successful medical management is contingent upon the identification of stone type and underlying metabolic abnormalities within the individual patient. Any stone fragments obtained at the time of surgical intervention or later by the patient at home when passing, the fragments should be collected and sent for chemical analysis, as there are a multitude of stone types, each of which may be most responsive to tailored medical and surgical therapies. In addition to stone analysis, metabolic

Table 22-2. Complete metabolic work-up for stone disease.

Stone analysis

Blood work

- CBC (complete blood count)
- BMP (basic metabolic panel)
  - Electrolytes
  - BUN/creatinine
- Calcium
- Phosphorus
- Magnesium
- Alkaline phosphatase
- Uric acid
- Intact parathyroid hormone (iPTH)

Urine studies

- Urinalysis with pH
- Urine for microscopy
- Urine culture
- 24-hour urine collection
  - Volume
  - Creatinine
  - Calcium
  - Phosphorus
  - Magnesium
  - Oxalate
  - Sodium
  - Uric acid
  - Citrate
  - Cystine

evaluation consists of a combination of blood and urine studies. Please refer to Table 22-2 listing the components of a complete metabolic work-up. The pH of urine is important to know, as certain types of stone will only form in the presence of a particular acid–base balance. Urine microscopy can reveal the presence of crystals that may provide a clue as to stone type (Figure 22-7). Hexagonal crystals are synonymous with cystinuria. Rhomboids are associated with uric acid, coffin lids with magnesium ammonium phosphate (struvite), envelopes or octahedrals with calcium oxalate dihydrate, dumbbells with calcium oxalate monohydrate, and

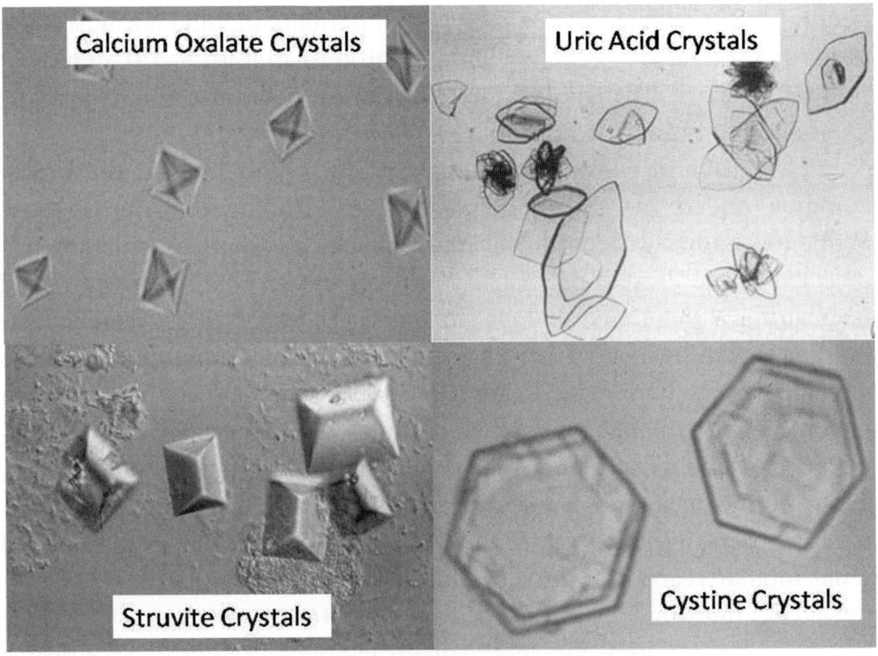

Figure 22-7. Common urinary crystal seen on centrifuged urine sediment.

needles with calcium phosphate. Urine culture is significant to determine the presence of bacteria, which may be a source for the stone but which may also lead to sepsis at the time of intervention, and should be treated appropriately. A 24-hour urine collection should be obtained while the patient is conforming to his/her standard diet and fluid consumption. Ideally, it is collected several weeks following surgical intervention and clearance of the stone.

First-line medical therapy in all patients is to increase fluid consumption. With increased fluid intake, the urine will be less saturated with solutes, and, with a greater volume of urine passing through the urinary tract, there should be less stasis. In adolescents, the goal is to drink two litres of fluid a day. Younger children should be instructed to drink enough fluid that their urine is almost colourless. It is often difficult for patients to comply long-term with such instructions, but efforts should be made, and, as such, children may need notes for school allowing them to carry water bottles throughout the school day. Other general dietary recommendations for all patients include a low sodium diet (2–3 grams/day), a low animal protein diet (0.8–1.0 grams of protein/kg/day), low oxalate diet, moderate calcium intake, and the avoidance of high doses of vitamins C and D.

Hypercalciuria (urinary calcium excretion > 4 mg/kg/day) is the most common underlying metabolic abnormality leading to stone disease. While it is known to occur in 4% of the general paediatric population, it is detected in one-third of paediatric stone formers. In children with isolated haematuria without any obvious stone disease, underlying hypercalciuria is often discovered and as much as 20% of these children will go on to develop stones within five years if no preventive steps are taken. Often patients with hypercalciuria without stones will experience urinary frequency dysuria syndrome. Hypercalciuria can be categorised as being either normocalcaemic or hypercalcaemic. Normocalcaemic hypercalciuria can be classified as either idiopathic renal leak (due to the impaired renal tubular reabsorption of calcium) or absorptive renal leak (due to the excess intestinal absorption of calcium). Renal leak should be treated with thiazide diuretics, but such patients should be monitored for resultant hypokalaemia and may need potassium supplementation. Absorptive hypercalciuria can be treated with thiazide diuretics, but the benefits will not be sustained beyond six months. The thiazides can be discontinued for six months, during which time the patient takes cellulose sodium phosphate to bind the calcium in the gut, and the thiazides then resumed for another six months. Additionally, orthophosphate can be taken to inhibit 1, 25-OH vitamin D synthesis, thereby reducing calcium absorption in the gut. Both cellulose sodium phosphate and orthophosphate can cause gastrointestinal distress with diarrhoea, and both are contraindicated in renal insufficiency due to their high phosphate content. Hypercalcaemic hypercalciuria is also known as resorptive hypercalciuria, in which there is increased calcium resorption from the bone. This can occur following prolonged immobilisation, particularly after a bone fracture, or can occur in the setting of primary hyperparathyroidism, which requires parathyroidectomy for successful treatment. Other less common causes of hypercalciuria include vitamin D toxicity, sarcoidosis, distal renal tubular acidosis, enteral formulas high in calcium, milk alkali syndrome, osteolytic metastases, and loop diuretics, particularly in premature infants.

Hyperoxaluria can be found in 20% of paediatric stone formers. Oxalate is excreted primarily in the urine and comes from both exogenous sources in the diet, as well as endogenous sources from liver production, as a byproduct in the metabolism of ascorbic acid (vitamin C) and certain amino acids. Underlying abnormalities leading to hyperoxaluria are classified as either enteric hyperoxaluria or primary hyperoxaluria. Enteric hyperoxaluria is due to the excessive absorption of oxalate in the gut. This occurs in the setting of malabsorptive states, such as Crohn's disease, ileal resection, and jejuno-ileal bypass. In these cases, the malabsorbed fatty acids bind the intra-luminal calcium, leaving the oxalate available for absorption. Additionally, the increased concentration of bile salts in the intestinal lumen damages the intestinal epithelium, which is leading to further oxalate absorption. Moreover, the chronic diarrhoea these patients experience can cause a metabolic acidosis, leading to a reduction in urinary citrate levels, and dehydration, leading to a reduction in urine volume, further increasing their risk for stone disease. This cause of hyperoxaluria can be treated by addressing the underlying disorder, in the case of inflammatory bowel disease, and with oral calcium supplementation to bind the oxalate and oral cholestyramine to bind the bile salts. These patients should also consume a low-fat and low-oxalate diet and maintain good hydration. Primary hyperoxaluria is a rare autosomal recessive disorder associated with a defect in the liver enzyme alanine:glyoxylate aminotransferase, which leading to an increased production of oxalate, which is then deposited in the kidneys (nephrocalcinosis) and other soft tissues. Individuals with this disorder will often experience renal failure at a young age. The diagnosis is confirmed with a liver biopsy. Successful treatment requires hydration, pyridoxine supplementation, and a low-oxalate diet, but definitive treatment requires liver transplantation and often concomitant renal transplantation.

Hyperuricosuria is found in 8% of children with stones. Uric acid results from purine metabolism. When excreted in acidic urine with a pH of < 5.8, it will precipitate out as urate crystals. These children will form not only uric acid stones, but also calcium oxalate stones due to epitaxis and heterogeneous nucleation. Idiopathic hyperuricosuria is familial and inherited in an autosomal dominant fashion. Hyperuricosuria can also be due to the overproduction of uric acid, as seen in inborn errors of purine metabolism, such as Lesch–Nyhan syndrome and type I glycogen storage disease, and also seen in myeloproliferative disorders and the other causes of rapid cell breakdown and turnover. Additionally, children with epilepsy treated with a ketogenic diet are prone to uric acid stones due to very acidic urine. Treatment fundamentals include hydration and urine alkalinisation to a pH of > 6.5 with potassium citrate or sodium bicarbonate. When such treatment measures fail or when high cell breakdown or turnover is expected, as in cases of myeloproliferative disorders, the xanthine oxidase inhibitor allopurinol may assist in the treatment.

Cystinuria accounts for 2% of paediatric urolithiasis. It is an autosomal recessive condition in which renal tubules fail to absorb the amino acids cystine, ornithine, lysine, and arginine, but only cystine has poor solubility in the urine. Homozygotes are likely to begin forming stones in childhood and form recurrent stones throughout their lifetime. Heterozygotes are also capable of forming stones. Cystine stones are extremely hard and resistant to ESWL; therefore, treatment is aimed at prevention. Hydration with a goal of urine volume production of 50 mL/kg/day is key. The patient's diet should be low in sodium and methionine, which are found in meats, milk, eggs, and wheat, as they are a precursor to cystine. Urine alkalinisation to a pH of > 7.5 with potassium citrate will keep the cystine soluble. If these measures fail, then patients can be given the chelating agents D-penicillamine and alpha-mercaptopropionyl glycine (Thiola), which function to cleave cystine and make it more soluble. These drugs are commonly associated with severe side effects, including fever, rash, pancytopenia, nephrosis, and epidermolysis, and patients taking them should be monitored closely.

Hypocitraturia can be associated with stone disease, as citrate is a known inhibitor of stone formation. It can occur in isolation or in association with other abnormalities, such as hypercalciuria, hyperoxaluria, and hyperuricosuria. Hypocitraturia can be found in conjunction with chronic metabolic acidosis, distal renal tubular acidosis, chronic diarrhoea, and hypokalaemia. Potassium citrate can be taken to increase the citrate level in urine. Hypocitraturia often is associated with hypomagnesuria. Magnesium helps to inhibit stone formation as well by increasing the solubility of calcium. The levels of magnesium in the urine can be increased by taking supplementary magnesium.

Struvite stones contain magnesium ammonium phosphate and calcium phosphate apatite and are found in the setting of chronic infection. Certain bacteria, such as *Proteus*, *Klebsiella*, *Pseudomonas*, *Serratia*, *Streptococcus*, *Staphylococcus*, *Candida*, and *Mycoplasma*, produce urease, which leads to an alkaline urine pH, which promotes the formation of struvite stones. Over half of the children with struvite stones have a genitourinary anomaly, predisposing them to recurrent UTIs. These stones rapidly propagate and often form staghorn calculi. Treatment should be aimed at correcting any underlying genitourinary anomaly and removing all stone fragments present in order to eradicate the source of infection, as just antibiotics alone will not clear the infection. Patients with augmented bladders are at particular risk for struvite stones and require regular catheterisation and irrigation, and sometimes prophylactic antibiotics. Even non-augmented patients may require long-term preventive antibiotics, sometimes in conjunction with urease inhibitors, such as acetohydroxaminic acid (AHA) and hydroxyurea, but urease inhibitors can have gastrointestinal and neurologic side effects. In addition, in select patients, stones can be dissolved using haemosiderin irrigation.

The successful management of existing stones and the prevention of future stones depends upon thorough surgical intervention as performed by the paediatric urologists, in conjunction with a complete metabolic evaluation and appropriate medical treatment as determined in conjunction with a paediatric nephrologist.

PROGNOSIS AND LONG-TERM COMPLICATIONS

Similar to the adult stone-forming population, paediatric patients with a history of urolithiasis are at risk of recurrence. Unlike the adult population, children with stones are at even greater risk owing to the prevalence of predisposing metabolic abnormalities. One-third to one-half of paediatric stone patients with a metabolic cause will form another stone, making them five times more likely to form recurrent stones than the patients without a metabolic abnormality. This predisposition emphasises the need for a complete metabolic evaluation in children.

Long-term complications are related not only to the disease process of urolithiasis itself but also to the potential for side effects from medical and surgical treatments. As noted previously, certain conditions such as primary hyperoxaluria are known to be associated not only with stone disease but with renal failure. In addition, as mentioned above, the medical treatment can have serious side effects, such as D-penicillamine and Thiola potentially leading to myelosuppression and epidermolysis. Furthermore, the surgical intervention for stones can have theoretical implications on future renal function, such as the concern for renal scarring and hypertension following ESWL. While short-term studies have not demonstrated significant deleterious effects of surgical intervention for stones, long-term studies are necessary to more thoroughly eliminate these concerns. Given the immediate and lifelong serious implications of stone disease on a child, it is important that such patients be cared for by surgical and medical stone specialists.

CURRENT CONTROVERSIES

In general, there is little controversy regarding paediatric urolithiasis. It seems to be a disease that most would agree the needs of active treatment and prevention. While some surgeons may prefer one approach over another, all forms seem to be relatively effective in children with minimal morbidity. As mentioned previously, there still exist concerns as to the long-term ill effects of some forms of surgical intervention, and this will require long-term prospective studies to fully assuage these apprehensions. Other areas in need of investigation include epidemiologic studies to determine the explanation for the universal rise in urolithiasis. Given this escalating trajectory of disease incidence, medical practitioners increasingly will need to familiarise themselves with the diagnosis and management of urolithiasis.

COMMENT FROM THE EDITORS

This excellent review highlights the state of the art in the management of urolithiasis in children. Paediatric urolithiasis was rare in the Western world for most of the 20th century but its incidence is rapidly increasing. The incidence has always been higher in developing countries. The challenge in paediatrics is to adapt the techniques developed by adult urologist to the smaller urinary tract of infants and children. This chapter should provide an excellent guide to manage this challenging problem.

FURTHER READING

Ather MH, Noor MA. Does size and site matter for renal stones up to 30-mm in size in children treated by extracorporeal lithotripsy? *Urology* 2003; **61**:212–215; discussion 5.

Coll DM, Varanelli MJ, Smith RC. Relationship of spontaneous passage of ureteral calculi to stone size and location as revealed by unenhanced helical CT. *AJR Am J Roentgenol* 2002; **178**:101–103.

Dawaba MS, Shokeir AA, Hafez AT, *et al.* Percutaneous nephrolithotomy in children: early and late anatomical and functional results. *J Urol* 2004; **172**:1078–1081.

Durkee CT, Balcom A. Surgical management of urolithiasis. *Pediatr Clin North Am* 2006; **53**:465–477, vii.

Fowler KA, Locken JA, Duchesne JH, Williamson MR. US for detecting renal calculi with nonenhanced CT as a reference standard. *Radiology* 2002; **222**:109–113.

Gofrit ON, Pode D, Meretyk S, *et al.* Is the pediatric ureter as efficient as the adult ureter in transporting fragments following extracorporeal shock wave lithotripsy for renal calculi larger than 10 mm? *J Urol* 2001; **166**:1862–1864.

Jackman SV, Docimo SG, Cadeddu JA, Bishoff JT, Kavoussi LR, Jarrett TW. The "mini-perc" technique: a less invasive alternative to percutaneous nephrolithotomy. *World J Urol* 1998; **16**:371–374.

Kurzrock EA, Huffman JL, Hardy BE, Fugelso P. Endoscopic treatment of pediatric urolithiasis. *J Pediatr Surg* 1996; **31**:1413–1416.

Lattimer JK, Hubbard M. Pediatric urologic admissions. *J Urol* 1951; **66**:289–293.

Milliner DS, Murphy ME. Urolithiasis in pediatric patients. *Mayo Clin Proc* 1993; **68**:241–248.

Patlas M, Farkas A, Fisher D, Zaghal I, Hadas-Halpern I. Ultrasound vs. CT for the detection of ureteric stones in patients with renal colic. *Br J Radiol* 2001; **74**:901–904.

Pietrow PK, Pope JC 4th, Adams MC, Shyr Y, Brock JW 3rd. Clinical outcome of pediatric stone disease. *J Urol* 2002; **167**:670–673.

Sheafor DH, Hertzberg BS, Freed KS, *et al.* Nonenhanced helical CT and US in the emergency evaluation of patients with renal colic: prospective comparison. *Radiology* 2000; **217**:792–797.

Stapleton FB. Idiopathic hypercalciuria: association with isolated hematuria and risk for urolithiasis in children. The Southwest Pediatric Nephrology Study Group, University of Texas, Southwestern Medical Center, Dallas, 1990.

Stapleton FB. Childhood stones. *Endocrinol Metab Clin North Am* 2002; **31**:1001–1015, ix.

Stapleton FB. Nephrolithiasis in children. *Pediatr Rev* 1989; **11**:21–30.

Yilmaz S, Sindel T, Arslan G, *et al.* Renal colic: comparison of spiral CT, US and IVU in the detection of ureteral calculi. *Eur Radiol* 1998; **8**:212–217.

Chapter 23

Bladder Exstrophy

Rita Gobet

DEFINITION

Bladder exstrophy (BE) (Figure 23-1) belongs to the category of lower abdominal midline malformations. This category includes a wide range of malformations, from the mildest form being a minor glanular epispadias (Figure 23-2) to the severest form cloacal exstrophy (Figure 23-3) often also referred to as OEIS (omphalocele, exstrophy, imperforate anus, and spinal defects) complex. The prevalence ranges from 1:30,000 (BE) to 1:100,000 (epispadias) to 1:200,000–400,000 (cloacal exstrophy). Note the unusual fact that the severer form of the malformation BE is commoner than the milder form epispadias. The male-to-female ratio ranges from 2:1 to 4:1.

The characteristic defects of BE include the urinary system (bladder, urethra, and ureterovesical junction), the musculoskeletal system (pelvis, pelvic floor, and abdominal wall), the genitalia, and rarely the spine and the anus. The bladder is not formed into the normal hollow organ but is part of the abdominal wall as a plate. Additionally, the urethra is not developed into the normal tubular structure, but again lies as the so-called urethral plate dorsally of the malformed corpora cavernosa. In females, the mons pubis, the labia, and the clitoris are split in the midline and the vagina lies horizontally but is otherwise normal. The pelvic ring is ventrally wide open; all patients have a significant

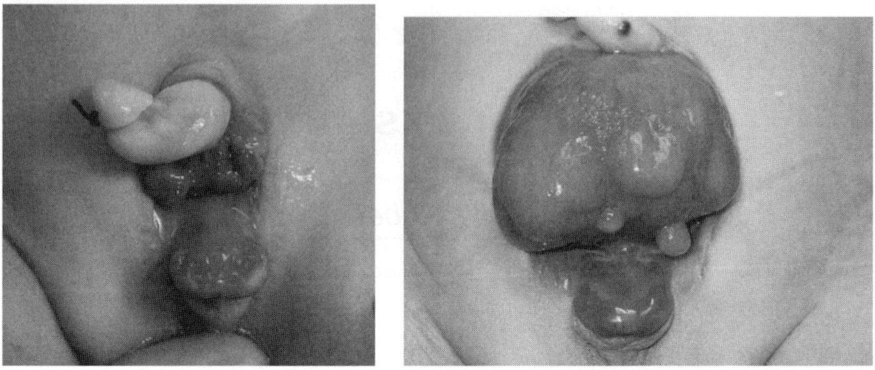

Figure 23-1. Classical BE in males. On the left, a newborn with a small bladder plate and on the right, one with a large bladder plate.

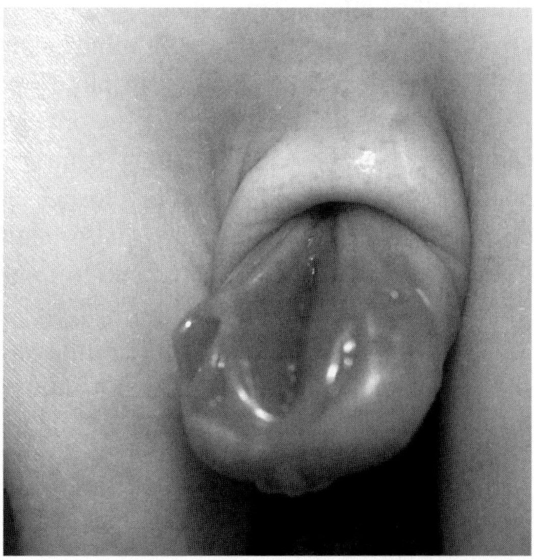

Figure 23-2. Male penile epispadias.

symphyseal diastasis (Figure 23-4) and therefore also an abnormally developed pelvic floor. Specifically, the urinary muscular continence mechanism is maldeveloped. External genitalia in both female and male patients are abnormal.

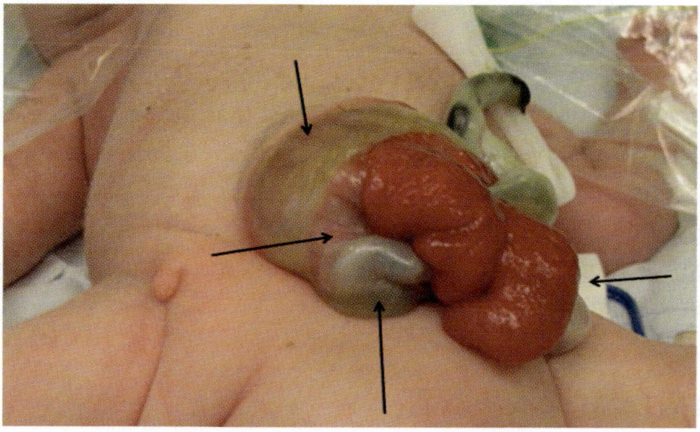

Figure 23-3. Cloacal exstrophy. The upper arrow points at the omphalocele, the right arrow to the intestinal herniation, the one on the left to the right hemibladder, and the one below to the umbilical cord.

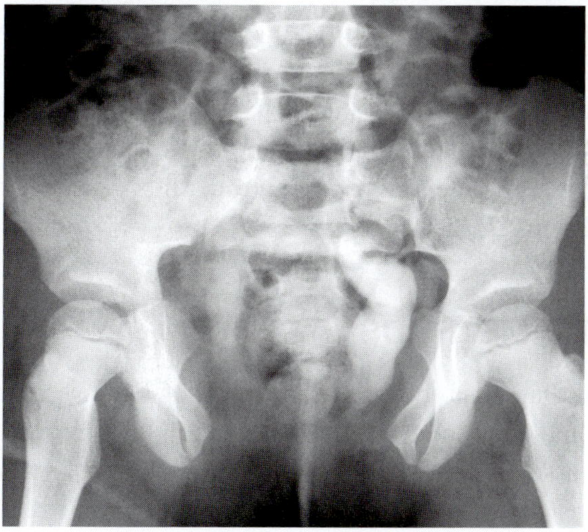

Figure 23-4. Plain roentgenogram of the abdomen showing pubic diastasis usually associated with bladder and cloacal exstrophy and proximal epispadias.

AETIOLOGY

The aetiology and embryology of this malformation are not completely understood. The most popular theory states that the reinforcement of the cloacal membrane by lateral mesenchymal ingrowth is somehow prevented. This mesenchyme usually gives rise to pelvic bones and abdominal muscle. The premature rupture of the "thinned" cloacal membrane exposes the bladder wall and prevents the normal development of the lower abdomen.

PRESENTATION

Usually BE is diagnosed at birth. Prenatal diagnosis is possible, but due to the rarity of the malformation and its subtle ultrasound findings, it is quite difficult to make. Prenatal ultrasound reveals the absence of a full bladder, small external genitalia, and a low set umbilicus. Prenatal diagnosis is the prerequisite for adequate prenatal counselling. The birth of an undiagnosed child with BE seems to be specially traumatic not only to the parents but also to the unacquainted medical team. Some countries allow the termination of pregnancy in the case of the prenatal diagnosis of BE, but there are no data in all available outcome studies to support this form of management.

Female patients with epispadias sometimes present with incontinence, since without careful genital examination, this malformation might be overlooked (Figure 23-5).

DIAGNOSTIC METHODS

BE is a visual diagnosis. In the classic form of BE, associated malformations are rare and BE occurs in otherwise healthy newborns. An abdominal ultrasound to assess upper urinary tracts at birth is usually normal.

MEDICAL AND SURGICAL MANAGEMENT

After birth, the exposed mucosa of the bladder plate should be protected; this is achieved most effectively by a soft plastic coverage (i.e. Saran wrap). The child should be transferred, as soon as possible, into a centre

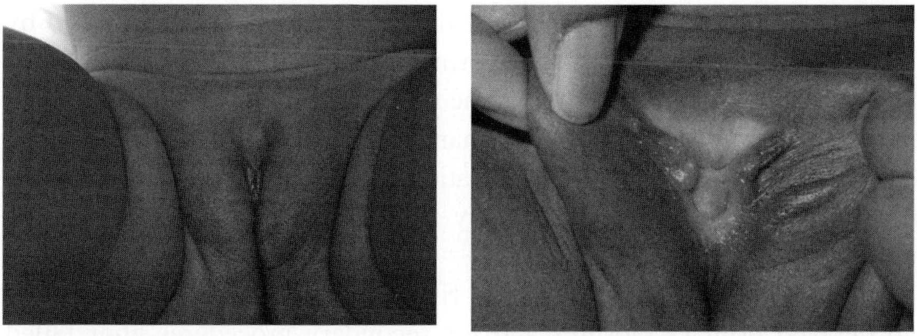

Figure 23-5. Female epispadias. On the left, apparently normal external genitalia. On the right, typical appearance after spreading the labia majora showing the bifid clitoris, the gaping urethra, and the anteriorly positioned vaginal introitus.

acquainted with the management of this malformation. The optimal time point for the surgical treatment of BE is within the first 48–72 hours of life. The usually healthy baby had time to adapt well to postnatal life, the pelvic bones are still malleable, and the bladder plate remains pink and healthy looking. The surgical procedure and postoperative management should be performed by an experienced team, since favourable long-term outcome parameters such as urinary continence and good quality of life are directly related to the outcome of primary bladder reconstruction.

Modern surgical strategies include staged reconstructions, complete primary repair, or primary urinary diversion.

The strategy of staged reconstruction begins with the bladder and abdominal wall closure; the approximation of symphysis without formal osteotomy within the first 72 hours of life. This is feasible for most patients since most patients are born with a reasonably sized bladder plate, allowing folding in easily. At this point, it is important to free the bladder plate and bladder neck extensively to allow the placement of bladder deep into the pelvis. This operation leaves the patient with an epispadiac penis, which will be repaired between the ages of six and 12 months.

Epispadias repair achieves the tubularisation of the urethral plate and the correct placement of the neourethra from its dorsal to a ventral position underneath the corpora cavernosa. In addition, the always substantial dorsal curvature (dorsal chordee) of the epispadiac penis is corrected by rotating the corpora cavernosa. In primary, complete repair of both steps are performed at the same time in the newborn patient.

Delayed primary closure or primary urinary diversion (ureterosigmoidostomy) is possible solutions for patients with a small and rigid bladder plate judged inadequate for primary repair or the occasional very sick patient.

Osteotomies to close the pelvic ring are generally recommended for all delayed primary closures and for secondary procedures after failed primary repairs by many authors at convenient times to improve prerequisites for urinary continence and improved cosmesis.

Almost all male patients and many female patients after staged reconstructions need further surgery to achieve continence, since the normal continence mechanism is defective. Increasing bladder outlet resistance without compromising normal voiding is the goal of these procedures. Many patients need, in addition to bladder neck-tightening procedures, to increase bladder capacity (enterocystoplasty). This is incompatible with normal voiding in most cases and requires bladder emptying by clean intermittent catheterisation. Complete primary reconstruction in the newborn period is hoped to diminish the need for these procedures by allowing a more normal bladder development from early on. If the yields of this concept are improved, enduring results remains to be seen.

Even more complex is the reconstruction of patients who are born with cloacal exstrophy. Associated malformation such as omphalocele, myelomeningocele, and short bowel syndrome have to be taken into consideration in almost all patients for immediate medical management. In medically stable patients, the separation of the intestinal tract from the two hemibladders is the first step of the highly individualised reconstruction plan. Most importantly, the hindgut remnants should be preserved and used for reconstruction.

Epispadias is most commonly associated with incontinence in both female and male patients. Therefore, the goals of surgical treatment are the same as in the BE to achieve urinary continence and to reconstruct functionally and cosmetically adequate external genitalia. In more distal forms (penile and glandular epispadias), the continence mechanism might be intact.

PROGNOSIS AND LONG-TERM COMPLICATIONS

Self-reported quality of life, generally speaking, is good. Good familial and professional psychosocial support allows most patients to lead a satisfying life, despite the repeated demanding surgical and medical procedures impressed on patients and their families by this severe malformation.

Renal function at birth is normal in most patients, and the primary objective of surgical and medical managements is to prevent renal damage. Incomplete bladder emptying, iatrogenic obstructive uropathies, and UTI should be avoided, since all ureterovesical junctions in BE are abnormal and allow VUR.

The rates of urinary continence with normal voiding vary significantly among surgeons, reconstruction or diversion type, and treatment centres (50–60%). Augmentation is reported to be necessary in between 0 and 80% of patients after primary staged repair.

Sexual functions in males are reported impaired mainly because of the residual uncorrected dorsal curvature of the penis. This interferes mechanically with vaginal intercourse. Erection is usually normal, although the penis is shorter and wider as normal. Ejaculation is very often retrograde or missing. Fertility in male patients is abnormal presumably due to several problems, including repeated epidydimitis and abnormal sperm maturation. In female patients, fertility is normal. The bifid clitoris can be surgically joined, but this seems not to be important for orgasmic capacity. Vaginal introital stenosis needs to be addressed in many patients to allow satisfactory vaginal intercourse. Uterine and vaginal prolapses are a major problem in many patients, presumably due to the weakened pelvic floor and the horizontally running vagina. Many female patients have Müllerian abnormalities such as partial or complete duplications.

CURRENT CONTROVERSIES

Despite impressively refined surgical and medical skills, BE remains a major challenge both for the medical team and for the patient and his or her family. Even the most experienced surgical team has to work hard to meet the expectations. A well-functioning bladder enduring a whole life, normal looking, and normal functioning of external and internal genitalia are not the average result achieved by current methods. Early urinary continence might be achieved on the costs of impaired fertility, upper urinary tract impairment, and/or bladder dysfunction during young adulthood. Whether complete primary reconstruction yields better results has to be seen.

COMMENT FROM THE EDITORS

BE and epispadias, though infrequent, possess a formidable challenge to the best of surgeons. To improve care, the centres of excellence need to be developed throughout the world where these children receive their treatment since birth. Often a poorly performed initial closure will doom all future attempts to failure. Inexperienced surgeons should work closely with experienced colleagues to avoid mistakes for which the child will pay for the rest of his/her life. This chapter makes the point clear.

FURTHER READING

Gargollo PC, Borer JG. Contemporary outcomes in bladder exstrophy. *Curr Opin Urol* 2007; **17**(4):272–280 (Review).

Gargollo PC, Borer JG, Diamond DA, *et al.* Prospective follow-up in patients after complete primary repair of bladder exstrophy. *J Urol* 2008; **180**(4 Suppl):1665–1670.

Shnorhavorian M, Grady RW, Andersen A, *et al.* Long-term follow-up of complete primary repair of exstrophy: the Seattle experience. *J Urol* 2008; **180**(4 Suppl):1615–1619.

Woodhouse CR, North AC, Gearhart JP. Standing the test of time: long-term outcome of reconstruction of the exstrophy bladder. *World J Urol* 2006; **4**(3):244–249.

Chapter 24

Urethral Obstruction Sequence or Prune Belly Syndrome

Ricardo González

DEFINITION

The Eagle-Barrett syndrome, triad syndrome, or prune belly syndrome (PBS) are equivalent terms used to describe the association of poorly developed abdominal wall musculature, urinary tract dilatation, and undescended testes. The bladder is usually much distended at birth; after decompression, the abdominal wall acquires a wrinkled appearance that led Osler to coin the term "prune belly syndrome". There are often associated anomalies that may include Potter's facies, club feet and other lower limb anomalies, dimples in the knees, and the other signs of oligohydramnios. Internally, there is a common mesentery for the small bowel and the colon with the lack of attachment of the colon to the posterior parietal peritoneum (universal mesentery); the spleen may not be attached to the abdominal wall (wandering spleen). In addition to hydronephrosis, the kidneys exhibit a certain degree of parenchymal dysplasia and the lungs may be hypoplastic due to the oligohydramnios and the elevation of the diaphragm caused by the distended urinary tract or ascites. The lower chest wall is flared (Figure 24-1).

PATHOGENESIS

In the past, it has been theorized that a defect in the migration of the mesenchyma was responsible for the hypoplastic or absent anterior abdominal

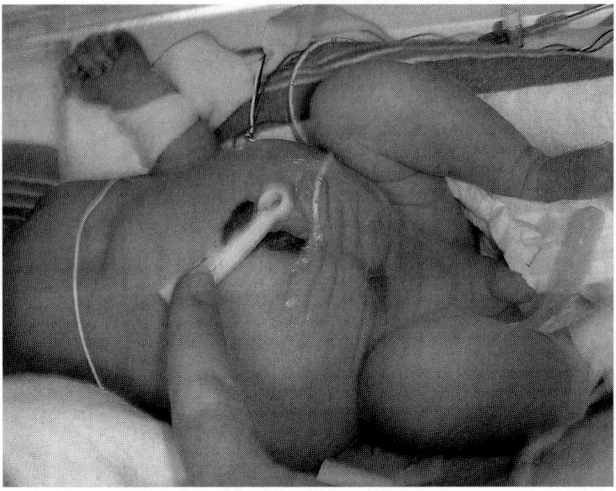

Figure 24-1. Classic appearance of a newborn with PBS. In this case, there was urethral atresia and the urachus was patent. There is a small polyethylene catheter in the urachus to drain the bladder. This child was treated successfully by progressive antegrade urethral dilatation.

musculature and the dilatation of the upper tracts. However, the autopsy studies by Pagon *et al.* (1979), the experimental studies in fetal sheep by González *et al.* (1990), and other observations in prenatal ultrasonography clearly demonstrated that significant and early urethral obstruction with a massively distended bladder can explain all the features of the syndrome. The abdominal wall muscles undergo atrophy due to ischemia; the distended bladder blocks testicular descent and can obstruct the iliac arteries resulting in the occasionally observed lower limb necrosis. The urinary ascites commonly seen in high-grade obstruction prevents coalescence of the colon to the posterior peritoneum, thus the universal mesentery. The remaining features of the syndrome can be attributed to oligo- or anhydramnios. Of course, high-grade and early fetal urethral obstructions explain the renal dysplasia, vesicoureteral reflux, and the massive dilatation of the ureters as well as the bladder wall changes.

Detractors of this hypothesis point out that urethral obstruction is rare in children with PBS. On the other hand, high-grade urethral obstruction is incompatible with extrauterine life because of lung hypoplasia. Only fetuses in whom the obstruction resolves spontaneously through the growth of a hypoplastic prostatic urethra, the rupture of the transverse urethral membrane, the spontaneous development of a vesicoamniotic fistula, or through a patent urachus survive the newborn period and are seen in clinical practice.

The urethra invariably shows dilatation, most commonly in the prostatic region but occasionally also extending distally. Fusiform megalourethra is commonly associated with PBS. Urethral atresia is also rarely seen. Only children who developed a fistula between the bladder and the amniotic cavity or have undergone successful prenatal decompression by vesicoamniotic shunting or repeated vesicocentesis will survive this condition.

Although predominantly seen in males, the association of obstructive lower urogenital anomalies with upper tract changes and atrophic abdominal wall muscle has been described in females as well. The abdominal features of PBS have been described in females with large congenital ovarian masses.

PRESENTATION

The diagnosis is often suspected on prenatal ultrasonography (see Chapter 1) (Figures 24-2A and 24-2B) or established at birth during the newborn examination (Figure 24-1). The most important thing after birth is the assessment of respiratory function and providing the necessary assistance if needed.

DIAGNOSTIC STUDIES

The determinations of the level of serial serum creatinine starting on the third day of life are needed to assess glomerular filtration. Abdominal ultrasonography allows assessment of the urinary tracts and kidneys. Eventually, a renal scan is needed to determine individual renal function.

A voiding cystourethrogram is needed to assess the bladder, urethra, and the presence of vesicoureteral reflux (Figures 24-3 and 24-4).

The evaluation of all other organ systems and karyotype are recommended since associated anomalies are common.

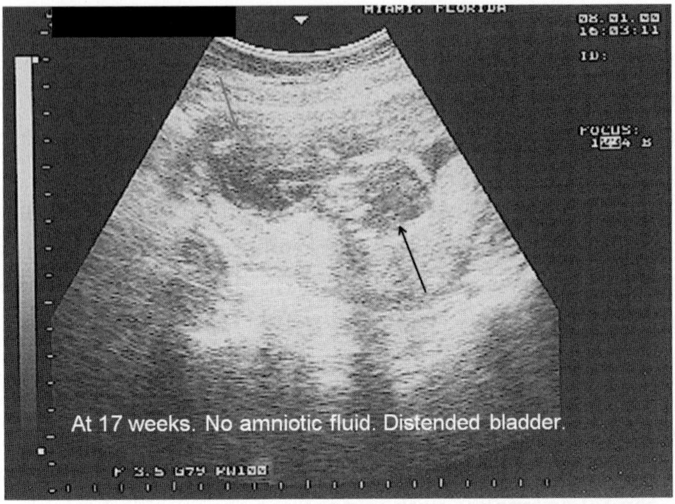

(A)

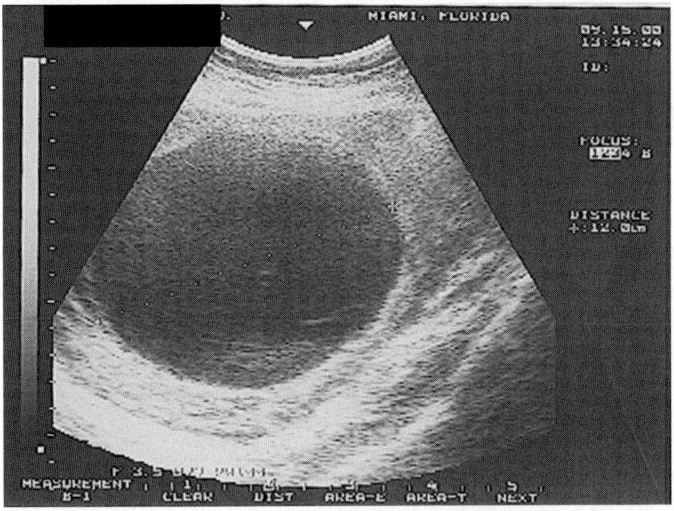

(B)

Figure 24-2. (**A**) Prenatal ultrasound at 17 weeks showing a much distended bladder (left arrow). The right arrow points to the head. Notice the absence of amniotic fluid. (**B**) At 19 weeks, the bladder measures 12 cm in diameter. The following week, a patent urachus developed, the amniotic fluid volume became normal, and the bladder distention resolved. At 10 years of age, this child has a solitary functioning kidney with normal function.

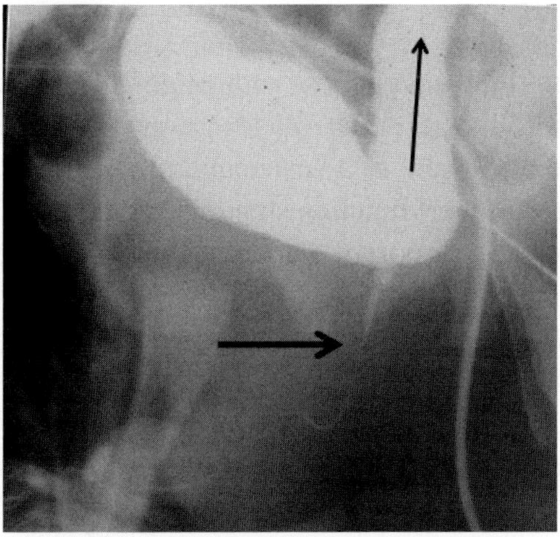

Figure 24-3. Simultaneous retrograde and antegrade contrast study done though the urachal fistula and the urethral meatus showing a transverse obstructing membrane at the level of the distal prostatic urethra, marked anterior urethra hypoplasia (thick arrow). There is massive right vesicoureteral reflux (upward pointing arrow) (same case as in Figure 24-2).

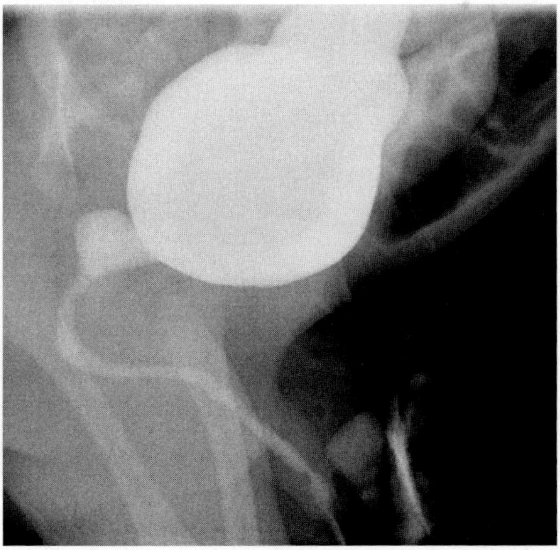

Figure 24-4. A more typical appearance of the urethra in PBS, showing the dilatation of the prostatic urethra but no evidence of postnatal obstruction.

MANAGEMENT

On occasions, urethral obstruction with oligo- or anhydramnios can be treated by amnioinfusion, serial bladder taps to assess potential renal function, and the placement of a vesicoamniotic shunt.

After birth, respiratory function should be addressed first. If the serum creatinine is elevated, temporary bladder catheter drainage will assess the role of infravesical obstruction or bladder dysfunction in the impaired renal function. A temporary vesicostomy will provide relief until more definitive treatment is possible. Antibacterial prophylaxis is important to prevent UTIs.

When children are stable, it is preferable to plan a major reconstructive procedure by six months of age. The procedure consists of an abdominoplasty (Monfort technique), bilateral orchiopexy, and, if needed, ureteral reimplantation (Figure 24-5).

The advantage of early orchidopexy for these high intra-abdominal testes is that at this age, it can usually be accomplished in one stage. When the orchidopexy is done later in life, a staged procedure is usually needed (see Chapter 18).

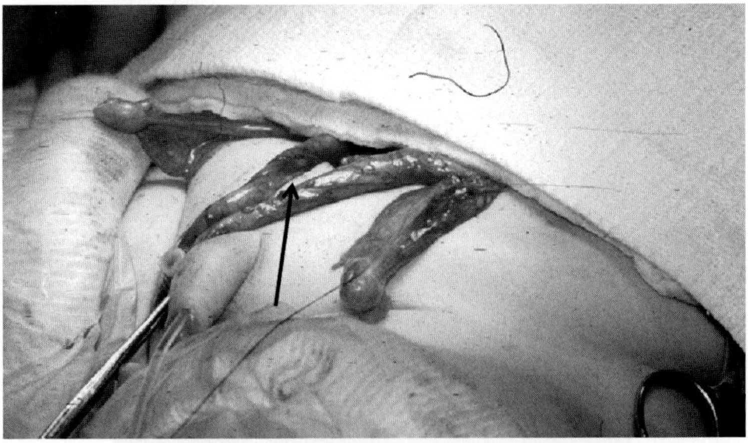

Figure 24-5. Intraoperative photograph of a boy undergoing complete reconstruction of PBS. Notice the well-mobilised testes that will reach the scrotum without tension and the dilated ureters (arrow) that will be reimplanted in the bladder.

The advantages of abdominoplasty are mostly cosmetic but it may also favorably affect pulmonary and voiding functions.

Cases with urethral atresia can be treated in the newborn period with progressive dilatation. Although the urethra distal to the obstructive membrane is much hypoplastic, it responds well to gentle progressive dilatation one over a period of weeks. The patent urachus or vesical fistula should then be closed to allow urethral refunctionalization.

As children begin to walk, an abdominal brace is usually needed and it may be useful throughout childhood, particularly during sport activities.

LONG-TERM OUTCOME

For children who survive the neonatal period, close follow-up during childhood is necessary. Bladder emptying and renal function should be evaluated at 6–12 months intervals.

The development of scoliosis due to the lack of anterior abdominal musculature is possible and regular follow-up visits with an orthopedic surgeon are recommended.

End-stage renal failure will develop in about 1/3 of patients. Renal transplantation can be successfully done. Infertility is the rule due to prostatic abnormalities and cryptorchism.

SUMMARY

Although the incidence of PBS in many places is decreasing because of the prenatal diagnosis and interruption of pregnancy, this rare condition presents challenges to the clinician and has taught us much about the abnormal development of the urinary tract.

FURTHER READING

Dénes FT, Arap MA, Giron AM, Silva FA, Arap S. Comprehensive surgical treatment of prune belly syndrome: 17 years' experience with 32 patients. *Urology* 2004; **64**(4):789–793.

Freedman AL, Johnson MP, Smith CA, González R, Evans MI. Long-term outcome in children following antenatal intervention for obstructive uropathies. *Lancet* 1999; **354**:374–377.

Galati V, Beeson JH, Confer SD, Frimberger D, Campbell JB, Ramji FG, Kropp BP. A favorable outcome following 32 vesicocentesis and amnioinfusion procedures in a fetus with severe prune belly syndrome. *J Pediatr Urol* 2008; **4**(2):170–172.

González R, Reinberg Y, Burke B, Wells T, Vernier RL. Early bladder obstruction in fetal lambs induces renal dysplasia and the prune-belly syndrome *J Pediatr Surg* 1990; **25**:342–345.

Moerman P, Fryns JP, Goodeeris P. Prune belly syndrome, a secondary urethral functional obstruction due to prostatic hypoplasia. *J Genet Hum* 1984; **32**(2):141–143.

Pagon RA, Smith DW, Shepard TH. Urethral obstruction malformation complex: a cause of abdominal muscle deficiency and the "prune belly". *J Pediatr* 1979; **94**(6):900–906.

Perez-Aytes A, Graham JM, Hersh JH, Hoyme HE, Aleck K, Carey JC. Urethral obstruction sequence and lower limb deficiency: evidence for the vascular disruption hypothesis. *J Pediatr* 1993; **123**(3):398–405.

Reinberg Y, Chelimsky G, González R. Urethral atresia and the prune belly syndrome. Report of six cases. *Br J Urol* 1993; **72**:112–114.

Reinberg Y, Manivel JC, Pettinato G, González R. Development of renal failure in children with the prune belly syndrome. *J Urol* 1991; **145**:1017–1019.

Reinberg Y, Shapiro E, Manivel JC, Manley C, González R. Prune belly syndrome in females: a triad of abdominal musculature deficiency and anomalies of the urinary and genital systems. *J Pediatr* 1991; **118**:395–398.

Chapter 25

Acute and Chronic Renal Failure

José Alberto Ramírez

ACUTE RENAL FAILURE

Definition

Acute renal failure (ARF) is the clinical syndrome that results from an abrupt and potentially reversible reduction in glomerular filtration rate (GFR). The primary function of the kidneys is the regulation of the volumen and the composition of the extracellular fluid; clinically significant ARF exists when the GFR is reduced sufficiently to cause adverse changes in one or both of these. A persistent rise in the concentration of serum creatinine (SCr) above 50% from baseline value, associated or not with the decrease in urine output to less than 0.5–1.0 ml/kg/h, is considered the feature of ARF in pediatrics.

Severe ARF is life threatening. However, recent evidence suggests that even a mild increase in the concentration of SCr is a risk factor for mortality and costs in hospitalized patients. When faced with clinical situations where ARF could be present, the role of nephrologists is to diagnose the presence of ARF and identify the modifiable and non-modifiable risk factors, followed by patient-specific management.

Epidemiology

Until recently, studies describing ARF epidemiology have used a wide variety of definitions, ranging from mild changes in the level of SCr and the output of urine, to the need for renal replacement therapy (RRT).

Table 25-1. Pediatric RIFLE criteria.

	Estimated creatinine clearance	Urine output
Risk	Decreased by 25%	< 0.5 ml/kg/h for 8 hours
Injury	Decreased by 50%	< 0.5 ml/kg/h for 16 hours
Failure	Decreased by 75% or eCrCl < 35 ml/min/1.73 m^2	< 0.3 ml/kg/h for 24 hours or anuric for 12 hours
Loss	Persistent failure > 4 weeks	
End-stage	End-stage renal disease (persistent failure > 3 month)	

The incidence of ARF is generally less than 1% when the requirement of RRT defines ARF. However, a requirement for the provision of RRT is the strictest definition of ARF, when less strict definitions for ARF are used, such as doubling of SCr, the incidence increases.

Based on the RIFLE (risk, injury, failure, loss, end-stage kidney disease) criteria for defining acute kidney injury (AKI) in adults, a proposed pediatric-modified RIFLE (pRIFLE) is shown in Table 25-1. Using pRIFLE criteria, ARF is seen in 82% of the most critically ill children those are admitted to the pediatric intensive care unit (PICU). Although the criteria are not currently applicable in the medical setting, they provide a useful research tool to develop descriptive and outcome studies of ARF and also allow clinicians and intensivists to speak the same language when discussing the presence of ARF.

Etiology

Single cause of ARF is unusual in the critical care setting. In the noncritical care setting, such as the emergency room or hospital wards, it is more likely to find a single important etiology. ARF can be classified into three major groups: prerenal failure, intrarenal/renal parenchymal disease, and postrenal/obstructive.

In prerenal failure, renal function is decreased owing to renal hypoperfusion secondary to volume contraction or a decrease in effective blood volume. Prerenal failure can progress to intrinsic ARF if predisposing cause or causes persist to the point at which hipoxic-ischemic injury occurs.

The diseases of renal tissue (intrarenal) are classified into: (a) tubular, (b) glomerular, (c) vascular, (d) interstitial, and (e) congenital renal diseases (renal dysplasia/hypoplasia and cystic renal disease), according to the renal anatomy most affected by the disorder.

Postrenal/obstructive, such as (a) urethral obstruction, (b) obstruction of solitary kidney urinary tract — congenital or acquired: stones, mass, and (c) bilateral ureteral obstruction — mass, stones, may mimics ARF in its presentation.

Renal hypoperfusion events are extremely common in the critical care unit, resulting from excessive blood loss, sepsis with capillary leak, cardiac dysfunction, vomiting, inadequate fluid replacement, and burns. Therefore, a detailed fluid balance history is necessary to determine the extent, to which renal hypoperfusion may be contributing to the ARF episode. Additionally, a fluid balance history is invaluable to evaluate whether a positive fluid balance is occurring, which may suggest more severe ARF, i.e. acute tubular necrosis (ATN). A detailed medication history will elucidate whether medication — induced nephrotoxicity — may be contributing to the current ARF episode.

Acute glomerular disease such as acute nephritic syndrome and hemolytic uremic syndrome (HUS) are clearly diagnosed at presentation. Gross hematuria, hypertension, and decreased GFR are the hallmark of acute glomerular disease, while "microangiopathic" hemolytic anemia, thrombocytopenia, and ARF caused by endothelial damage are the principal clinical manifestations of severe HUS, which follows an episode of bloody diarrhea because of hemorrhagic colitis.

Vascular insults such as renal artery and renal vein thrombosis can result in ARF if bilateral or if either occurs in patients with only one kidney. For the most part, renal vascular thrombosis can be a complication in neonatal ICU patients with umbilical catheters or in the neonates or children those are severely dehydrated.

In postrenal ARF, the kidney function is initially normal, but obstruction to urine flow causes ARF. This type of ARF is important to identify quickly because it typically reverses with relief of obstruction. However, postrenal ARF can also progress to intrinsic renal damage, if not corrected promptly.

Diagnosis

Evidence of a reduced GFR is essential for the diagnosis of ARF, whether or not oliguria is present. Estimating baseline kidney function will help determine the severity of kidney injury, and can be assessed by reviewing previously drawn levels of SCr over the previous three to six months to determine a patient's true baseline level of SCr. If previous SCr levels are unavailable, the normal creatinine level for each individual can be calculated using the formulas below:

$$\text{SCr (mg/dl)} = 0.18 + 0.032 \text{ age (years)},$$

$$\text{SCr (mg/dl)} = 0.004 \times \text{length (cm)}.$$

Estimate GFR (eGFR) by means of the Schwartz formula (in ml per min per 1.73 m^2) can then be calculated and confronted with the GFR at a normal level of SCr.

Schwartz formula from the first two years of life to the early adolescent age is equal to 0.55 by length (cm) divided by SCr in mg/dl.

As an example, a four-year-old boy, who is 100 cm tall, has a level of SCr of 1.0 mg/dl. eGRF in ml/min/1.73 m^2 is 55, while his normal baseline eGFR is 137.5 ml/min/1.73 m^2. Our patient is in severe AKI with 40% of kidney function remaining.

Other typical changes in the biochemical values of serum are summarized in Table 25-2.

Urinalysis and Urinary Indices in the Diagnosis of ARF

Urine examination is normal in prerenal ARF, while abnormalities are present in intrarenal disease and in postrenal ARF when infection is present.

Hematuria and the casts of red blood cell and white blood cell with proteinuria are seen in glomerular disease. Nephrotic proteinuria (40 mg/kg/day of urine protein or urine protein/creatinuria index of two) is the hallmark of heavy proteinuria. Patients with ATN may have granular or muddy brown casts.

The oliguria of prerenal failure is a physiologic response to renal under perfusion, which is leading to the production of urine of high

Table 25-2. Typical changes in serum values in ARF.

Substance	Direction of change from normal
Creatinine	↑
Urea	↑
Uric acid	↑
Sodium	↓
Potassium	↑
Chloride	↓ ↑
Hydrogen ion	↑
Bicarbonate	↓
Calcium	↓
Inorganic phosphate	↑

Hyponatremia is dilutional in oliguric renal failure, but may reflect sodium depletion in non-oliguric renal failure. The chloride level may be low, reflecting dilution or salt depletion, but may be paradoxically raised, as a result of metabolic acidosis.

osmolality, high concentration of urea and creatinine, and low concentration of sodium. The oliguria of ATN results from the passage of a small amount of "poor-quality" urine, i.e. urine similar in composition to glomerular filtrate because of the inability of the damaged tubules to modify it appropriately. The analysis of the composition of the urine, therefore, allows a degree of differentiation between prerenal failure and ATN (Table 25-3).

The most discriminating test is the measurement of the fractional sodium excretion (FE_{Na}) and the fraction of sodium filtered by the glomeruli that are excreted in the urine:

$$FE_{Na}(\%) = UNa \div SNa/UCr \div SCr \times 100,$$

where U and S refer to the concentrations of urine and serum and Na and Cr to sodium and creatinine, respectively.

The diagnosis of prerenal failure is confirmed by an improvement in urine flow and renal function in response to fluid repletion. Provided there is no clinical evidence of circulatory overload, a "fluid challenge" of isotonic saline 10 ml/kg, should be given intravenously over one hour. Failure to respond confirms ATN as the diagnosis.

Table 25-3. Typical values for biochemical indices in prerenal failure and acute tubular necrosis.

	Prerenal failure	Acute tubular necrosis
Urine specific gravity	> 1.025	1.010
Urine osmolality	> 500 mOsm/kg	300 mOsm/kg
Urine/plasma osmolality	> 2	=1
Urine sodium	< 10 mEq/L	> 20 mEq/L
Urine/serum urea	> 10	Low
Urine/serum creatinine	> 40	Low
FENa (%)		
Children	< 1	> 2
Neonates	< 3	> 3
FE uric acid (%)	< 12	> 20
FE urea (%)	< 35	> 35

Low FENa is not unique to prerenal ARF, since it can occur in acute glomerulonephritis, vasculitis, some cases of acute interstitial nephritis, acute or chronic renal failure, and myo- or hemoglobinuric renal failure.

Blood Biochemical Studies

Besides BUN, SCr, electrolytes, and blood gases, the analysis blood should cover those directed to the causes of intrarenal ARF such as hemoglobin and platelets, coagulation profile, albumin, complement fraction, and autoimmune work-up.

Imaging Studies

Imaging studies serve to distinguish between congenital intrarenal disease and postrenal ARF on the one hand and prerenal failure and intrinsic ARF on the other hand. Renal ultrasound (US), voiding cystourethrogram, renal vessel Doppler study, and radionucleoisotope scan are the most useful screening studies.

Renal US in the diagnosis of the cause of ARF can document the presence of (a) dilated pelvicalceal systems with or without calculi, (b) large echobright kidneys suggestive of an acute process, and (c) small kidneys or cysts: ARF on chronic kidney disease.

Renal Biopsy

Renal biopsy is indicated as soon as possible when the renal function is deteriorating and the etiology is not certain with nephritic and nephrotic presentations. These features are suggestive of rapidly progressive crescentic glomerulonephritis, which needs urgent treatment to prevent long-term renal damage.

Conservative Management of ARF

A range of factors must be addressed in the conservative management of IRA.

Fluid Balance

Meticulous attention to fluid balance is essential. Once intravascular volume is re-established, fluid intake should be restricted to 400 ml/m^2 per day (5% dextrose in water) and should restrict urinary output and extrarenal losses if the child has a urinary output of at least 1 ml/kg per hour. This formula accounts for insensible water loss from the lungs, skin, and GI tracts, as well as from excretory losses.

Electrolytes

Frequent electrolyte abnormalities seen in ARF that must be corrected include hyponatremia, hyperkalemia, acidosis, and hypocalcemia/hyperphosphatemia.

Hyponatremia in an anuric or oliguric patient is generally associated to extracellular volumen expansion; therefore, fluid restriction is mandatory. If this is severe, dialysis should be considered. In nonoliguric patient, hyponatremia may be secondary to the losses of urine sodium and its replacement should be prescribed. Occasionally, the correction of the serum sodium is necessary when hyponatremia is severe (below 120 mEq/L) and the patient is symptomatic. Infusion of 3% sodium chloride, at 3.5 ml/kg/dose in less than one hour, would raise serum sodium in 3 mEq/L. This should only be done if there are symptoms such as altered mental status or seizures.

Hyperkalemia is a life-threatening abnormality in ARF that must be treated aggressively and quickly. Hyperkalemia is defined as mild-to-moderate when the concentration of potassium is between 6.0 and 7.0 mEq/L and severe when the concentration is greater than 7.0 mEq/L with any electrocardiographic changes. The treatment of hyperkalemia should be initiated in patients whose potassium values are 6 mEq/L or higher as well as in those who have peaked T waves, weakness, paresthesias, or tetany.

The treatment of hyperkalemia includes: the infusion of 10% calcium gluconate 0.5–1 ml/kg/dose through a central venous line to stabilize the membrane potential; the infusion of sodium bicarbonate 1 mEq/kg to shift the potassium intracellularly; the infusion of insulin (0.1 to 0.2 U/kg) plus 10–25% glucose at 0.5 g/kg as a continuous infusion over 2–3 hours to allow the uptake of potassium from the extracellular space to the intracellular space; Salbutamol by inhalation (nebulizer) at a dose of 2.5 mg if weight is less than 25 kg or 5.0 mg if it is greater than 25 kg; and the administration of sodium polystyrene sulfonate (1 g/kg rectally or orally) to exchange sodium for potassium in the colonic mucosa. Once administered, the resin takes a few hours to be effective.

If these attempts do not correct the patient's hyperkalemia, dialysis should be initiated, especially if anuria is present. Once the decision to begin dialysis has been made, the previously noted measures should be continued until dialysis is available.

Metabolic acidosis in the acute setting can be corrected by administering sodium bicarbonate intravenously if the acidosis is severe (bicarbonate $\leq$ 8 mEq/L). Calculation for the amount of bicarbonate to be administered to correct the acidosis is: mEq of bicarbonate = half of the base deficit $\times$ kg body weight $\times$ 0.3. If correction cannot be achieved within the fluid allowance, in the case of severe and persistent acidosis, dialysis should be considered.

Hypocalcemia/hyperphosphatemia in ARF can be caused by hyperphosphatemia, vitamin D deficiency, parathyroid hormone resistance, and hypoalbuminemia. Usually, it is mild and it responds to the correction of hyperphosphatemia by the addition of oral calcium carbonate to feeds at a dose of 50 mg/kg/day. Calcium between meals should not be given until the plasma phosphate level has been reduced to normal, otherwise ectopic calcification may occur.

Nutrition

Nutrition is an important consideration in ARF and may be severely limited by the imposed fluid restriction. A relatively high caloric intake of 80–100 cal/kg/day must be provided to promote anabolism and prevent catabolism, which potentiates hyperkalemia, hyperphosphatemia, and acidosis. Protein intake recommended is 1.0 g/kg/day in children and 0.8 g/kg/day for older teenagers. An inability to meet nutritional needs because of fluid that can be given is an indication for dialysis.

Hypertension

Hypertension in ARF usually is due to volume overload or changes in vascular tone. If volume overload is present, diuresis with furosemide in nonoliguric patient or dialysis in anuric ARF should be initiated to return the patient to hemodynamic stability.

If increased vascular tone is the cause of hypertension, oral or intravenous antihypertensive treatment may be necessary. Intravenous antihypertensive medications should be used if the patient cannot take oral medications or if severe hypertension exists (systolic or diastolic blood pressures at least at the 99th percentile for age, sex, and height).

Sodium nitroprusside is an effective antihypertensive IV drug, but its use requires monitoring of thiocyanate concentrations because the kidney cannot excrete this by-product of metabolized nitroprusside. Recommended continuous IV infusion is 0.3–10 mcg/kg per minute. In cases where hypertension is not as severe, short-acting PO nifedipine can be administered at 0.25–1 mg/kg/dose (maximum 10 mg/dose or 3 mg/kg per day).

Management by Dialysis

Because of the complexity of ARF with associated volume status issues and metabolic derangements, dialysis is often the management strategy of choice to rapidly restore fluid and electrolyte homeostasis. The indication and choice of the specific mode of dialysis depend on patient requirements/limitations, facility experience, and local resources. Common indications for dialysis in ARF are (a) failure to improve with conservative management, and (b) to make room for nutrition and drug administration.

Dialysis is the removal of small solutes across a semipermeable membrane by diffusion down their concentration gradient. The membrane may be the peritoneum, or synthetic, as in hemodialysis. This process differs from ultrafiltration, in which there is convective removal of plasma water and small solutes, because of a pressure gradient across a highly permeable membrane. Treatments can consist of pure dialysis, pure filtration, or more often, both.

Peritoneal Dialysis

Peritoneal dialysis (PD) is the modality of choice in most neonates, the advantages are being the relative ease of access and the technical simplicity in comparison with hemodialysis (HD). The preferred means of access to the peritoneal cavity for dialysis is via a biologically inert silastic Tenckhoff catheter inserted using sterile technique by a surgeon experienced in the procedure. In low birth weight infants, in whom the insertion of this type of catheter is not feasible, PD can be carried out via an angiography catheter or a thoracic drain.

Extracorporeal Renal Replacement Therapy

There are occasions on which PD fails or is contraindicated, necessitating the use of hemofiltration and/or HD. Although it is preferable to perform these techniques continuously in order to avoid swings in intravascular volume and biochemistry, intermittent hemodialysis has been successfully used. Access-related problems are the most vexing aspects of extracorporeal dialysis therapy. Suggested size and the selection of hemofiltration vascular access for pediatric patients is shown in Table 25-4.

Intermittent hemodialysis and continuous modalities such as continuous venovenous hemofiltration (CVVH), continuous venovenous hemodialysis (CVVHD), or continuous venovenous hemodiafiltration (CVVHDF) may be used to provide enhanced solute clearance and ultrafiltration. Data have demonstrated that small molecular weight solute clearance, such as urea, is similar with CVVH and CVVHD. However,

Table 25-4. Suggested size and selection of hemofiltration vascular access for pediatric patients.

Patient weight	Catheter size	Site of insertion
Neonate	Single-lumen 5 F	Femoral artery or vein
	Dual-lumen 7.0 F	Femoral vein
3–6 kg	Dual-lumen 7.0 F	Internal/external jugular, subclavian, or femoral vein
	Triple-lumen 7.0 F	Internal/external jugular, subclavian, or femoral vein
6–30 kg	Dual-lumen 8.0 F	Internal/external jugular, subclavian, or femoral vein
> 15 kg	Dual-lumen 9.0 F	Internal/external jugular, subclavian, or femoral vein
30 kg	Dual-lumen 10.0 F	Internal/external jugular, subclavian, or femoral vein

larger molecular weight compounds have improved clearance with CVVH (connective clearance) than with CVVHD (diffusive clearance).

Review of the pediatric nephrology literature over the past decade has demonstrated an overall trend toward CVVH when continuous RRT is indicated.

In critically ill patients with severe sepsis or multiorgan dysfunction syndrome or those requiring extracorporeal membrane oxygenation, the use of CVVH with high replacement fluid rates has demonstrated improved solute and cytokines clearance.

Prognosis

Recovery from ARF may take days to weeks, a period that requires frequent and careful patient assessment. If renal failure continues for several weeks, transition to chronic care may be necessary. Over the last 15 to 20 years, improvement in the care of very ill children has led to a better prognosis for those who have ARF. Prognosis depends on several factors, including the need for dialysis, the time between onset of illness and presentation to medical care, and the underlying disease. Patients who present at a younger age and have multisystem organ failure appear to have worse prognoses. Therefore, early identification of patients who have ARF and early intervention are necessary to improve the current rate of mortality from 10 to 60% associated with these risk factors.

Of particular interest is the long-term renal outcome of patients who have hospital-acquired ARF. Up to 60% of children who had hospital-acquired ARF had some form of renal abnormality at the 3–5 years follow-up evaluation, defined as hematuria, hypertension, microalbuminuria, low GFR, or high GFR; all of them evidence of chronic kidney injury. Routine evaluation of all pediatric ARF survivors is recommended to determine who is at risk for long-term renal complications.

CHRONIC RENAL FAILURE IN CHILDREN

Introduction

Prior to 2002, the term chronic renal insufficiency was used to characterize patients who had progressive decline in renal function, defined as a glomerular filtration rate (GFR) of less than 75 mL/min per 1.73 m^2 body surface area. Chronic kidney disease (CKD) is the new term defined by the National Kidney Foundation Kidney Disease and Outcome Quality Initiative (KDOQI) Group, to classify any patient who has kidney damage lasting for ≥3 months, as defined by the structural or functional abnormalities of the kidney, with or without a decreased GFR, manifested by one or more of the following features:

- abnormalities in the composition of the blood or urine,
- abnormalities in imaging tests, and
- abnormalities on kidney biopsy.

Alternatively, if any patient has a GFR <60 mL/min per 1.73 m^2 for ≥3 months, with or without kidney damage; it denotes the presence of CKD. In 2003, these guidelines were reviewed and recommended for the same use in children with CKD.

The KDOQI Group classified CKD into five stages (Table 25-5). GFR values for CKD staging are for children older than two years of age, because the GFR values for younger children are low, due to

Table 25-5. DOQI stages of CKD.

Stage	Description	GFR (ml/min/1.73 m^2)
1	Kidney damage with normal or increased GFR	≥90
2	Kidney damage with mildly decreased GFR	60–89
3	Moderate decrease in GFR	30–59
4	Severe decrease in GFR	15–29
5	Kidney failure (ESRD)	≤15 (or on dialysis)

Table 25-6. Normal glomerular filtration rates (GFR) values in pediatrics.

Age	GFR (ml/min/1.73 m^2)
One week	40.6 ± 14.8
2–8 weeks	65.8 ± 24.8
>8 weeks	95.7 ± 21.7
2–12 years	133.0 ± 27.0
13–21 years (males)	140.0 ± 30.0
13–21 years (females)	126.0 ± 22.0

ongoing maturation. The normal range of GFRs at different ages is given in Table 25-6.

GFR provides the best measure of overall kidney function. However, the correct interpretation of GFR values in individual patients, especially children and adolescents, requires a clear understanding that the normal level of GFR varies according to age, gender, and body size. The normal GFR in young adults is ~120–130 ml/min/1.73 m^2, whereas the normal level of GFR is much lower than this in early infancy, even when corrected for body surface area, and subsequently increases in relationship to body size for up to two years (Table 25–7).

Etiology

CKD has a prevalence of 1.5 to 3.0 per 1,000,000 among children who are younger than the age of 16 years. The commonest causes of CKD in

Table 25-7. **GFR by Schwartz equation.**

Age (gender)	Constant	Equation
1 week (males–females) Preterm	0.33	0.33 × length/SCr
2–8 weeks (males–females) Term	0.45	0.45 × length/SCr
>8 weeks (males–females)	0.45	0.45 × length/SCr
2–12 years (males–females)	0.55	0.55 × length/SCr
13–21 years (males)	0.70	0.70 × length/SCr
13–21 years (females)	0.55	0.55 × length/SCr

Length in centimeters; SCr: serum creatinine in mg/dl.

children are urologic abnormalities (30–33%) and glomerulopathies (25–27%). These two abnormalities are account for more than 50% of the reported causes of end-stage renal disease (ESRD) in children. The other major causes are hereditary nephropathies (16%) and renal hypoplasia and dysplasia (11%). CKD in typical HUS patients is ~20%. Histologic similarities among the various causes of CKD are many and possible common mechanisms accounting for similarities include cell-specific damage, the role of growth factors, and the effects of metabolic factors. Ultimately, these mechanisms could lead to some degree of healing or to additional sclerosis (scarring).

The incidence and prevalence of CKD are greater in males than in females. Two-thirds of patients were males in the chronic renal insufficiency registry of the North American Pediatric Renal Trials and Collaborative Studies (NAPRTCS), which includes patients below 21 years of age, with a CrCl less than 75 mL/min per 1.73 m^2. The increased risk in males is due to the higher incidence of congenital anomalies of the kidney and urinary tract (CAKUT), including obstructive uropathy, renal dysplasia, renal hypoplasia, and prune belly syndrome.

Diagnosis

The clinical presentation of CKD is dependent upon the severity of renal impairment and the underlying disorder. Patients presenting during the early stages, such as Stages 1 or 2 of CKD, are typically asymptomatic. As CKD progresses and renal function deteriorates, patients become symptomatic.

Patients with CKD may present in a variety of ways:

- The symptoms and signs of direct kidney injury such as nephritic-nephrotic syndrome: edema, hypertension, hematuria, and proteinuria. Polyuria may be an early presenting finding, because many congenital anomalies of the kidney and urinary tract, inherited disorders, and tubulointerstitial disorders are associated with reduced concentrating ability. The impairment in renal concentration, generally, precedes a significant reduction in GFR.
- Incidental findings of an elevation in the concentration of SCr and/or abnormalities on urinalysis. Persistently increased protein excretion is usually a marker of kidney damage.
- The detection of congenital or structural anomalies by imaging studies, particularly prenatal ultrasonography.
- *Poor growth*: The age of CKD onset is correlated with the degree of growth retardation, because the average birth length of 50 cm in a normal child increased by about 50% by the end of the first year and the length has been doubled by the age of four years.
- Acute failure on CKD precipitated by infection or dehydration.
- The symptoms and/or signs of severe renal impairment begin to appear in some patients with Stage 3 and are present in those with Stages 4 and 5. Anemia, osteodystrophy, and poor nutrition are the commonest features.

Estimation of GFR and Assessment of Proteinuria

In children and adolescents, the GFR should be estimated from prediction equations that take into account the concentration of SCr and the height and gender of the patient. Of the various prediction formulas that have been developed, the Schwartz formula has gained widespread use. The equation and the constant to be used in infants, children, and adolescent boys and girls are shown in Table 25-8.

Table 25-8. Relative contraindications for pre-emptive kidney transplantation.

1. Conditions requiring native nephrectomies prior to transplant:
   - uncontrolled hypertension,
   - chronically infected urinary tract with stasis, and
   - persistent nephrotic syndrome.
2. Patient non-compliance with medications, follow-up visits, and general ability to follow instructions.
3. Catastrophic presentation with ESRD.
4. Inadequate time to assess patient and family for pre-emptive transplant.
5. Problems with the potential live donor:
   - health problem identified in the donor,
   - live donor pregnancy, and
   - the potential recipient is allosensitized to the donor.

The measurement of creatinine clearance using timed (for example, 24-hour) urine collections does not improve the estimate of GFR over that provided by prediction equation. A 24-hour urine collection to determine GFR, however, is more reliable in patients with an unusual dietary intake — e.g. vegetarian diet or creatinine supplements, in those with decreased muscle mass — e.g. amputation, malnutrition, muscle wasting, in the assessment of diet and nutritional status, and to prescribe the need to start dialysis.

Increased excretion of albumin is a sensitive marker for CKD attributed to glomerular disease and hypertension. The increased excretion of low molecular weight globulins is a sensitive marker for some types of tubulointerstitial disease. The term "proteinuria" refers to the increased urinary excretion of albumin, other specific proteins, or total protein, the term "albuminuria" refers specifically to increased urinary excretion of albumin, and the term "microalbuminuria" refers to albumin excretion above the normal range, but below the level of detection by dipstick for total protein.

The most frequently used screening method for proteinuria is the urinary dipstick, which primarily detects albumin. Negative or trace in a concentrated urine (specific gravity ≥ 1020) is the normal range, while 1+ (≈ 30 mg/dl), 2+ (≈ 100 mg/dl), and 3+ (≈ 300 mg/dl) are abnormal and deserved further confirmation.

Under most circumstances, untimed ("spot") urine samples should be used to detect and monitor proteinuria in children and adolescents. It is usually not necessary to obtain a timed urine collection (overnight or 24-hour) for these evaluations. First morning specimens are preferred, but random specimens are acceptable if first morning specimens are not available.

Accordingly, the urine protein/urine creatinine is often used to estimate protein excretion in children. This ratio has been shown to reflect 24-hour urine protein excretion quite accurately, particularly since first morning specimen eliminate the possibility of postural proteinuria. The normal range for the ratio is: <0.2 mg/mg in children those are more than two years old and <0.5 in those are 6–24 months old. Quantitation or proteinuria in a documented 24-hour urine collection normal range is <100 mg/m^2/24 hours or <4 mg/m^2/hour.

The creatinine content should be measured to determine whether the specimen is truly 24-hour collection. The urine content of creatinine is estimated as 15–20 mg/kg ideal body weight in females and 20–25 mg/kg ideal body weight in males. Normal range microalbuminuria is <30 mg urine albumin/g creatinine on first morning urine or <30 mg/24 hours in a timed urine collection.

Other Laboratory Tests

The other laboratory tests that are used for the evaluation of a child with CKF include the following.

Electrolytes and arterial blood gases are used to detect abnormalities such as hyponatremia, hyperkalemia, and metabolic acidosis, which can be hypercloremic in early stages and with high anion gap in Stages 4 and 5.

Complete blood count with red blood cell indices and reticulocyte count to detect normocytic and normochromic anemia usually characterize the anemia of CKD.

The level of serum calcium, phosphorus, and parathyroid hormone is used to detect any abnormalities in bone mineral metabolism.

Fasting lipid profile is used to detect the presence of dyslipidemia.

Imaging may be useful in identifying the underlying cause. Findings on renal ultrasonography help determine the loss of renal parenchyma, cysts, renal size, the presence of hydronephrosis, or calculi (with and without nephrocalcinosis) may be enough to provide a diagnosis and will guide further investigation as necessary.

Renal biopsy may be necessary if the cause of CKD is not clear, but should be avoided in advanced CKD when the kidneys are small (<5 cm bipolar length), as there is a significantly increased risk of bleeding and histology may show ESRD without being able to identify the cause.

Complications and Management of CKD According to KDOQI Stages

Electrolyte and Acid–Base Abnormalities

Hyponatremia can occur because of excess free water ingestion in a patient with severe reduction in GFR or reduced salt intake in a salt-losing nephropathy. A salt-losing syndrome and hyperkalemia with tubular resistance to aldosterone can occur in infants and children with urinary tract malformations and acute pyelonephritis.

Sodium chloride should not automatically be restricted in CKD unless there is hypertension, edema, or volumen expansion. Electrolyte wasting in CKD4 and CKD5 is reported to be four times greater than in CKD1. Some patients in the early stage of CKD with impaired ability to concentrate urine and polyuria are at risk of hypernatremia, when output is not matched by water intake.

Hyperkalemia is the result of reduced GFR, metabolic acidosis, inactivation of the renin–angiotensin–aldosterone system, reduced flow rate of distal tubular fluid, and medications such as angiotensin-converting enzyme inhibitors. Hyperkalemia plays a pivotal role in potassium homeostasis in CKD by stimulating potassium excretion. When extracellular K^+ rise to the level needed to stimulate excretion, a new steady state develops where its excretion again matches intake. When this new steady state is achieved, serum K^+ remains stable, unless dietary intake increases, GRF falls or drugs disrupt the new balance. Patients with CKD and hypokalemia must not be given bolusses of potassium, because the serum concentration may increase too quickly.

The risk of hyperkalemia in CKD patients increase significantly from CKD1 to CKD4 and CKD5.

Metabolic acidosis is expected in CKD, caused mainly by a failure of renal excretion of acid, to keep pace with the daily production of fixed acid from dietary intake (±3 mEq/kg/day). Typically, the anion gap is increased because the renal excretion of phosphate, sulfate, and organic acids is insufficient to maintain balance for these anions. When CKD is mild, the anion gap may be normal, because at this stage the renal excretion of the above-named anions can still keep pace with their production.

As the patient approaches CKD3 to CKD4, the plasma bicarbonate concentration gradually falls to stabilize at 12–20 mEq/L. Although hydrogen ions continue to be retained, a further reduction in the plasma bicarbonate is prevented by buffering of the excess H^+ by bone, with a negative impact on growth and bone mineralization.

Therapy with sodium bicarbonate or its precursors, such as sodium citrate, should target maintaining a plasma bicarbonate of 20–22 mEq/L. In children with CKD, the treatment of osteodystrophy is more effective, if the acidosis is corrected.

Calcium-Phosphate Metabolism

Abnormalities in mineral metabolism and bone structure are almost a universal finding with progressive CKD. The bone disease of CKD, referred to as renal osteodistrophy, is a result of several factors: firstly, the decreased renal clearance of phosphorus results in its retention and the elevation of serum parathyroid hormone (PTH); secondly, the decreased production of calcitriol. The normal kidney converts 25-dihydroxyvitamin D_3 (calcidiol) into 1,25-dihydroxyvitamin D_3 (calcitriol) when stimulated by hypocalcemia, PTH release, and the decreased dietary intake of phosphate. In renal disease, 1,25-dihydroxyvitamin D_3 production decreases, the intestinal absorption of calcium decreases, and hypocalcemia develops. This series of events, in turn, causes an increase in PTH formation. Finally, a decreased availability of calcidiol may indicate generalized vitamin D deficiency. The prevalence of metabolic bone disease is as high as 47% in CKD3 and 100% in CKD4 and CKD5.

The goal of the therapy of renal osteodystrophy is to normalize the growth and prevent the development of bony deformity, extraskeletal calcifications, and marked secondary hyperparathyroidism. This goal can be achieved through the use of calcium supplements, calcium-acetate phosphate binders, 1,25-dihydroxyvitamin D_3, alkali therapy, and dietary control.

Serum total calcium and phosphorus should be maintained in the 9- and 4.5-mg/dl range, respectively, while for PTH, it has been suggested that levels three to four times the upper limits of normal, may provide the best defense against adynamic bone disease and hyperparathyroid-induced renal osteodystrophy. The product of $Ca \times P < 40$ mg/mg is required to prevent soft tissue calcification.

Anemia in CKD is mainly caused by the decreased renal production of the glycoprotein erythropoietin. Anemia, generally, becomes manifest at a GFR below 35 mL/min/1.73 m^2, but may develop earlier in some forms of renal disease such as nephronophthisis (medullary cystic disease). In addition to overcoming the anemia, the treatment with recombinant human erythropoietin (rhEpo) eliminates the need for blood transfusions, thus reducing the potential risk of blood-borne infections and human lymphocyte antigen sensitization.

The goal of rhEpo therapy, presently, is to maintain the hematocrit at 33–36%. Current recommendations suggest that therapy with rhEpo should be instituted when the hematocrit falls below 30%. The starting doses of rhEpo range from 50 to 150 U/kg per dose, given one to three times a week. rhEpo may be given subcutaneously or intravenously, although studies suggest that it may be more effective when given by the subcutaneous route. Although the maintenance dose of rhEpo necessary to keep the hematocrit in the desirable range varies greatly among patients, most of them appear to require doses between 100 and 200 U/kg/week.

The concomitant use of iron supplementation is almost always necessary when rhEpo treatment is prescribed. If adequate iron stores cannot be maintained with oral therapy, intravenous iron therapy should be instituted. Iron studies, including serum ferritin and transferrin saturation, should be performed to detect the onset of functional iron deficiency (e.g. the presence of iron in sufficient quantity in storage tissues but with erythroid precursor cells unable to efficiently access the iron). The goal should be to maintain serum iron levels in the normal range, transferrin saturation greater than 20%, and the serum ferritin at greater than 150 ng/mL.

Possible reasons for a less than expected response to rhEpo treatment include: iron deficiency, occult blood loss, occult chronic infections, the deficiency of vitamin B_{12} or folate, and severe bone marrow fibrosis.

Hypertension prevalence estimates in children with CKD range from 20–80% depending on the degree of renal dysfunction and underlying renal disease. Hypertension, systolic and/or diastolic, is defined as the presence of ≥95th percentile in 54% of children and adolescent with CKD Stage 3. The European Study Group for Nutritional Treatment of Chronic Renal Failure in Childhood demonstrated that in CKD children, an SBP greater than 120 mmHg was associated with a significantly faster GFR decline.

The Kidney Disease Outcomes Quality Initiative (KDOQI) guidelines on BP control in CKD children adopted the recommendations of the task force that target blood pressure should be <90th percentile for normal values adjusted for age, gender, and height percentile. The integrity of the normal diurnal blood pressure pattern may play a significant role in renal failure progression, in addition to and independent of the absolute BP level.

"Non-dipping", a well-known independent cardiovascular risk factor and common characteristic of renoparenchymal hypertension, is associated with more rapid progression of renal failure in adult CKD patients, and non-dipping is believed to reflect sympathetic hyperactivation in CKD. Whereas the different classes of antihypertensive agents are comparable with respect to their blood pressure-lowering efficacy, they differ markedly regarding their effects on proteinuria and CKD progression.

Antagonists of the renin-angiotensin system (RAS), such as angiotensin-converting enzyme inhibitors (ACEs) and, more recently, angiotensin II type I receptor blockers (ARBs), have become pharmacotherapeutics of first choice in adults as well as children with CKD by virtue of their pharmacological properties. They significantly reduce BP as well as urinary protein excretion. RAS antagonists suppress the local angiotensin II tone (ACEs) or action (ARBs). This results in a reduction of intraglomerular pressure and proteinuria, the diminished local release of cytokines and chemokines, and the alleviated activation of inflammatory pathways, with consequently attenuated glomerular hypertrophy and sclerosis, tubulointerstitial inflammation, and fibrosis, as well as in a normalized central nervous sympathetic tone by reduced renal afferent nerve stimulation.

Combined RAS blockade, using ACEs and ARBs concomitantly, has only a minor effect on BP (3–4 mmHg vs. monotherapy), but increases the antiproteinuric effect of ACEs or ARBs monotherapy by 30–40%. Bedtime administration of ACEs tends to restore the dipping pattern. The restoration of the dipping pattern will result in long-term clinical benefit for cardiovascular health, in general, and for renal function preservation in CKD. The recommended doses of ACEs and ARBs are shown in Table 25-7.

Growth Failure

Although growth failure has long been recognized in children with CKD, it is only now recognized that these children are surviving to adulthood with severe short stature, which has emerged as one of the most significant long-term sequelae of ESRD in childhood. Sixty two percent of boys and 41% of girls who developed ESRD during childhood had final adult heights below the normal range. The similar incidence of short stature is seen in adults who received a renal allograft as a child.

The degree of growth failure has been correlated with the age of onset of CKD. The cause of growth failure is believed to be multifactorial, including growth hormone (GH) and insulin-like growth factor-I (IGF-I) function, nutritional status, acid–base balance, and bone mineralization. Despite the recognition and treatment of all these factors, most children still do not reach their genetic height potential despite optimal management and almost half of them are less than the third percentile for height at the onset of dialysis.

The use of recombinant human growth hormone (rhGH) is for children with CKD of all ages, who have a height standard deviation score (SDS) of ≤ 2SD and a height velocity SDS of ≤ 1SD below the mean, but only after adequate nutrition has been established, metabolic abnormalities have been corrected, dialysis adequacy has been ensured, and steroid therapy has reduced to a minimum.

Nutrition Deficiency

It is present in CKD for several reasons, including anorexia, nausea, and vomiting from the uremia and an abnormal sense of taste. Young children, in particular, need sufficient caloric intake for growth. Protein intake should be optimized to allow the maintenance of nitrogen balance and the preservation of lean body mass.

The optimal caloric requirement for children with CKD and those in ESRD treated with dialysis has not been defined. However, a positive correlation between caloric intake and growth has been shown in children with CKD and ESRD treated with both HD and PD.

In children and infants, the energy intake should be at least 100% of the recommended daily allowance (RDA) for age. Because many of these patients are anorexic, special strategies may be required to achieve this goal. These may include high-density caloric supplements, transpyloric or nasogastric feedings, or even gastrostomy feedings.

Adolescents also have very high energy requirements. Caloric supplementation should be given; therefore, the adolescent boy receives at least 44–55 kcal/kg/day and the adolescent girl receives at least 40–50 kcal/kg/day.

The current recommendations for dietary protein intake are:

- infants and children younger than three years of age: 2.5–3.0 g/kg/day,
- children with an age of three years to puberty: 2.0–2.5 g/kg/day,
- pubertal patients: 2.0 g/kg/day, and
- postpubertal patients: 1.5 g/kg/day.

To achieve salt and water balance in these patients, the intake must often be exactly quantitated.

Renoprotection — Strategies to Slow Down CKD Progression

CKD commonly progresses toward ESRD, largely independent of the underlying disorder, once a critical impairment of renal function has occurred. The efficient control of BP and the minimization of proteinuria appear as the two most important measures to preserve residual kidney function.

However, information on the natural course of CKD progression in children is still limited. The prospective population-based ItalKid registry, including almost 1200 CKD children with various renal diseases over a 10-year period, reported a prevalence of 23% of patients suffering from severe kidney disease with CKD4. The incidence of renal replacement therapy was 7.3 per year per 100 patients with CKD5 and the risk of developing ESRD by the age of 20 was 68%.

The European Study Group for Nutritional Treatment of Chronic Renal Failure in Childhood first demonstrated in 200 children with CKD Stages 3–4 that proteinuria and hypertension are major independent determinants of GFR that decline in pediatric nephropathies. The decline of renal function is not linear but rather characterized by a sharp decline during puberty and at early postpubertal age. RAS antagonists preserve kidney function not only by lowering blood pressure but also by their antiproteinuric, antifibrotic, and anti-inflammatory properties.

Intensified BP control, probably aiming for a target BP below the 75th percentile and protein and salt restriction to reduce proteinuria as much as possible, ideally to <300 mg/m^2/day, may slow down the progression to the level of "very slow", which is ≤ 2 ml/min per 1.73 m^2 per year.

Other factors contributing in a multifactorial manner to renal disease progression include dyslipidemia, anemia, and the disorders of mineral metabolism. The measures to preserve renal function should, therefore, also comprise the maintenance of the levels of hemoglobin, serum lipid, and calcium-phosphorus ion product in the normal range.

Management of ESRD

Dialysis Therapy

The indications for initiating dialysis treatment in children with ESRD depend on a combination of the biochemical and clinical characteristics of the patient. Whenever possible, dialysis should be initiated early enough to prevent the development of severe malnutrition and uremic symptomatology. Whereas there is no definitive level of blood urea nitrogen or serum creatinine that mandates the institution of the dialysis: the dialysis has historically been initiated when the creatinine clearance has declined to a value between 5 and 10 ml/min/1.73 m^2.

The presence of fluid overload resulting in systemic hypertension or cardiovascular instability is the indication for dialysis. Dialysis should be initiated also if the fluid intake must be restricted so severely that adequate nutrition cannot be provided. Uncontrolled hyperkalemia, hyperphosphatemia, or acidosis is the objective indication for dialysis. Subjective indications include fatigue, drowsiness, and general weakness, especially, if these symptoms result in school absenteeism.

Pediatric dialysis programs in North America currently favor the use of chronic peritoneal dialysis (PD) by 2:1 over chronic hemodialysis (HD). Whereas virtually all infants on dialysis receive PD and a nearly equal percentage of adolescents receive PD and HD.

PD can be provided either as continuous ambulatory peritoneal dialysis (CAPD) or delivered as one of several automated therapies with a cycler. Current practice favors cycler or automated peritoneal dialysis (APD) over CAPD by more than two to one, because APD techniques allow for the delivery of the higher doses of dialysis than CAPD. As more experience is gained in tailoring the PD prescription, to the individual child's peritoneal transport characteristics, the need to provide adequate dialysis will further impact recommendations for dialysis delivery. Thus, the optimal pediatric dialysis program must provide both CAPD and APD options.

HD is provided almost to all pediatric patients in the in-center setting. Although it is technically feasible, few infants currently receive maintenance HD. However, these babies may require HD for extended periods if peritoneal catheter and infection problems arise. Thus, the optimal pediatric dialysis program must be able to provide maintenance dialysis for infants as either PD or HD.

Peritoneal Dialysis

A single- or double-cuffed Tenckhoff Catheter® for chronic used is inserted if more than seven days of dialysis are anticipated. Three sizes of catheter are available: neonatal (<3 kg), pediatric (3–10 kg), and adult (>10 kg). The exit site must face inferolaterally in order to minimize the risk of exit-site infection. When double-cuffed catheters are used, the second cuff must be at least 2 cm from the exit site in order to prevent cuff extrusion. A partial omentectomy is recommended in all children to prevent catheter obstruction.

The PD prescription should be individualized, taking into account the patient's body surface area (BSA), the peritoneal membrane solute transport membrane characteristics, and the residual renal function (RRF) (determined by the average of urea and creatinine clearance of the patient) into account.

To maximize solute clearance, the maintenance exchange volumes should be 1100 to 1500 ml/m^2 BSA, as tolerated by the patient. Although increasing the total dialysate volume will commonly increase solute clearance, it is usually most effective to increase the exchange volume and not the number of exchanges.

Usual dialysis prescription take into account: (a) exchange volumes of 20–50 ml/kg, (b) inflow-dwell times between 30 and 60 minutes, (c) total cycle number of 8–10, and (d) dialysate dextrose concentration, according to the amount of ultrafiltration that is required (1.5, 2.5, and 4.25% solutions). Adequacy of APD is assessed using actual ultrafiltration, weekly Kt/V of urea of 1.7 (where Kt = clearance of urea and V = the distribution volume of urea, which is total body water), and a total weekly creatinine clearance of at least 45 L/1.73 m^2.

Hemodialysis

Since the first clinical report of HD in a preadolescent patient with ESRD in 1966, enormous technical progress has been made in adapting HD for children of all ages. These advances include the developments in the field of vascular surgery and techniques in vascular access for dialysis, the availability of low-primming hollow fiber dialyzers, and the small blood lines for dialysis.

While short-term and acute HD therapies are technically feasible in infants and young children, chronic HD is generally avoided in this age group because of the problems associated with long-term vascular access.

Additionally, HD in infants requires technical known-how and specialized dialysis equipment, which is usually available only in tertiary-care pediatric facilities.

Access for chronic HD is tunneled by single or double venous-cuffed catheters in infants and children aged less than six years. Arteriovenous fistulae (AVF) are the preferred method of vascular access in children and adolescents. When AVF placement fails, grafts (Gortex®) or double venous cuffed catheter can be used. Tunneled access is superior to non-tunneled lines but inferior to an a-v fistula. The internal jugular vein is the preferred site. Lines should preferably not be sited in the subclavian veins, as this may lead to vascular stenosis and, therefore, inability to create a fistula in the future.

To provide the desired quantity of dialysis, the dialysis variables that must be considered include: (a) the dialyzer type, (b) the blood flow, (c) the dialysate flow, (d) the duration of the dialysis treatment, and (e) the ultrafiltration requirements of the patient.

Dialyzer, arterial, and venous lines are selected on the basis that the children can tolerate 10% of their total blood volume (80 ml/kg dry weight) in the extracorporeal circuit and the surface area of the dialyzer should be equal to, but not exceed, that of the child's. Thus, a 10-kg child with 0.47 m^2 of BSA would use a Fresenius F3 with a 0.4 m^2 of membrane SA.

The blood flow is calculated to provide a urea clearance of 3 ml/kg/min for the first session of the week and 5–6 ml/kg/min by the end of the week. The speed at which the blood is pumped out of the child and around the circuit is equivalent to its extracorporeal volume total. Thus, a 10-kg child with a total blood volume of 80 ml/kg and extracorporeal circuit of 80 ml can have the blood speeds of up to 80 ml/min. The flow rate of dialysis solution is usually fixed at 500 ml/min, rarely it is up to 700 ml/min. The length of session for standard chronic HD is four hours and is usually performed three times a week.

Ultrafiltration is individualized, but as a general rule, 5% of the loss of body weight is recommended in four-hour dialysis. The measures of HD adequacy in terms of small solute clearance have not been defined in pediatric patients, but consensus standards propose that they should be equal to or better than adult recommendations of $Kt/V > 1.2$ and a urea reduction ratio (URR) (predialysis urea — postdialysis urea ÷ predialysis urea − 100%) of >65% during each treatment session.

Conclusions

Irrespective of the choice of dialysis modality, hemodialysis vs. peritoneal dialysis, the efficacy of dialysis should be measured regularly and the prescription of dialysis should be designed to achieve target clearances. Attention to the adequacy of dialysis, the control of osteodystrophy and nutrition, and the correction of anemia are mandatory, because all may influence patient outcome in terms of growth, cognitive development, and school performance. Finally, the availability of a multidisciplinary team of pediatric specialists is desirable to provide all facets of pediatric ESRD care, including renal transplantation, in an optimal manner.

Pediatric Renal Transplantation

Renal transplantation is accepted as the therapy of choice for children with end-stage renal disease (ESRD). This is based upon the belief that successful transplantation not only ameliorates symptoms of CKD but also allows for significant improvement, and often the correction of delayed skeletal growth, sexual maturation, cognitive performance, and psychosocial functioning. The child with a functional graft can lead a life of superior quality, when compared with that achieved with available dialysis. Improvements in pediatric renal transplantation are attributed to better age-appropriate clinical and surgical cares, histocompatibility matching, and newer immunosuppressive therapy.

Indications and Timing of Renal Transplantation

There is no absolute minimum age for the transplantation of pediatric kidney. Once the child is in Stage 4 CKD, it is the time to start preparing the child and the family for renal replacement therapy. The outcome of renal transplantation in children has improved over the last decades so that, even infants with ESRD may be suitable candidates for renal transplantation. Many centers still prefer an age of above two years and a weight of

≥15 kg at the time of transplantation, but infants aged six months and weighing 5 kg have been successfully transplanted.

The 2002 annual report of NAPRTCS showed that, between 1987 and 2001, a total of 7247 children received 7951 transplants. The mean age of transplant recipients was 10.9 years; 46% aged were over 12 years, 34% were 6–12 years old, 15% were between two and five years, and only about 5%, were less than two years.

In the US, more than 50% of the kidneys transplanted in children are from living donors (LD). Of these donors, 82% were parents (56% mothers and 44% fathers). In the Eurotransplant region (Austria, Belgium, Croatia, Germany, Luxemburg, The Netherlands, and Slovenia), this percentage is 20%, but is increasing.

What is clear is that an increasing number of families are opting for LD, presumably because of the information showing its superior results, at least over the first five years, the increasing understanding of the complications of dialysis, and the ability to plan the timing of the transplantation.

Long-Term Outcome after Renal Transplantation in Childhood

Patient Survival

Overall patient survival

As noted from the 2004 NAPRTCS data, five-year patient survival ranged between 97 and 99% in children 1–10 years of age who received LD allografts; among those who received deceased donor kidney (DD), the survival was 90–97%, respectively. Data from the same cooperative study group in 2006 showed that seven-year patient survival exceeded 90% in all recipients of LDs or DDs, other than 0–1-year-old recipients of DD kidneys.

Recipient age

Recipient age is an important factor that has been demonstrated to affect patient survival, although there is evidence that its effect has declined in recent years. Early reviews showed a mortality rate of 21% in young children, and particularly, in those under two years of age at transplantation. However, more recently, the survival rates of over 98% have been reported. The increased risk of death was also seen to extend up to an age of five years at transplantation; however, a reduction in the rate of mortality has occurred in this age range too, with a five-year survival rate of over 97% in those under six years old, a 10-year survival rate of 91% in those weighing <15 kg, and 15-year survival of 87% in those weighing <11 kg.

Donor source

All reports have shown a small but consistent benefit of LD on mortality at all ages up to five years after transplantation. LD has a particular benefit for the very young child: five-year patient survival rates for recipients less than two years old was 86% following LD and 70% following DD transplantation.

Benefits with LD include the following: the incidence of ATN is lower, cold ischemia is shorter, long-term survival is longer, and the most important is that the period on dialysis can be shortened because the time of transplantation is decided in advance. Despite these advantages, the proportion of LDs varies greatly among countries and regions. Several factors may explain these differences. These include the activity of the cadaver transplant program, cultural variations, and the manner in which parents are solicited for donation.

Transplant Survival

Overall graft survival

LD graft survival rates at one, three, and five years are 92, 86, and 81%, respectively. By comparison, DD graft survival rates at one, three, and five years are 84, 75, and 67%, respectively. Graft survival of repeat transplants has been reported as being equal to, or slightly reduced, that of first grafts. When DD were used for the repeat transplants, the survival rates at one, three, and five years were 74, 60, and 47%, respectively, compared to 86, 78, and 72% for repeat LD transplants.

In a report from the NAPRTCS in 2008, children in whom the transplant fails within 10 years were more likely to be older and non-Caucasian, had a history of focal segmental glomerulosclerosis (FSGS), receive a DD kidney, and were less likely to have obstructive uropathy.

In addition to the efficacy of newer immunosuppressive regimens, other general factors implicated in the success or failure of a renal graft in children include the following:

- recipient age,
- donor age,
- donor source,
- HLA compatibility and sensitization,
- immunosuppression,
- bladder voiding disorders,
- pre-emptive transplant,
- delayed graft function,
- acute rejection episodes,
- infections,
- compliance with therapeutic regimens, and
- recurrent diseases.

Recipient age

Age has an important influence on the transplant as well as on patient survival. Some data suggest that young children have excellent long-term allograft survival. In the 2004 US Scientific Registry of Transplant Recipients, five-year graft survival rates among LD recipients were 90–91% for children 1–5 years of age and 6–10 years of age, respectively. For DD recipients, the survival rates at five years were 78 and 77%, respectively. While graft survival in recipients below 11 years is superior to that of all other age groups, the Registry provides continued evidence of the disappointing long-term graft survival rates of adolescent transplant recipients, which are presumably a manifestation of poor compliance with medications and the subsequent development of chronic allograft nephropathy. Adolescents, as a group, have the worst graft survival rate of all ages; in addition, they have a high percentage of late acute rejection episodes and relatively poor rejection reversal outcomes, compared to the other age groups.

Donor age

Kidneys from DDs aged 11–17 years do best with a 73% five-year survival rate. Some studies have warned of the increased risk of graft thrombosis and primary non-function in young patients when young donors, particularly under five years of age, are used. However, in the Scientific Registry of Transplant Recipients, five-year allograft survival from the donors are those younger than one year of age and one to five years of age was approximately 60 and 70%, respectively.

A comparison of graft survival of 1175 single transplants from pediatric donors and 24,530 single kidney transplants using "ideal" DDs kidney between the ages of 19 and 36 years demonstrated that the recipients of kidneys from pediatric donors were at a significantly increased risk for graft loss. On the other hand, double "en bloc" transplanted kidneys from the youngest donor group have similar graft survival as "ideal" donors. Therefore, it may be that the use of small kidneys is appropriate in selected patients.

Donor source

Allograft survival is higher in children with LD grafts compared to those with DD grafts. The 2006 data of NAPRCTS reveal that five-year graft survival is 80% with LDs as compared to 66% with DDs grafts. LD is of particular benefit to the recipient under two years of age. Five-year graft survival for recipients under two years old was 86% following LDs and 38% following DDs transplantation. It has been calculated that a 10-year-old child who received a renal transplant in 2000 and is receiving cyclosporine-based immunosuppression can expect a transplant half-life of 13.1 years from an LD and 10.8 years from a DD, although for LD recipients with no acute rejection episodes, half-life has been calculated to be as high as 37.6 years.

dHLA matching and sensitization

In children as well as adults, superior HLA matching between recipient and donor, whether DD or LD is associated with improved outcomes. Worst outcome has been observed for two HLA-DR mismatched grafts, while 000 and favorably matched kidneys (100, 010, 110 HLA-A, -B, -DR mismatches) survived the longest. Optimal HLA matching is, therefore, preferred, particularly for young recipients, retransplantation and transplantation in sensitized patients. However, the maximization of HLA matching is not entirely beneficial because sharing kidney based upon such matching increases the cold ischemia times and the rate of delayed graft function, which in turn, may affect long-term graft survival.

Sensitized patients [panel reactive antibodies (PRA) >40%] also have a poorer outcome, and donor antigen-specific hyporeactivity correlates with better graft function. The incidence of graft survival at one year is higher in patients with negative anti-human globulin cross-match test, compared with those with a positive reaction. The significance of a positive B-lymphocyte cross-match when T-lymphocyte cross-match is negative is controversial. It is probably harmful in patients who are candidates for retransplantation.

Immunosuppression

There have been considerable changes in the use of immunosuppression over the years. NAPRTCS has reported that the use of cyclosporine A (CsA) has decreased from 82.3% in 1996 to 20.7% in 2003. In contrast, the use of tacrolimus has increased from 5.5 to 67.1% over the same period. There has also been a move away from azathioprine (AZA), from 56.4 to 1.9%, toward mycophenolate mofetil (MMF); the use of which is now approximately 57.4%. Antibody induction has also moved away from OKT3 to antithymocyte globulins (ATGs) in DD transplant and to anti-IL2 receptor blockers in LD transplant. The use of steroid-sparing regimens is also becoming common.

There is evidence that the use of MMF in association with CsA is associated with better outcome in five years than a similar regimen using

AZA; the transplant survivals being 90.7% for MMF and 68.5% for AZA patients.

There is also evidence that tacrolimus is more effective than CsA: a randomized trial of steroids and AZA with either tacrolimus or CsA demonstrated that tacrolimus was significantly more effective than CsA in both preventing acute rejection and maintaining graft function, with a four-year transplant survival rate of 86 and 69%, respectively, and glomerular filtration rates of 71.5 ml/min/1.73 m^2 and 53.0 ml/min/ 1.73 m^2 body surface area, respectively.

Bladder voiding disorders

Transplantation into an abnormal urinary tract is associated with a high incidence of urological and infectious complications, and residual voiding disorders also jeopardize late graft function. It has been suggested that bladder reconstruction should be performed before transplantation when clinically indicated. Because of the high urological complication rates, the careful surveillance of lower urinary tract function by urodynamic evaluation is essential before transplantation. Reflux does not need to be corrected before transplantation, unless it is causing symptoms or infection.

Pre-emptive transplant

Pre-emptive kidney transplantation, or transplantation without prior dialysis, has been associated with a survival advantage compared with transplantation that is performed following dialysis, in both children and adults. NAPRTCS data show that transplant survival is improved in patients receiving a pre-emptive transplant compared with those undergoing PD and HD. Graft loss resulting from vascular thrombosis is commoner in children who undergo PD than in those who were on HD. Eurotransplant found a difference in graft survival between those not on dialysis and those on dialysis of 82 and 69%, respectively, at six years post-transplantation.

The Australia and New Zealand Dialysis and Transplant Registry (ANZDATA), in their analysis of data from transplant recipients less than

30 years of age, confirm that the overall risk of graft failure is increased in recipients 10–19 years of age and that graft survival in these adolescents is better among those who receive an LD kidney than among those who receive a kidney from a DD. Most striking, however, was the finding of a nearly 50% reduction in the risk of LD graft failure in adolescents who received a pre-emptive transplant compared with those who received a graft after 6–24 months of dialysis. In fact, there was a trend toward a benefit of pre-emptive transplantation in the entire group of LD kidney recipients. Marked improvement in outcome could be the result of a selection bias for pre-emptive transplantation toward patients who have characteristics associated with better graft survival, such as a social background that promotes adherence.

Conditions that preclude patients from undergoing pre-emptive transplant are shown in Table 25-8. Children are often perfect candidates for pre-emptive transplantation, they frequently have slowly advancing CKD because of a congenital kidney disorder, and young healthy parents willing to serve as kidney donors.

Delayed graft function

Small children present a difficult challenge in the operating room. The relatively large size of the graft may result in longer anastomosis times, a longer ischemia time, and subsequently higher rates of early graft dysfunction (DGF). DGF, defined by the requirement for dialysis within the first week of transplantation, occurs in about 5% of LD and 20% of DD transplantation, and is associated with a reduced graft survival. In children with DGF, the three-year graft survival rates are reduced by 30 and 20% in recipients of DD and LD donor kidneys, respectively.

Kidney transplantation in children below 10 kg of body weight is often done through a midline incision and the graft is placed into the peritoneal cavity. The donor vein is anastomosed to the vena cava of the recipient. Immediately after the venous anastomosis has been completed, the donor artery is either anastomosed with the distal aorta, to obtain the best arterial inflow or with one of the common iliac arteries if the size allows it. The ureter is cut and shortened to obtain the best vascularization of the anastomosis.

The commonest cause of graft failure in young recipients in the first year after transplantation is graft thrombosis. This complication results in almost universal graft loss. Its incidence in children is between 2 and 3%, but may be as high as 10% in children younger than five years. The risk of graft thrombosis is further associated with previous treatment of PD, DD source, prior transplantation, and prolonged cold ischemia time.

Differential diagnoses of DGF are:

- ATN,
- ureteral obstruction — perirenal fluid collection, lymphocele, hematoma, and abscess,
- urinary leak,
- renal arterial or venous thrombosis,
- intravascular volume contraction,
- Nefrotoxicity,
- acute rejection, and
- infection.

Acute rejection episodes

Acute rejection is responsible for 13% of graft failures in children. In patients who received DD grafts, the estimated graft half-life is shorter in patients who had acute rejection episodes than those who did not (6.6 vs. 12.5 years). The beneficial effects of improved immunosuppressive regimens and optimal HLA matching on allograft survival are in part because of their role in lowering the risk of acute rejection. In addition, acute rejection episodes markedly increase the risk of developing chronic rejection, thereby enhancing possible allograft loss over time. Chronic rejection is the cause of graft loss in 33% of transplanted children, while primary non-function, accelerated rejection, and technical problems are 2.3, 1.7, and 1.4%, respectively.

Infections

Cytomegalovirus (CMV) infection is associated with an increased risk of rejection. Prophylaxis of CMV infection may improve graft survival.

Polyomavirus, mainly BK virus, affect 3–8% of children with renal allografts and may be responsible for allograft nephropathy and graft failure. Risk factors for BKV infections are intense immunosuppression and acute rejection.

Compliance with therapeutic regimens

Non-compliance with therapeutic regimens is a difficult problem to deal with. It affects patients and families at all ages, but particularly so in adolescence. Non-adherence to immunosuppressive treatment, which occurs in more than 30% of children and adolescents, is a major cause of acute and chronic rejection.

Recurrent diseases

The risk of disease recurrence following renal transplant is becoming relatively high, due to increased immunosuppression and reduced acute rejection. Disease recurrence has a greater prevalence in children than in adults, thereby increasing patient morbidity, graft loss, and sometimes, mortality rates. Indeed, the current overall graft loss to acute rejection in children is 13% vs. 7–8% to disease recurrence, mainly due to primary glomerulonephritis (70–80%) and inherited metabolic diseases.

The risk of recurrence in a first graft is 14–50% with a risk of graft loss of 40–60%; while the risk of recurrence in a second graft after a first graft loss to recurrence is 60–100%. The spectrum of recurrence is rather wide and mainly depends on the primary disease itself, ranging from the recurrence of the full disease with various risks of graft loss, to the recurrence of specific features of the disease. Structural abnormalities such as reflux, posterior urethral valves, and congenital kidney disease have a better outcome than ESRD caused by FSGS, membranoproliferative glomerulonephritis type 2 (MPGN 2), or atypical hemolytic uremic syndrome (HUS). The percentage is adversely affected by young age at presentation, and rapid progression to ESRD. In half of the patients with recurrence the graft fails. Therefore, the five-year graft survival in recipients with FSGS is approximately 10% less than in other pediatric transplant recipients.

MPGN 2 recurs in most patients with a significantly worse five-year graft survival than other pediatric transplant recipients: 50% vs. 74%, respectively. Recurrence of HUS is reported in 20–80% of the transplanted patients particularly in atypical, no diarrheal HUS. Moreover, there is a relatively high incidence of early arterial or venous thrombosis so that in 50% of patients with HUS, graft loss will occur within a year after transplantation. The recurrence rate of primary disease after the first renal transplantation and graft loss due to recurrence is shown in Table 25-9.

Contraindications to transplantation

Most children with ESRD qualify as candidates for renal transplantation. Although there is no clear agreement on the contraindications to renal transplantation in children, the general practiced absolute and relative contraindications to renal transplantation are listed in Table 25-10. Patients with childhood malignancies should be free of recurrence for a period of 2–5 years, based on the site and type of malignancy. Children with oxalosis should be considered for a combined liver and kidney transplant. Patients with hepatitis C should be evaluated by a hepatologist prior to considering an LD or DD transplantation. Children with multiple congenital anomalies, or severe mental retardation, pose an ethical dilemma, where a multidisciplinary team is necessary in weighing the option of renal transplantation.

Table 25-9. Recurrence of primary disease after the first renal transplantation.

Primary disease	Recurrence rate (%)	Graft loss to recurrence (%)
FSGS	14–50	40–60
Atypical HUS	20–80	10–83
MPGN type 1	30–77	17–50
MPGN type 2	66–100	25–61
SLE nephritis	0–30	0–5
IgA nephritis	35–60	7–10
Henoch Schönlein nephritis	31–100	8–22
Primary hyperoxaluria type 1	90–100	80–100

Table 25-10. Contraindications to renal transplantation in children.

Absolute contraindications	Relative contraindications
HIV infection	Multiple congenital anomalies
Untreated malignancy	Untreated hepatitis C infection
Oxalosis	Severe mental retardation
Multiorgan failure	Poor compliance with medical regimens
Progressive neurologic illness	
Active infective state	
Chronic hepatitis B infection	

Table 25-11. Pretransplant evaluation and preparation of the recipient.

1. History and physical examination:
   - determine the cause of ESRD, if possible,
   - identify comorbidities,
   - GU, lower spine, perineum, and neurologic examination,
   - nutrition evaluation and optimization, and
   - age-appropriate immunizations.
2. Psychosocial evaluation and counseling of the child and family.
3. Immunologic evaluation: ABO and HLA typing and screening for anti-HLA antibodies.
4. Evaluation for exposure to infections: antibodies to viral infections (CMV, EBV, HSV, HIV, varicella zoster virus, and hepatitis B and C); hepatitis B surface antigen; serologic tests for syphilis; chagas; chest X-ray; and tuberculin testing.
5. Urologic evaluation: urinalysis and urine culture; ultrasonography, including postvoid images of the bladder, voiding cystourethrogram; voiding diary; uroflow; urodynamics; and rarely cystoscopy in patients with complicated urologic problems.
6. Optional: neurocognitive evaluation; hematologic evaluation if suspected of being at risk for thrombosis; cardiac, pulmonary, dental, and ophthalmologic examinations, as indicated.
7. Financial screening and counseling.

Pretransplant evaluation of the recipient

The goal of pretransplant evaluation is aimed to ensure and enhance the patient's suitability as a transplant recipient. Table 25-11 lists the principles of pretransplant evaluation applicable to children. Pretransplant evaluation should be aimed at identifying clinical, physiological, psychological, and socioeconomic conditions that may impact the successful outcome of a renal transplant.

Patients should be screened for chronic infections, which may be regarded as contraindications to renal transplantation. Native nephrectomies for chronic infection of the kidneys, severe nephrotic syndrome (congenital or idiopathic FSGS), polyuria with severe fluid and electrolyte wasting, polycystic kidneys, intractable hypertension, large renal masses, or nephrolithiasis may be necessary in some children.

NAPRTCS data suggest that about 25% of children undergo native nephrectomies in preparation for renal transplantation. Establishing the cause of ESRD is important, since many diseases have the potential for recurrence in the transplanted kidney. This includes FSGS, atypical HUS, and MPGN. In such cases, strategies should be developed to optimize the timing of transplant and to monitor for the recurrence and treatment. The potential for the recurrence of primary glomerular diseases is not considered a contraindication to transplantation, but some centers do not use living donors if the risk of recurrence is high.

Age-appropriate immunizations, including hepatitis B, varicella, pneumococcal, and influenza vaccines, should be provided to children prior to transplantation procedure.

Pretransplant evaluation of the donor

Living renal transplant donation can be from either an individual who is related to the child (parents or siblings older than 18 years of age) or an unrelated person with a significant emotional bond with the child. An outline of donor work-up is shown in Table 25-12.

Perioperative transplant management

Fluid and electrolytes

Some children may need to be dialyzed prior to renal transplantation in order to optimize fluid and electrolyte status, particularly if they are to

Table 25-12. Evaluation of living related donor.

1. Psychosocial screening and counseling.
2. Detailed history and physical examination.
3. Renal function tests, including 24-hour urine collection for protein and creatinine measurement, liver function tests, and screening diabetes.
4. Age-appropriate screening for cardiovascular health and malignancies.
5. ABO, Rh, and HLA typing.
6. Screening for infections: antibodies to viral infections (HIV, CMV, EBV, and hepatitis B and C); hepatitis B antigen; serologic tests for syphilis and chagas; chest X-ray; tuberculin testing, and screening for infection pertaining to geographic area of origin.
7. Renal and renovascular anatomy: renal ultrasound, renal angiography, or spiral CT scan or MRI of kidneys with MRA and MRV.

receive an organ from a DD; however, hypovolemia should be avoided. Except in polyuric children, preoperative intravenous fluids are not necessary in most cases. Close attention needs to be paid to intravascular volume in the operating room by infusion of crystalloid and colloid solutions. After vascular anastomoses, an adult kidney can sequester up to 250 ml of the recipient's blood volume. This may represent a significant proportion of total blood volume in an infant or a small child (blood volume 80 ml/kg). As a result, appropriate intraoperative fluid management is critical in infants and young children. Central venous pressure (CVP) should be maintained between 10 and 15 cm H_2O prior to the removal of the vascular clamps to ensure good blood flow to the allograft, as a low-flow state can promote allograft thrombosis. Pressor agents such as dopamine may be required in order to help maintain adequate blood pressure. Many centers use mannitol (0.5–1 g/kg) and furosemide in a dose of 1–2 mg/kg at the time of unclamping the vessels to induce diuresis in the transplanted organ. Sometimes, an intra-arterial vasodilator such as verapamil may also be given in order to overcome renal arterial vasospasm.

Postoperative fluid and electrolyte management includes the replacement of insensible losses and the replacement of urine output with an appropriately constituted fluid. Five percent dextrose solution can be used to replace insensible fluid losses and the replacement of urine output can be achieved with a solution with an electrolyte composition approximating that of urine electrolyte analysis. Further adjustments in the electrolyte composition of the replacement fluids should be based on serum and urine electrolyte analysis. In order to facilitate renal function of the allograft, CVP should be maintained in the range of 8–10 cm H_2O in the first 24 hours after transplantation. The status of fluid and electrolytes needs to be monitored and managed carefully in patients with delayed graft function. Need for dialysis should be considered carefully in such cases. Attempts at aggressive fluid removal during dialysis should be avoided, since this can result in hypovolemia and superimposed ATN, further impeding the recovery of function in these grafts.

Immunosuppressive management

The goal of immunosuppressive therapy is to prevent allograft rejection, while avoiding the complications of immunocompromise, such as infections and malignancy. Immunosuppressive therapy is most intense in the first few weeks to few months after renal transplantation. Most centers use some form of induction therapy at the time of transplantation. Induction regimens usually consist of monoclonal or polyclonal antibodies and are indicated in high-risk patients (highly sensitized retransplants and patients with delayed graft function). Infants and young children may have a propensity for more intense allograft-directed immune responses, and usually metabolize immunosuppressive medications at a faster rate than adults. Therefore, they may benefit from induction therapies.

CsA, tacrolimus, prednisone, AZA, MMF, and sirolimus are used in various combinations for the maintenance of immunosuppression and are initiated around transplant surgery. Steroids have been traditionally used in most transplant immunosuppression protocols. Intravenous steroids are often used intraoperatively and for the first few postsurgery days, followed by oral therapy, after adequate gastrointestinal function is achieved.

A combination of calcineurin inhibitor drugs (CsA or tacrolimus) and antiproliferative agents (AZA, MMF, or sirolimus) is initiated soon after transplantation. In order to avoid nephrotoxicity in patients with DGF, calcineurin inhibitors should not be initiated until satisfactory allograft function is established. The use of CsA as a primary immunosuppressive agent has been largely replaced by tacrolimus in recent years. Similarly,

MMF is used more widely now, in place of AZA. Sirolimus is also being selectively used in pediatric renal transplantation. Recent NAPRTCS data indicate that in one month after transplantation, 67% of children were receiving tacrolimus, 57% MMF, and 20% CsA.

Because of a high-toxicity profile associated with long-term steroid use, attempts have been made to curtail or eliminate steroid use in long-term maintenance immunosuppressive protocols. Steroid withdrawal in more recent studies has been more successful in protocols, especially using tacrolimus in combination with either MMF or AZA. The familiarity and experience of the physician and the transplant team often dictate the choice of immunosuppressive protocol used in any renal transplant center with the particular pharmacologic agents.

The immunosuppression protocol followed currently consists of a single preoperative dose of MMF in low-risk recipients, followed by the first dose of anti-IL-2R antibody (Daclizumab or Basiliximab) given intraoperatively. In high-risk transplants (patients with high PRA, retransplants, and in whom a DGF is anticipated), thymoglobulin is initiated either preoperatively or intraoperatively. Intravenous methylprednisolone (10 mg/kg) is given in the operating room. After establishing good renal function in the postoperative period, tacrolimus is started and MMF and steroids are continued. Anti-IL-2R antibody treatment is completed in patients in whom it has been started. Similarly, those receiving thymoglobulin induction complete their anticipated 3–7 doses based on the allograft function. Steroid dose is gradually tapered and by the end of three months, most children receive prednisone at 0.1 mg/kg/day. Common dose and side effects of immunosuppressive transplant medications are listed in Table 25-13.

Anti-infective prophylaxis

Anti-infective prophylaxis is important in preventing opportunistic infections. The American Society of Transplantation has published guidelines for the prevention and management of infectious complications of solid organ transplantation. Trimethoprim–sulfamethoxazole is used for prophylaxis against *Pneumocystis carinii* pneumonia infection and urinary tract infections.

Table 25-13. Immunosuppressive drugs.

Name of the drug	Dose	Side effects
Polyclonal antibodies	ATG 10–15 mg/kg/day Thymoglobulin 1.5 mg/kg/day	Leukopenia, thrombocytopenia, Fever, anaphylaxis, increased risk of infections, and PTLD.
Anti-IL-2R antibodies	Daclizumab: 1 mg/kg on day 0, 2, 4, and 6 and 8 weeks Basiliximab: <35 kg (10 mg/dose) and >35 kg (20 mg/dose) on day 0 and 4.	Side effects same as placebo.
Methylprednisone	10 mg/kg/day $\times 1$ for induction and 10 mg/kg/day for treatment of acute rejection.	Hypertension, hyperglycemia, and fluid overload.
Prednisone	2 mg/kg/day to be tapered to 0.5 mg/kg/day in two weeks, 0.1–0.15 mg/kg/day over six months.	Weight gain, hypertension, hyperglucemia, growth retardation, gastric ulceration, and cataracts.
Cyclosporine A	6–8 mg/kg/day at the onset; adjust dose according to levels.	Nephrotoxicity, hypertension, hirsutism, and gingival hyperplasia.
Tacrolimus	0.1–0.15 mg/kg/day; adjust dose according level.	Nephrotoxicity, tremors, and diabetes mellitus.
Azathioprine	2 mg/kg/day.	Myelosuppression and hepatotoxicity.
Mycophenolate mofetil	1200 mg/m^2/day to a maximum of 1500 mg bid.	Myelosuppression and diarrhea.
Sirolimus	Loading dose 6 mg/day, followed by 2–5 mg/day, adjust according to levels.	Hypertriglyceridemia, mucosal ulcers, trombocytopenia, and pneumonia.

Prevention of CMV infection is important on those most at risk which are antibody negative recipient (R–) of a positive donor (D+), although disease can also occur with R+D– and R+D+ combination, but not with R–D–, unless infection is acquired from a source other than the transplant. Oral ganciclovir, or valganciclovir, is adequate in most patients and is continued for 3–6 months. Valganciclovir is preferred, since it offers better absorption and bioavailability than oral ganciclovir. Herpes simplex virus (HSV) infections can be prevented by low-dose acyclovir in children who are not receiving ganciclovir or valganciclovir.

Complications of transplantation

Surgical complications, bladder-voiding disorders, delayed graft function, acute rejection episodes, and recurrent diseases are considered above as general factors implicated in the success or failure of a renal graft in children.

Infection

Infections constitute the commonest reason for hospitalization after renal transplantation. Infectious complications after transplantation usually follow a predictable pattern. In the first month after transplant, infectious complications are related to technical and mechanical problems, such as wound infections, UTIs, pneumonia, and fungal infections. Between one and six months post-transplant, common infectious events involve viral pathogens, such as CMV, Epstein–Barr virus (EBV), HSV, human herpes viruses (HHV), varicella-zoster virus (VZV), parvovirus (PV) B19, polyoma BK virus, and fungal infections.

Beyond six months, the patterns of infections in patients on stable maintenance immunosuppression and with good allograft function are similar to that seen in the general population. Patients who develop opportunistic infections more than six months post-transplant, are generally those who have higher serum creatinine and are receiving higher doses of maintenance steroids, or have had recurrent rejection episodes requiring intensification of immunosuppression.

Hepatitis B and C infections may become a clinical concern in long-term survivors of kidney transplants. This may be due to the reactivation of these viruses in the recipient or because of infection acquired in the peri-transplant period. Tuberculosis is a serious problem in developing countries due to high risk of exposure and the immunosuppressed state of these patients.

Malignancy

In children with ESRD, the probability of developing a malignancy within 25 years after renal replacement therapy is estimated at 17%. The majority of malignancies in renal pediatric transplant patients are skin cancers (40–50%), predominantly squamous cell carcinoma and post-transplant lymphoproliferative disorders (PTLD) in approximately 30% of the transplanted patients.

PTLD is promoted by Epstein–Barr virus (EBV) infection. EBV can also become more pathogenic in previously infected asymptomatic patients. The risk of PTLD depends on the age of the patient and on the immunosuppressive regimen and it is greatest in the first year post-transplantation.

The risk of malignancy can be reduced by the appropriate low dosing of immunosuppressive medication and by the use of less carcinogenic immunosuppressive agents such as sirolimus. Antiviral therapy to reduce PTLD in children after EBV-positive solid-organ transplantation seem logical but its value to prevent malignancy has not been proven.

Standard chemotherapy for non-Hodgkin lymphoma shows a high percentage of complete remission, but approximately 30% of the children still die within two years.

Hypertension

Fifty to 80% of pediatric kidney transplant recipients develop hypertension. In the immediate post-transplant period, hypertension may be related to fluid overload, high-dose steroids, and acute rejection. The presence of diseased native kidneys, the side effects of medications such as CsA, tacrolimus, and prednisone, acute and chronic rejection, recurrent glomerulonephritis, and renal artery stenosis may be the cause of hypertension when it is present beyond the first few weeks of post-transplantation.

Hypertension is managed with a low sodium diet and antihypertensive medications. The reduction of corticosteroid dose may also improve blood pressure control. Calcium channel blockers are particularly useful in the treatment of hypertension in the early post-transplant period, because of their ability to counteract the vasoconstrictive effects of CsA and tacrolimus. However, the use of calcium channel blockers may be associated with the development of significant edema. ACEs may be useful in the long-term management of hypertension and in prolonging the life of the allograft due to their inhibitory effect on expression of transforming growth factor-β and other growth factors, chronic tubulointerstitial scarring, and their ability to ameliorate proteinuria. Renal artery stenosis is best treated by percutaneous transluminal angioplasty or surgical correction.

Growth retardation

Even though an acceleration of growth velocity is commonly seen in the majority of children following successful renal transplantation, growth retardation may continue to be a clinical concern in some children. Post-transplant growth velocity is better in children who receive transplant at an early age (<5 years of age), those who have good allograft function, and those who are on minimal steroids (prednisone dose <0.15 mg/kg/day), no steroids, or alternate-day steroids. Children younger than four years have the largest benefits from transplantation. Their growth velocity increases more than 3 cm/year compared with children on dialysis. In children who receive a transplant postpuberty, the acceleration of growth velocity and adult height are much less than in children who are transplanted at younger age. Despite the positive influence of renal transplantation on growth velocity, the final adult height of children with ESRD remains less than that of the normal population.

Children with continued post-transplant growth retardation may benefit from rhGH. When rhGH therapy is used in transplanted children, linear growth is best in the first year of therapy, with a somewhat slower growth seen in the second and third years. The potential for increased incidence of acute rejection in children treated with rhGH has been seen in early clinical studies. However, larger studies have not been able to substantiate any increase in the incidence of acute rejection with rhGH use. Patients with one or more episodes of acute rejection prior to rhGH therapy may be at a higher risk for acute rejection. The close monitoring of renal function and the evidence for acute rejection are desirable after the initiation of rhGH therapy. The dose of CsA may need to be increased after the initiation of rhGH therapy. Treatment with rhGH can lead to glucose intolerance, slipped capital femoral epiphysis, and intracranial hypertension. However, the incidence of these complications is not higher than the control ESRD population.

LONG-TERM OUTCOME

Kidney transplantation only means a different stage (CKD-T) and not a complete cure from CKD. In children, as in adults, transplantation provides the substantially improved quality of life compared with dialysis, reduces the hazard of death by about 70%, and is clearly the optimal mode of renal replacement therapy. However, it is not a panacea; it does not remove the CKD state and mortality for transplanted children remains substantially higher than children who do not have CKD. The management of a child with a kidney transplant should include both the care of the graft and the care of the complications of CKD. Unfortunately, it remains largely speculative whether the correction of anemia, hypertension, and the metabolic disturbances associated with CKD improve long-term outcomes in children who have received a kidney transplant.

COMMENT FROM THE EDITORS

This comprehensive discussion of the management of renal insufficiency in children serves as an invaluable reference for those taking care of children with diminished renal function. Although one of the missions of the pediatric urologist is to prevent renal insufficiency, this goal is not always reached. The knowledge of the principles of management and working alongside with pediatric nephrologists will provide the best care for these patients. Not all pediatric urologists get involved in renal transplantation but even those who do not, are often called upon to perform pretransplantation reconstructions and to manage post-transplantation urological complications. This chapter provides the current knowledge needed to undertake this task.

Index